Handbook of
Home Health
Nursing
Procedures

MW01036219

Handbook of

Home Health Nursing Procedures

Robyn Rice, MSN-R, RN-C
Clinical Associate Professor
Barnes College of Nursing
The University of Missouri-St. Louis
St. Louis, Missouri;

Home Health Clinical Nurse Specialist
American Nursing Development
Maryville, Illinois

Second Edition

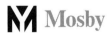 Mosby

St. Louis   Baltimore   Boston   Carlsbad
Chicago   Minneapolis   New York   Philadelphia   Portland
London   Milan   Sydney   Tokyo   Toronto

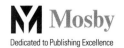
Mosby
Dedicated to Publishing Excellence

Editor-in-Chief: Sally Schrefer
Senior Editor: Loren Wilson
Developmental Editor: Nancy L. O'Brien
Project Manager: Deborah L. Vogel
Production Editor: Sarah E. Fike
Design Manager: Bill Drone
Cover Photograph: Jose L. Pelaez, Inc.-
The Stock Market

SECOND EDITION

NOTICE

Pharmacology is an ever-changing field. Standard safety precautions must be followed, but as new research and clinical experience broaden our knowledge, changes in treatment and drug therapy may become necessary or appropriate. Readers are advised to check the most current product information provided by the manufacturer of each drug to be administered to verify the recommended dose, the method and duration of administration, and contraindications. It is the responsibility of the licensed health care provider, relying on experience and knowledge of the patient, to determine dosages and the best treatment for each individual patient. Neither the Publisher nor the editor assume any liability for any injury and/or damage to persons or property arising from this publication.

Mosby, Inc.
A Harcourt Health Sciences Company
11830 Westline Industrial Drive
St. Louis, Missouri 63146

Printed in United States of America

International Standard Book Number 0-323-00911-5

99 00 01 02 03 CL/FF 9 8 7 6 5 4 3 2 1

FOR JACK

Contributors

Jo Jo Dantone, RD, LD, CDE
President
Nutrition Education Resources, Inc.
Grenada, Mississippi

Patricia E. Freed, EdD, RN
Assistant Professor
Barnes College of Nursing
The University of Missouri, St. Louis
St. Louis, Missouri

Lynn Garone, RN
Director of Operations-Infusion Pharmacy
PSA Healthcare Services
Charlotte, North Carolina

Sandra Lindquist, PhD, RN
Clinical Associate Professor
Barnes College of Nursing
The University of Missouri-St. Louis
St. Louis, Missouri

Donna Bridgman Musser, MSN, RN
Clinical Assistant Professor and Coordinator for Center of
    Technology
Barnes College of Nursing
The University of Missouri-St. Louis
St. Louis, Missouri

Robyn Rice, MSN-R, RN-C

Clinical Associate Professor
Barnes College of Nursing
The University of Missouri-St. Louis
St. Louis, Missouri;
Home Health Clinical Nurse Specialist
American Nursing Development
Maryville, Illinois

Anne Cahill Schappe, PhD, RN

Assistant Professor
School of Nursing
Webster University
St. Louis, Missouri

Joan Vernitte-Kohorst, BHS, RRT

Respiratory Care Practitioner
Apria Home Healthcare Services
St. Louis, Missouri

Pamela Becker Weilitz, MSN-R, RN, CS, AWP

Nurse Practitioner
St. Louis, Missouri

Clinical Consultant

Cindy Smith, RN
Clinical Director-Pharmacy Infusion Services
PSA Healthcare Services
Charlotte, North Carolina

Preface

As a practicing home health nurse, I believe it is crucial for home health agencies to have written clinical procedures that provide contemporary guidelines for practice. Moreover, such guidelines should be readily available as a resource to nurses who care for patients in the very challenging and sometimes isolating environment of the home milieu. Most important, such procedures are valuable as they serve as unifying standards of practice for the home health agency and reflect the quality of care rendered by each nurse. I have revised the second edition of the *Handbook of Home Health Nursing Procedures* to serve as a working resource for nurses in the field.

The handbook has been designed so that it is easy and convenient to use. It fits easily into most nursing bags and serves as a quick reference for care. The procedures in each section are listed alphabetically within each body system or grouping for ease of use. Each procedure generally adheres to the following simple and direct format:

Purpose
Equipment
General Information
Procedure (in a step-wise format)
Nursing Considerations
Documentation Guidelines

General Information provides background information useful for implementing the procedure. Nursing Considerations provide nursing alerts and patient education considerations to keep in mind when the procedure is implemented. Documentation Guidelines describe important aspects of the procedure to document on visit reports. The arrow and pencil symbols in the margins allow the user to quickly locate the Nursing Considerations and Documentation Guidelines for immediate reference.

This book is divided into 13 chapters. Chapter 1, Infection

Control in the Home, reflects current Occupational Safety and Health Administration regulations and Centers for Disease Control and Prevention guidelines for infection control that are tailored to home care concerns. Chapter 2, Assessment and Therapeutic Procedures, details assessment procedures and basic nursing care, such as Adult Head-to-Toe Assessment and Positioning and Seating the Immobilized Patient. The remaining chapters include information on cardiopulmonary care; head, eyes, ears, nose, throat (HEENT) care; dermatologic and wound care; gastroenterologic and ostomy care; intravenous therapy; medications; rehabilitation and palliative care; urologic and renal care; and procedures for specimen collection. All procedures have been updated. In addition, more than 35 new procedures (e.g., pain assessment and nephrostomy tube care) have been added. Also, a new chapter on nutrition has been added that lists nutritional recommendations based on disease process and physical needs.

A comprehensive bibliography organized by chapter appears at the end of the handbook. The handbook also features appendices that assist field staff. Appendix I, Dermal Wound Care Products, is an extensive table describing currently available wound care products. Appendix II, Laboratory Values, lists normal blood and urine values for laboratory tests. Furthermore, as a resource for home health nurses, Appendix III, which describes Internet sites relative to the needs of practicing home health nurses, has also been included.

The following points should be noted:

1. The term patient/caregiver is used throughout the handbook to denote the patient's family, friend, or significant other, who may assist the patient and the nurse in carrying out the procedure. Although most patients live at home with their families, some patients receive care and support from other sources. For this reason I have chosen to use the term **caregiver** to encompass the services of all who provide assistance.

2. The initials **HHA** stand for *home health agency.* This is not to be confused with **hha,** which is an abbreviation for *home health aide.*

3. It is understood that all procedures are to be implemented under the auspices of each state's nurse practice acts. In addition, it is expected that the nurse would obtain physician's

orders for all procedures and activities of daily living care before implementing them. Orders and the specifications of any procedure or treatment must be reviewed by the nurse before they are implemented.

4. As a primary component of patient education, clean technique is commonly taught in the home health setting today. Obtain physician's orders for clean technique as appropriate. Sterile technique, as it is assessed by the home health nurse, may be more appropriate for patients with certain diseases and active infections and for immunocompromised patients or patients who require certain invasive procedures. Keep in mind that infection control practices should provide safety for the patient, caregiver, and health care worker. **Please note the stop sign symbol in the Equipment section of most procedures.** This is the symbol used to signify that *Standard Precautions* should be followed. It alerts the nurse to refer to and follow recommendations regarding principles of infection control as described in Chapter 1.

The procedures in this book were written with goals of simplicity and ease of use in mind. In view of the enormous amount of documentation and paperwork that exists in home health, I have always valued relevant, as well as easily accessible, material. The content in this book, as reflected in the bibliography and reference section, is largely derived from evidence-based practice and from governmental regulations for care and includes current clinical practice guidelines from the U.S. Department of Health and Human Services Agency for Health Care Policy and Research. However, a couple of points should be made. First, research supporting clinical practice continues to expand. Also, governmental regulations influencing nursing practice frequently change. Therefore, it is expected that home health nurses and home health agencies keep-up-to date with and adhere to evolving clinical practice guidelines. Second, in my opinion, there is a danger in absolutism. Therefore, keep in mind that the basis of caring in the home is to promote the well-being of the patient. Hence, home health nurses should always use their best judgment when implementing any procedure.

The information in this handbook will assist home health nurses to carry out a vast array of procedures demanded by this area of nursing practice. It will increase the nurse's clinical understanding of procedural issues related to patient care, the importance of a multidisciplinary approach, and the importance of patient education when a procedure is performed in the home.

Nursing faculty, student nurses, and registered nurses new to the home health field will also benefit from the handbook. Most important, this book was written by a practicing home health nurse for practicing home health nurses. It is my sincere hope that it will serve as a helpful resource for my colleagues working out in the field.

Robyn Rice

Acknowledgments

I would like to take this opportunity to acknowledge and recognize the caring that home health nurses give to their patients and to their communities. Such devotion to duty and commitment to work are essential for maintaining the health of the American public today and tomorrow.

Contents

Box 1-1
OSHA TERMINOLOGY
1919-1030 Final Rule*

Bloodborne pathogens

   Pathogenic microorganisms that are present in human blood and can cause disease in humans. These pathogens include (but are not limited to) hepatitis B virus (HBV) and human immunodeficiency virus (HIV).

Contaminated laundry

   Laundry that has been soiled with blood or other potentially infectious materials or that may contain sharps.

Decontamination

   The use of physical or chemical means to remove, inactivate, or destroy bloodborne pathogens on a surface or an item so that it is no longer capable of transmitting infectious particles; the surface or item then is rendered safe for handling, use, or disposal.

Engineering controls

   Controls (e.g., sharps-disposal containers, self-sheathing needles) that isolate or remove the bloodborne-pathogens hazard from the workplace.

Exposure control plan

   A written plan designed to eliminate or minimize employee exposure (required of all employers whose employees have occupational exposure that is identified in a job description).

Exposure incident

   A specific contact with the eye, mouth, other mucous membrane, or nonintact skin or a parenteral contact with blood or other potentially infectious materials that occurs during the performance of an employee's duties.

---

*From Occupational Safety and Health Administration: 29 CFR, Part 1910, 1030, *Occupational exposure to bloodborne pathogens: final rule,* U.S. Department of Labor, Washington, DC, December 7, 1991.

Continued

> ## Box 1-1
> ## OSHA TERMINOLOGY—cont'd
> ### *1919-1030 Final Rule**
>
> **Occupational exposure**
>
> Reasonably anticipated skin, eye, mucous membrane, or parenteral contacts with blood or other potentially infectious materials that may occur during the performance of an employee's duties.
>
> **Personal protective equipment**
>
> Specialized clothing or equipment worn by an employee for protection against a hazard. General work clothes (e.g., uniforms, pants, shirts, or blouses) not intended to function as protection against a hazard are not personal protective equipment.
>
> **Universal precautions**
>
> An approach to infection control. According to the concept of universal precautions, all human blood and certain human body fluids are treated as if they are infectious for HIV, HBV, and other bloodborne pathogens.
>
> **Work practice controls**
>
> Controls that reduce the likelihood of exposure by altering the manner in which a task is performed (e.g., prohibiting the recapping of needles by using a two-handed technique).

*From Occupational Safety and Health Administration: 29 CFR, Part 1910, 1030, *Occupational exposure to bloodborne pathogens: final rule,* U.S. Department of Labor, Washington, DC, December 7, 1991.

    d. Masks, disposable cardiopulmonary resuscitation (CPR) masks, goggles, National Institute of Occupational Safety and Health (NIOSH)-approved respiratory protection devices, moisture-proof aprons or gowns, shoe covers, caps, and an extra uniform stocked in the car

---

Box 1-2

POTENTIAL SIGNS AND SYMPTOMS OF INFECTION

1. Changes in the skin: redness or rash, heat, swelling, weeping or drainage
2. Green or yellow exudates or drainage in the wound bed
3. Elevated temperature
4. Sore throat
5. Cough or change in sputum production or color
6. Fever, chills, or sweating
7. Nausea, vomiting, or diarrhea
8. Burning or painful urination
9. Clouds or filtrates in the Foley catheter bag
10. Tenderness or pain in a body part
11. Stiff neck or headache
12. Diminished breath sounds or wheezing on auscultation; labored respirations
13. Tachycardia or rapid pulse
14. Mental status changes

---

    e. Liquid soap (bacteriocidal), soap towelettes, dry hand disinfectants (bleach and alcohol based), hand lotion
    f. Paper towels
    g. Plastic bags with a seal and marked with a biohazard sign for use when transporting laboratory specimens
    h. Leak-proof and puncture-proof containers marked with a biohazard sign on the outside of the containers for use when transporting laboratory specimens
    i. Sharps containers
    j. Large plastic container or cardboard box to store nursing bag and supplies in trunk of field staff car
    k. Impermeable plastic trash bags for soiled dressings, etc.
    l. Sterile bottled water

PROCEDURE
Handwashing

    The hands should be washed before and after patient contact. The hands are to be washed during patient care if they become soiled. Wash the hands with liquid soap and water immediately after removing gloves. If soap and water are not available, antiseptic hand cleanser or towelettes may be used. The hands should then be washed with soap and water as soon as possible.

Gloves

Wear gloves if the possibility of contact transmission may occur. Change gloves between each patient procedure or when going from dirty to clean (e.g., multiple dressing changes). Wear disposable nonsterile nonlatex gloves when performing any clinical procedure that may expose you to the patient's blood or other body substances (e.g., during venipuncture or perineal care). Sterile disposable nonlatex gloves are to be worn during certain clinical procedures that require sterile technique (e.g., during certain dressing changes or when inserting a urinary catheter). Sterile and nonsterile nonlatex disposable gloves are to be disposed of after each use in a leak-resistant waste receptacle, such as a plastic trash bag.

Utility gloves are to be used to clean up equipment, the work area, or spills. Utility gloves are to be issued to each household. Utility gloves may be disinfected and reused. Dispose of and replace utility gloves that show signs of cracking, peeling, tearing or puncture, or other signs of deterioration.

Impermeable plastic trash bag

Place all soiled dressings, disposable gloves, etc. in an impermeable plastic trash bag, then secure it. Place the trash bag in the family trash. Follow federal, state, and local ordinances regarding disposal of biohazardous waste in the community.

Additional personal protective equipment

This type of equipment is provided to home health nurses by the home health agency for use in appropriate clinical circumstances and includes the following:
Blood spill kit. The blood spill kit travels with the nurse and should be kept in the car supply container. The kit should at least contain utility gloves, plastic trash bags, and paper towels. The kit should also contain a 1:10 bleach solution, bleach wipes, or an approved home health agency disinfectant for cleaning up blood or body substance spills in the patient's home. Make a new batch of bleach solution daily because chlorine deteriorates and loses efficacy over time.

Gowns, aprons, shoe covers, caps. Wear moisture-proof disposable gowns or aprons, shoe covers, and caps when there is a reasonable expectation that contact transmission may occur. After use, remove and dispose of personal protective equipment in an impermeable plastic trash bag in the work area.

Masks. Disposable face masks are to be worn whenever there is a reasonable expectation that droplet transmission may occur. Dispose of masks after each use.

When respiratory isolation is required, post a homemade **"STOP"** sign outside the patient's room. Instruct the family, caregivers, and/or visitors to wear masks when entering the room and/or when caring for the patient. The **STOP** sign should alert everyone, including children, of the necessity to wear a mask when entering the patient's room.

DISPOSABLE CPR MASKS

Use disposable CPR masks if artificial mouth-to-mouth or mouth-to-stoma ventilation is required. Most CPR masks are designed to be discarded after one use. Follow individual manufacturer's recommendations for usage and care.

RESPIRATORY PROTECTION DEVICES

Use a NIOSH-approved respiratory protection device when caring for patients and families with tuberculosis; fit-testing is required. Respirators must be cleaned according to the manufacturer's recommendations and discarded when excessive resistance, physical damage, or any other condition renders the respirator unsuitable for use.

GOGGLES OR FACE SHIELDS

Goggles or face shields are to be worn when there is a reasonable expectation that droplet transmission may occur to the eyes. Clean the goggles or shields according to the manufacturer's recommendations, and discard when physical damage or any other condition renders them unsuitable for use.

Sharp objects and needles

Place sharp objects and needles in a puncture-proof disposable container that can be sealed with a lid. A needle should not be bent, sheared, replaced in the sheath or guard, or removed from the syringe after use. Do not recap used needles unless using a capping device or one-hand scoop method (nursing staff should be inserviced on a one-hand method if this technique is approved by the home health agency).

Sharps containers. Sharps containers should have the following characteristics:
- Be puncture-proof
- Be red or opaque in color (do not use a clear container where needles can be easily identified)
- Be labeled or marked with a biohazard sign on the outside
- Be leak-proof

Never fill sharps containers so that the contents protrude out of the opening. *Do not fill sharps containers over two thirds full.* Store sharps containers out of reach of children (e.g., on the top shelf in a bedroom closet). Follow state and local ordinances regarding disposal of sharps containers.

Specimen collection

Wear gloves when handling specimens. Handle all specimens carefully to minimize spillage. Blood or other body substance specimens should be placed in a leak-proof plastic bag and secured in a puncture/leak-proof container during collection, handling, storage, and transport. Label specimens with the patient's name and identifying data. Place the puncture/leak-proof container on the floor of the car during transport.

In accordance with the home health agency policy, a courier service may be called to pick up laboratory specimens that have been left at the patient's home.

Uniform

Nursing and field staff are responsible for keeping an extra (clean) uniform secured in a water-resistant bag in their car. The extra uniform shall be stored in the supply container in the trunk of the nurse's car. If a uniform becomes soiled during patient care, change into the clean uniform as soon as possible. Place the soiled uniform in a leak-proof plastic bag, and launder according to individual home health agency policy. (If the home health agency purchases scrubs for nurses to wear or a uniform *specific* for contact with blood and/or body substances, then the agency is responsible for laundering the uniform. Contact your local OSHA representative with further questions on this subject.)

If nurses choose to launder their uniform or work clothes at home, it is recommended that clothing soiled with blood or body substances be washed separately from household laundry in extremely hot water for about 25 minutes (use a detergent and bleach that will not damage colored clothes). Uniforms or work clothes not soiled with blood or body substances may be routinely cleaned in the regular family wash. Store one dry uniform or set of work clothes in a plastic bag in the field staff car for possible future use.

Principles of cleaning, disinfecting, and sterilizing in the home

All equipment must be cleaned thoroughly to remove organic material before disinfection or sterilization. Review the procedures in this manual for specific guidelines. Modifications to routine disinfection practices in the home may include the use of the following:

- Bleach
- Hydrogen peroxide
- Boiling water
- Hot, soapy water
- Phenolic resin (e.g., Lysol)
- Isopropyl alcohol (70%)
- Acetic acid (white vinegar)

Patient/family laundry. Laundry should be handled as little as possible and with minimum agitation to prevent gross microbial contamination of the air and of the persons handling the linen. Place linens soiled with blood or body fluids in a leak-resistant bag at the location where care was given. Instruct the family to wash soiled linens in hot, soapy water with a bleach solution, separate from the family wash.

Personal. Eating, drinking, smoking, applying cosmetics or lip balm, and handling contact lenses are prohibited in patient care areas where there is reasonable likelihood of occupational exposure to blood or body substances. Food and drinks are not to be kept in patient care areas where blood or other potentially infectious materials are present.

Miscellaneous

All clinical procedures shall be performed in a manner that minimizes splashing, spraying, splattering, or generating droplets of blood or body substances. Mouth pipetting/suctioning of blood or other body substances is prohibited.

Immunizations

It is recommended that all staff involved in direct patient care (e.g., touching, working with patients/caregivers) be immunized against hepatitis B. In addition, ACIP strongly recommends that all staff be vaccinated against (or have documented immunity to) influenza, measles, mumps, rubella, and varicella.

Lastly, it is mandatory that all staff involved in direct patient care receive an initial two-step tuberculosis skin test (the Mantoux test with 5 tuberculin units of purified protein derivative [PPD]) at time of employment. Repeat skin testing is to be done annually. Previous bacille Calmette-Guérin (BCG) vaccination is not a contraindication for skin testing.

Exposure incident

In the event of eye or body contact with the patient's blood or body substances, including deep wound puncture from a needlestick, (1) irrigate the eye with water or wash the exposed body part with soap and water (use bottled sterile water stocked in the nursing bag or car as necessary), and (2) contact the home health agency Infection Control Director for follow-up instructions and care. In addition, report suspect exposure to *Mycobacterium tuberculosis* or any other infectious organism to the Infection Control Director.

OSHA regulations

Infection control standards and policies published by OSHA should be accessible to all home health staff for reference. A copy of these regulations should be placed in the Infection Control Manual or in the appropriate policy or procedure manual located in an easily accessible place at the home health agency. The home health agency is responsible for having an infection control program, including a staff infection–control exposure plan, that identifies patient risk for infectious organisms on admission to the home health agency and includes guidelines for clinical management.

NURSING CONSIDERATIONS

The nursing bag is to be handled and transported in as clean a manner as possible.

Instruct the patient/caregiver on infection control precautions.

Consider placing patients who have active infectious organisms, such as vancomycin-resistant *Staphylococcus aureus,* with an

"infection control care team" or specific case manager to reduce the risk of staff exposure and transmission of infectious
organisms to other patients. Try to visit these patients last or
at the end of the day. When possible, use disposable equipment or keep needed equipment in the home with these patients, and contact the local health department for further
surveillance/management guidelines.

Be aware that at the time of this writing, OSHA was proposing
new rules for staff protection against exposure to *M. tuberculosis,* including skin retesting every 6 months for all staff who
are at risk for exposure to sources of aerosolized *M. tuberculosis* or who come in contact with patients with suspected or
active *M. tuberculosis.*

DOCUMENTATION GUIDELINES

Document the following on the visit report:

- Any patient/caregiver instructions regarding infection
  control precautions and response to teaching, including ad-
  herence to recommendations
- Implementation of *Standard Precautions*
- Physician notification, if applicable
- Other pertinent findings

Update the plan of care.

CHAPTER 2

Assessment and Therapeutic Procedures

Adult Head-to-Toe Assessment

PURPOSE
- To obtain a data base to establish the plan of care
- To identify patient problems or needs on the patient care plan
- To establish a baseline physiologic status

RELATED PROCEDURES
- Mental Health Assessment
- Socioenvironmental Assessment

GENERAL INFORMATION
In conjunction with a health history, a review of all the patient's body systems is necessary at the time of admission to the home health agency. A baseline physiologic data base is established to evaluate deviations from normal findings.

Data from the health history and the physical assessment are both objective and subjective and are usually obtained from the patient. However, information may be supplemented from a secondary source, such as a caregiver, multidisciplinary team, or records from the referring institution.

PROCEDURE
1. Explain the interview and techniques of examination to the patient/caregiver.
2. Assess the following:

General
Usual weight, any recent weight change, weakness, fatigue, fever, appearance, and patient's/caregiver's major concerns;

identify and list all known allergies; ask the patient whether he or she can maintain normal daily activities

Head

Headache, head injury, dizziness, hair color and distribution, facial movement, symmetry, and surgeries

Eyes

Vision, glasses or contact lenses, most recent eye examination, pain, redness, excessive tearing, double vision, glaucoma, cataracts, pupil or conjunctive discoloration, abnormal eye movement, and surgeries

Ears

Hearing, tinnitus, vertigo, earaches, infections, discharge, and surgeries

Nose

Frequent colds, nasal stuffiness, hay fever, nosebleeds, sinus trouble, patency of nasal passages, discharge, and surgeries

Mouth and throat

Condition of teeth, gums, and buccal mucosa; bleeding gums; last dental examination; sores or lesions; frequent sore throat; hoarseness; gag reflex; swallowing difficulties; and surgeries

Neck

Masses, swollen lymph nodes, goiter, pain, stiffness, and surgeries

Skin

Rashes, masses, lesions, itching, dryness, color change, changes in nails, pustules, papules, turgor, dermal wounds (bedsores or ulcerations), and surgeries

Breasts

Masses, pain, nipple discharge, self-examination, mammogram, and surgeries

Respiratory

Wheezes or crackles, cough, dyspnea, orthopnea, paroxysmal nocturnal dyspnea, sputum (color and quantity), hemoptysis, wheezing, asthma, allergies, chronic obstructive pulmonary disease (COPD), pneumonia, tuberculosis, pleurisy, tuberculin test, last chest x-ray examination (dates and results), flu vaccination, tobacco use, and surgeries

Cardiac

Heart sounds, hypertension, rheumatic fever, murmurs, bruits, thrills, edema, jugular venous distention, chest pain, palpitations, irregular heart rate, shortness of breath (SOB) or poor activity tolerance, capillary refill, last electrocardiogram, cardiac procedures, and surgeries

Neurologic

Level of consciousness, orientation, reflexes, strength, coordination, balance, sensation, fainting, blackouts, seizures, paralysis, local weakness, numbness, tingling, tremors, memory, speech, perceptual disturbances, sleep, and surgeries

Peripheral vascular

Clubbing, capillary refill, intermittent claudication, color, temperature, pulses, cramps, varicose veins, and thrombophlebitis, and surgeries

Gastrointestinal

Diet, height, difficulty in swallowing, heartburn, appetite, nausea, indigestion, excessive belching or passing of gas, food intolerance, caffeine and alcohol use, vomiting of blood, frequency of bowel movements, change in bowel habits, diarrhea, laxative use, bowel sounds, abdominal pain, hemorrhoids, jaundice, liver or gall bladder disease, hepatitis, ostomy, gastrointestinal or drainage tubes, ulcers, cirrhosis, masses, tenderness, rectal bleeding, and surgeries

Fluid and electrolyte

Dehydration, central/peripheral edema, fluid and diet restrictions, intravenous therapy, serum electrolyte panel (SMA-7), blood urea nitrogen (BUN), input and output, and surgeries

Musculoskeletal

Range of motion (ROM), strength, tenderness, crepitus, pain, swelling, redness, heat, arthritis, osteoporosis, deformities (kyphosis, scoliosis, and barrel chest), amputation, gait, paralysis, and surgeries

Endocrine

Endurance; thyroid disease; diabetes mellitus; steroids; insulin management; excessive thirst, hunger, or sweating or frequency of urination; and surgeries

Hematologic

Easy bruising or bleeding, anemia, HIV infection, AIDS, past transfusions and any reactions, complete blood cell (CBC) count, blood cultures, and surgeries

Urinary

Urgency, hesitancy, dribbling, incontinence, urinary tract infection, frequency of urination, polyuria, nocturia, dysuria, hematuria, kidney stones, urinary catheterization, ileostomy, dialysis, kidney disease, urinalysis, and surgeries

Genitoreproductive

Male

Discharge from or sores on penis, history of sexually transmitted disease and treatment, hernias, testicular pain or masses, frequency of intercourse, libido, sexuality, last prostate examination, and surgeries

Female

Age at menarche; regularity, frequency, and duration of menstrual periods; amount of bleeding; bleeding between menstrual periods after intercourse; last menstrual period; dysmenorrhea; age of menopause; menopausal symptoms; postmenopausal bleeding; discharge; itching; sexually transmitted disease and treatment; last Papanicolaou smear; number of pregnancies; number of deliveries; number of abortions (spontaneous and induced); complications of pregnancy; birth control methods; frequency of intercourse; libido; sexuality; and surgeries

Psychiatric

Depression, mood changes, memory loss, obsessive compulsions, hypochondriasis, dementia, schizophrenia, grief, suicide attempts, anxiety, drug abuse, agitation, nervousness, eye contact, unusual affect or communication patterns, sleep and eating disturbances, unusual dress and behavior, impaired socialization, and any previous hospitalizations

Medications

Identify medications currently prescribed, and elicit information about compliance; include over-the-counter medications

Functional learning limitations

Ambulation, transfers, reading, attention span, dressing, toileting, personal hygiene, housekeeping, and cooking

NURSING CONSIDERATIONS

Pay particular attention to the specific disease pathology and to any abnormal findings noted on the physical examination.

A brief inquiry into the family history of diseases, such as cancer, tuberculosis, cardiac complaint, or diabetes, is appropriate.

Deviations from normal findings should be reported to the physician (as appropriate) and should be reflected in the patient care plan.

A referral to social services, rehabilitation services, or specialty nursing services may be required.

DOCUMENTATION GUIDELINES

Use the data base to implement the plan of care and to develop the patient care plan. Identified problems on the patient care plan should then be a focus of the visit report. Document *Standard Precautions* on the visit report. Update the plan of care to reflect the current patient status.

Blood Pressure

PURPOSE
- To assess systolic and diastolic arterial blood pressure

EQUIPMENT
1. Sphygmomanometer with cuff
2. Stethoscope

 3. Antiseptic wipes and an impermeable plastic trash bag (see *Infection Control*)

PROCEDURE
1. Explain the procedure to the patient/caregiver.
2. Assemble the equipment at a convenient work area.
3. Expose the patient's arm above the elbow. Instruct the patient to relax his or her arm. Support the patient's forearm at his or her side during the procedure.
4. Determine the proper cuff size to obtain an accurate reading. (The width of the cuff should be 40% of the circumference at the midpoint of the limb on which the cuff is to be used: 20% wider than the diameter. The length of the bladder should be approximately twice the recommended width.)
5. Adjust the cuff by placing a compression bag over the inner aspect of the arm, approximately 1 inch above the elbow. Center the arrows marked on the cuff along the brachial artery. (Before the cuff is applied, squeeze out the excess air.)
6. Strap the Velcro sleeve band, and firmly secure it. Position the manometer at eye level.
7. Palpate the brachial artery at the bend of the elbow (antecubital area).
8. Tighten the pressure valve or screw that is located on the bulb.
9. Squeeze the bulb to inflate the pressure cuff until the brachial artery can no longer be palpated. Then inflate the cuff to a mercury reading of 20 to 30 mm Hg above the point where the pulse disappeared.

10. Place the bell (or diaphragm) of the stethoscope over the patient's brachial artery where the pulse was palpated. (The bell of the stethoscope transmits low-pitched arterial blood sounds more effectively than the diaphragm.)
11. Insert the tips of the stethoscope in your ears, with the tips pointing down and forward.
12. Slowly release the pressure valve on the inflation bulb, allowing the mercury to fall at a rate of 2 to 3 mm Hg a second. Listen for pulse sounds.
13. Take the reading when the first sound is heard; this is the systolic pressure. Continue to release the pressure slowly, until the last pulsation is heard; this is the diastolic pressure.
14. Allow the pressure to fall rapidly to zero, and remove the cuff.
15. If you repeat the procedure, wait 30 seconds.
16. Provide patient comfort measures.
17. Clean the bell of the stethoscope with an antiseptic wipe to prevent cross-contamination. Discard disposable items according to *Standard Precautions.*

NURSING CONSIDERATIONS

At the initial assessment, take the patient's blood pressure while the patient is sitting and again while he or she is standing to evaluate for orthostatic hypotension.

During the first visit, take blood pressure readings on both arms. Thereafter, take blood pressure readings on the patient's arm that shows the highest reading while the patient is in a sitting position to ensure accurate measurements. If the patient is unable to sit, always take the blood pressure reading in the same position/arm for consistency in readings.

Avoid taking blood pressure readings on an injured arm, an arm with a shunt, an arm that is being infused with an intravenous solution, or on the arm on the affected side of the mastectomy patient because blood flow may be compromised.

DOCUMENTATION GUIDELINES

Document the following on the visit report:
• Vital signs, including systolic *and* diastolic blood pressure readings
• Correlate the blood pressure readings with medications,

and notify the physician about abnormal findings or deviations from the baseline status
- Physician notification, if applicable
- *Standard Precautions*
- Other pertinent findings

Update the plan of care.

Edema

PURPOSE
- To assess cardiopulmonary status
- To provide a uniform and objective approach to measuring the central, peripheral, and abdominal edema for baseline evaluation
- To evaluate the effect of diuretic administration
- To evaluate the patient's adherence to prescribed medications, diet, and activity regimen

RELATED PROCEDURE
- Weight

EQUIPMENT
1. Scale
2. Tape measure

PROCEDURE
1. Explain the procedure to the patient/caregiver.
2. Assemble the equipment at a convenient work area.
3. Assist the patient to a sitting or comfortable position.
4. Assess the cardiopulmonary status.
5. Notify the physician about signs of central circulatory overload, such as crackles or wheezes on auscultation, dyspnea, mental status changes, or deviations from the patient's baseline status.
6. Assess the patient's adherence to prescribed medications, diet, or activity regimen.

7. Weigh the patient at each visit.
   a. Notify the physician if a 3- to 4-pound weight gain occurs in 1 week because such a weight gain may indicate progressive heart failure or noncompliance with prescribed medication, diet, or activity regimen.
   b. Instruct the patient to weigh himself or herself each morning before breakfast and after the first voiding and to record the weight. Instruct the patient to notify the physician of a 2-pound weight gain in 1 day.
8. Assess and evaluate edema. (Dependent edema may be located in the feet, legs, or hands. Edema at the sacral area may be found in bedridden patients. Abdominal edema may be found in bedridden and ambulatory patients, particularly patients with congestive heart failure and with liver or renal disease.)
9. Measure the edematous area each visit. If edema is present, the area should be measured for an objective comparison with the patient's normal body measurements. Measurements should be taken in the following manner:
   a. *Pedal edema measurement.* Measure above bony prominences, such as over the dorsum of the foot, above the ankle, and at midcalf. On the visit report, note the number of inches from the knee the edema is located for uniform calf measurements (Fig. 2-1).
   b. *Hand edema measurement.* Measure between the phalangeal joints, over the dorsum of the hand, and at the wrist (Fig. 2-2).
   c. *Abdominal edema measurement.* Measure abdominal girth, and then record the measurement above, across, or under the navel (Fig. 2-3).
10. Palpate the edematous area to assess whether pitting is present. Palpate the area over the bony surface at the ankle, the tibia, the foot, the sacrum, and the hand (or bones of the wrist). Use one of the following to describe the pitting edema:
    a. Pitting is 1+ if the area can be depressed 1 cm; it is 2+ if a 2 cm depression can be made. This procedure continues until 4+ is reached. Identify the area where the pitting edema is assessed. For example: pitting 3+, left foot.

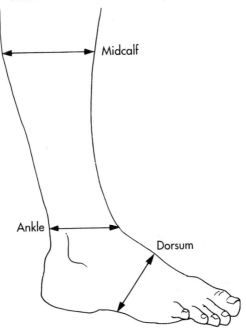

Fig. 2-1 Measurement of pedal edema.

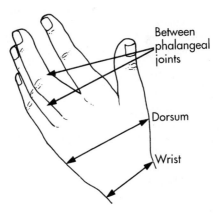

Fig. 2-2 Measurement of hand edema.

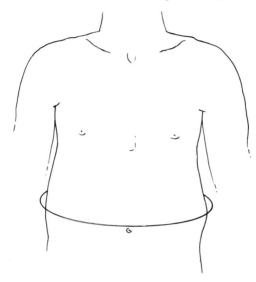

Fig. 2-3   Measurement of abdominal edema.

b. Depress the edematous area, and note the time that is required for the area to return to normal. If the time is greater than 15 seconds, record: >15 seconds. Identify the areas where pitting edema is assessed. For example: pitting edema is 10 seconds, ankle to midcalf.

11. Provide patient comfort measures.

NURSING CONSIDERATIONS

Instruct the patient about the signs of fluid retention, such as sudden shortness of breath at night, shoes or clothes that suddenly do not fit, wheezing, and chest pain.

Instruct the patient about when to call the physician and when to go to the emergency room.

DOCUMENTATION GUIDELINES

Document the following on the visit report:
• The procedure and patient toleration
• Cardiopulmonary status, including auscultatory findings
• Weight

- Measurements of edematous areas, assessed in centimeters
- Description of pitting edema as appropriate
- Any patient/caregiver instructions, including response to teaching
- Physician notification, if applicable
- *Standard Precautions*
- Other pertinent findings

Update the plan of care.

Foot Care

PURPOSE
- To promote personal hygiene
- To prevent infection of the feet
- To promote self-care in the home

EQUIPMENT
1. Large basin
2. Bath thermometer if available
3. Soap, lotion, nail clipper, emery board, and toilette items
4. Bath towel and washcloth
5. Plastic sheeting or towel
6. White cotton socks, shoes, or slippers
7. Disposable nonsterile gloves and an impermeable plastic trash bag (see *Infection Control*)

PROCEDURE
1. Explain the procedure to the patient/caregiver.
2. Assemble the equipment at a convenient work area.
3. Fill a basin half full of soapy water, leaving sufficient space for rinse water. Make sure the temperature does not exceed 105° F.
4. Place plastic sheeting under the basin to prevent the floor from getting wet.
5. Assist the patient in placing his or her feet in the basin of soapy water.

6. Rinse the soapy solution from the patient's feet with clear water.
7. Assist the patient in removing his or her feet from the basin, taking care not to get the floor wet.
8. Dry the patient's feet thoroughly, especially between the toes. Examine the patient's feet carefully for evidence of slight discoloration or lesions.
9. Encourage foot care and inspection as part of the morning routine after bathing.
10. Apply lotion to the patient's feet.
11. Perform nail care for the patient, as needed. Use lamb's wool, as needed, when there is overlapping of the toes or when maceration between the toes is evident.
12. Put white cotton socks on the patient to minimize dryness and infections. Discourage the patient from wearing garters or nylon hose that may constrict circulation.
13. Make sure the patient's shoes fit properly to avoid rubbing or blisters. (Three quarters of an inch of space between the great toe and the widest part of the shoe should exist when the patient is standing.)
14. Provide patient comfort measures.
15. Clean and replace the equipment. Discard disposable items according to *Standard Precautions.*

NURSING CONSIDERATIONS

Assess the type of shoe worn as appropriate for level of ambulation and safety.

Patients with diabetes may have peripheral neuropathies, causing decreased sensation. Therefore, instruct patients with diabetes to examine their feet for blisters, cracks, or sores each day and immediately report any problems to the physician.

DOCUMENTATION GUIDELINES

Document the following on the visit report:
• The procedure and patient toleration
• The condition of the patient's feet and toenails
• Any patient/caregiver instructions regarding foot care and response to teaching, including the ability to care for feet
• Physician notification, if applicable
• *Standard Precautions*
• Other pertinent findings

Update the plan of care.

Home Improvisation of Equipment

PURPOSE

- To use equipment for patient care made from materials or resources that are found in the home
- To promote self-care in the home

EQUIPMENT

1. Improvised household resources

PROCEDURE

1. Explain the procedure and the use of improvised equipment to the patient/caregiver.
2. Assess the household resources, and assemble the materials.
3. Examples of improvised household items include the following:
    a. *Linen protectors*—plastic trash bags
    b. *IV pole*—attach the bag of IV fluids through the hook of a coat hanger; slip one of the triangular ends of the coat hanger onto the coat hook of the bedroom door
    c. *Transfer belt*—use the patient's belt
    d. *Call bell*—a soda can filled with small stones, or a dinner bell
    e. *Shawl*—fold a large bath towel into a triangle; place it on the patient, and secure it with a safety pin
    f. *Robe*—find a blanket; make the collar by making a fold along the length of the blanket; adjust it on the patient's shoulder, with the center of the collar at the back of the neck; bring the blanket around to the front, and pin it; make the sleeves by centering the width of the blanket and draping it across the wrists; turn back the cuff, and pin the sides of the blanket to make the sleeves and sides of the robe
    g. *Bed table*—use a clean, heavy cardboard carton; remove the bottom; cut out the sides to allow the table to fit over the patient's lap; cut small holes in the short ends for hand holds to use in lifting the table; draw a picture on top or color with crayons to personalize; the long end

of an ironing board adjusted over the patient/s lap may also be used as a bedside table; a book can also be used to make a firm surface

h. *Backrest*—pillows or card table propped against the head of the bed, tied securely, and padded

i. *Backrest*—pillows or card table propped against the head of the bed, tied securely, and padded

j. *Bed cradle*—make a bed cradle by using the instructions for the bed table in step *g;* place it over the feet, and bring the covers over the cradle

k. *Medicine organizer and dispenser*—egg carton, muffin tray, envelopes, check-off chart of daily or weekly medicines made from poster board or a large piece of paper

l. *Foot towel*—tape a washcloth around the bottom of a yard stick; the patient may use this to dry the feet or between the toes if he or she has difficulty bending over or reaching the feet

m. *Diabetic tray*—place a glucose meter and supplies in a large bowl or container for easy access to supplies (bath or personal care supplies may also be organized in this manner)

n. *Sharps container*—use a heavy-duty plastic laundry detergent bottle with a screw-on lid and attach a label that indicates it as a sharps container. When the bottle is two-thirds full, tape on the lid with duct tape. Store out of reach of children (consider bedroom closet shelf)

NURSING CONSIDERATIONS

Home-improvised equipment should be inexpensive, safe, easy to use, and practical.

DOCUMENTATION GUIDELINES

Document the following on the visit report:
• Equipment needed and provided
• Any patient/caregiver instructions and response to teaching, including ability to safely use home-improvised equipment
• Other pertinent findings
Update the plan of care.

Intake and Output (I/O)

PURPOSE
- To measure the patient's liquid and solid intake and output
- To maintain an accurate record of the patient's fluid status

RELATED PROCEDURE
- Edema

EQUIPMENT
1. Home health agency intake and output record sheet
2. Bedpan, urinal, or drainage bag
3. The following individualized measuring utensils:
   a. Graduated measuring cylinder
   b. Commode urine collection hat
   c. Reference charts
      (1) 1 cup = 120 ml
      (2) 1 large glass = 240 ml
      (3) 1 ounce = 30 ml
      (4) 1 tablespoon = 15 ml
      (5) 1 teaspoon = 5 ml
      (6) 1 soup bowl = 180 ml
STOP 4. Disposable nonsterile gloves (see *Infection Control*)

PROCEDURE
1. Explain the procedure to the patient/caregiver.
2. Assemble the equipment to measure the patient's I/O.
3. Keep a record of the patient's I/O in the following manner:
   a. Use graduated cylinders or other measuring utensils to measure the I/O.
   b. Total liquid and solid intake on an I/O record sheet for an 8-hour period.
   c. Record the totals of three 8-hour periods to equal one 24-hour period.
4. Estimate and measure the following other forms of I/O:
   a. Vomitus
   b. Blood
   c. Wound drainage
   d. Ostomy drainage

   e. Nasogastric (NG) or gastrostomy tube output

   f. Excessive perspiration

   g. The number of formed stools

   h. The number of times and the estimated amount that the patient was incontinent with urine or diarrhea

5. Assess I/O records, and evaluate the patient's fluid status in relation to the disease process, medication regimen, diet, and activity orders on subsequent visits.

6. Provide patient comfort measures.

7. Clean and replace the equipment. Discard disposable items according to *Standard Precautions.*

NURSING CONSIDERATIONS

Instruct the patient/caregiver in the procedure.

Explain, establish, and demonstrate measurements to the patient/caregiver that are to be used for both intake and output.

Ice cubes, gelatin, and ice cream are considered liquid intake.

Instruct the patient/caregiver in record keeping. If the patient has difficulty in understanding or reading standard units of measure, make him or her an I/O sheet that is easy to use (use recognized drinking glasses or bowls as units of measurement for the patient to check off, and instruct the patient to measure output by number of times he or she voids).

Elicit feedback and a return demonstration from the patient/caregiver.

DOCUMENTATION GUIDELINES

Document the following on the visit report:

- The procedure and patient toleration
- Patient I/O
- Any patient/caregiver instructions and response to teaching, including the ability to measure and record I/O
- Physician notification, if applicable
- *Standard Precautions*
- Other pertinent findings

Complete the home health agency I/O record sheet, with 8- and 24-hour totals.

Update the plan of care.

Mental Health Assessment

PURPOSE
- To obtain a data base to establish the plan of care
- To identify the patient's mental health needs
- To lessen or diminish symptoms of patient distress or anxiety
- To promote self-care in the home

RELATED PROCEDURES
- Adult Head-to-Toe Assessment
- Socioenvironmental Assessment

GENERAL INFORMATION
The mental status assessment should be completed when the patient has a psychiatric diagnosis, or when during physical assessment or care, the nurse discovers that an in-depth mental status examination is warranted. If such is the case, the psychiatric home health nurse would be best qualified to implement the assessment.

Collect both subjective and objective information from the patient. Supplementary information, however, may be contributed by secondary sources, such as the spouse, other family members, caregiver, other members of the health care team, and/or records obtained from the referring institution.

PROCEDURE
1. Explain the interview and techniques to the patient/caregiver.
2. Gather information during the course of establishing the nurse-patient relationship.
3. Attain a brief summary of past psychiatric admissions or a history of psychiatric treatment.

Assessment of the patient should include the following:

General appearance
Grooming and manner of dress, general behavior, affect, facial expression, communication, posture, and gait; note any distinctive feature that would identify the individual immediately, would suggest a deviation from the expected norms for

the patient's age, or would compromise relationships with others.

Current medication

Identify medications that are currently prescribed, and elicit information about the patient's compliance; include over-the-counter medications.

Concurrent drug/alcohol use

Assess smoking and illicit drug and alcohol use.

Emotional status

Range: Limited, narrow, wide, or expansive; stable or labile (fluctuating)
Intensity: High- to low-energy investment in verbalizations/expression
Type: Emotional category congruent or incongruent to context

Thought processes

Reality testing: Realistic goals, perceptions, and ideas or illusions, hallucinations, and delusions
Orientation: Knows self, place, and time or is disoriented
Memory: Good to poor recall, short- and long-term memory
Attention and concentration: Focused, easily distracted, or noninvolved
Thinking: Good to poor performance on cognitive tasks such as categorization, serial sevens, or interpretation of proverbs
Integration: Expresses appropriate or inappropriate content, needs, desires, and wants in context; volunteers information and cooperates or is guarded and suspicious
Judgment: Satisfactory to unsafe expressions of actions in real or hypothetical situations and reflection versus impulsiveness
Insight: Recognizes or fails to recognize own role and responsibilities toward illness and identifies or does not identify behaviors that may be beneficial

Patterns of interaction

Goal direction content: Logical, sensible, focused, realistic to themes
Volume: Loudness or softness of voice

Rate: Speed of speech; pauses, blocks, pressured rates, or complaints of racing thoughts

Tone: Full range, monotone, booming, tedious, or monotonous

Productivity: None to minimal and brief answers; detailed or elaborate answers, neologisms, clang associations of echolalia (persecution, nihilism, and grandeur), ideations, repetitions, or incomprehensible language

General lifestyle

Methods of coping

a. When the problem began and when the symptoms that the patient is experiencing began

b. The effects of the symptoms on daily living and social functioning

c. How the patient has attempted to cope with the current situation

d. The presence of defense mechanisms and their effectiveness in reducing anxiety; the degree to which the defense mechanisms are dysfunctional

e. Community resources and support systems that are available to the patient, including the assistance of a competent caregiver

Manner of relating: Note the social and relational manner of behaving toward others and toward the nurse in the home setting

Activity: Usual patterns or changes in activities, basic need patterns, and high to low levels of energy and motivation

Satisfaction: High to low levels of involvement and expression of life satisfaction and self-worth

Level of autonomy: Appropriate interdependency as opposed to dysfunctional levels of dependency; independence, passivity, or aggressiveness

NURSING CONSIDERATIONS

Sudden changes in behavior, affect, or patterns of thinking may represent an acute health-threatening situation and should result in appropriate referral to emergency services or facilitated admission into the hospital.

Indications of new-onset depression, self-threat, threat to others, or behaviors that threaten health status, as well as evidence of delirium requires *immediate* physician evaluation.

Use the data base to develop and implement the plan of care.

 DOCUMENTATION GUIDELINES

Problems identified in the patient care plan should be a focus of the visit and visit report. Update the plan of care to reflect the current patient status.

——————

Author: Patricia E. Freed, Ed.D., R.N.

Pain Assessment

PURPOSE

- To assess the patient's level of pain
- To identify factors that exacerbate the patient's pain
- To identify factors that relieve the patient's pain
- To promote comfort and well-being

RELATED PROCEDURES

- Administration of Medications: General Guidelines (see Chapter 9)
- Pain Management (see Chapter 11)

GENERAL INFORMATION

A thorough pain assessment that includes physical and psychosocial considerations should precede any intervention for pain management. See the procedure for *Pain Management* in Chapter 11.

PROCEDURE

1. Explain the procedure to the patient/caregiver.
2. Assess the following when the patient has complaints of pain:
   a. Location (identify location of the patient's pain)
   b. Pain increases with (identify action or circumstance)
   c. Pain decreases with (identify action or circumstance)

    d. Quality of the patient's pain (circle as appropriate)—
dull, intermittent, constant, stabbing, other _____

    e. Symptoms caused by the pain (circle as appropriate)—
nausea, vomiting, diaphoresis, tachycardia, dyspnea,
other _____

    f. On a scale of 1 to 10, patient rates pain at _____

    g. How the pain affects the patient's physical and social
functioning

    h. Any history of prior pain medication and its effective-
ness in controlling the pain

       (1) Any history of possible drug abuse/misuse

    i. The following psychosocial implications for chronic
pain:

       (1) The meaning of the pain to the patient/caregiver

       (2) The patient's typical coping responses to the
pain

       (3) Changes in the patient's mood as a result of the
pain

3. Discuss pain management options and therapies with the
patient/caregiver. Assess the patient's preferences for and
expectations about pain management (accommodate and
recognize cultural considerations as well as individual
health beliefs).

4. Identify the treatment or medication currently used to
control the patient's pain.

5. Evaluate the effectiveness of treatment or medication currently used to control the patient's pain.

6. Continue to assess pain:

    a. At regular intervals after starting the treatment plan

    b. With each new report of pain

    c. At a suitable interval after each nonpharmacologic or
pharmacologic intervention (for example 15 to 30
minutes after parenteral drug therapy and/or 1 hour
after oral administration)

7. Instruct the patient to report changes in his or her pain or
any new pain so that appropriate reassessment and
changes in the treatment plan can be initiated.

NURSING CONSIDERATIONS

Be aware that many older patients in home care more often experience chronic pain as related to long-term disease processes, co-morbidities, and/or functional disability.

Perceptions of pain in the elderly may be diminished. Disorders such as dementia or stroke may interfere with the patient's ability to report the chronology and character of the pain. Use questions that are very specific and related to activities, such as "what happens to the pain when you lean forward or stand up?"

Patients who have diabetes may have decreased sensations/ reports of pain as related to disease process. It is especially important for patients in this group to visually check their legs and feet for signs of ulceration or tissue necrosis, because they may not feel pain in their lower extremities. Patients who have diabetes can also experience a painless myocardial infarction and should be regularly assessed for signs of heart failure.

DOCUMENTATION GUIDELINES

Document the following on the visit report:
- Patient vital signs and overall health status
- Location of the patient's pain
- Factors that increase and decrease the patient's pain
- Quality of the patient's pain
- Patient self-rating of pain
- Any treatment used to control the patient's pain
- Patient expectations of and response to pain therapy
- Physician notification, if applicable
- Other pertinent findings

Document medications on the medication record.
Update the plan of care.

Positioning and Seating
the Immobilized Patient

PURPOSE

- To prevent skin breakdown
- To reduce contracture formation and skeletal deformities
- To enhance internal organ functioning
- To maximize patient comfort
- To promote self-care in the home

RELATED PROCEDURE

- Skin Care (Chapter 4)

GENERAL INFORMATION

Home care patients probably spend a majority of their waking hours sitting up in some kind of chair: a wheelchair, a recliner, or a couch or sofa.

Be aware that standard living room furniture typically is made for generic comfort and is not structured enough to provide positioning support for patients experiencing weakness, paralysis, or contractures. For example, it is easier to support patients in a more upright chair, such as a wheelchair. Many patients have a tendency to sit in a slouched position with their hips placed forward on the seat, back curved, knees lower than the hips, and feet unsupported. Therefore, in assisting patients to maintain an upright, neutral body position, the home health nurse must address patient seat, back, foot, and leg supports.

PROCEDURE

1. Explain the procedure to the patient/caregiver.
2. To promote a correct sitting position for the patient, do the following:
   a. Assess the patient from the side (the keystone in proper positioning is pelvic control).
      (1) Position the patient so that his or her hips are back on the seat as close to the backrest as his or her body structure will allow. (Securing the pelvis in this position will help the patient sit upright. This prevents a

slouched position, which is damaging to the patient's skin and uncomfortable over time.)

(2) Use a seat cushion that promotes pelvic control by cradling the ischials and blocking them from sliding forward on the seat.

3. To promote correct positioning of the patient's back, do the following:

   a. Instruct the patient not to slouch his or her back (if the back is allowed to slouch, the hips will tend to push forward away from the backrest and the pelvic control gained by the seat cushion will be lost).

   b. Position the patient so that the patient's back and lumbar (lower back) curves are as upright as his or her body allows (again, this keeps the patient's pelvis in a neutral position).

4. To promote correct positioning of the patient's feet, do the following:

   a. Position the patient's feet so that the weight of the legs does not drag the patient forward out of position.

   b. Provide enough foot support so that the knees and hips are on the same level (i.e., the thigh is parallel to the floor). (This can be accomplished in a wheelchair by raising the footrests or in a piece of living room furniture by providing a stool of the proper height.)

5. To promote correct positioning of the patient's legs, do the following:

   a. Assess the patient from the front.

      (1) Align the thighs so that they are pointing straight ahead rather than rolling together or falling away from each other (it may be necessary to use support between or along the side of the thighs as needed).

      (2) Prevent leaning of the trunk by using a trunk brace or support.

   b. Assess the patient from the side and front.

      (1) Keep the pelvis as close to the backrest as possible by providing a seat cushion that keeps the ischials from sliding forward.

      (2) Prevent a slouched back posture and a pelvis that rolls backward by providing back support to maintain the natural lumbar curve.

(3) Bring the patient's knees to the same level as the hips by providing foot support.

NURSING CONSIDERATIONS

Be aware that wheelchairs typically have a sling-type upholstery that encourages a slouched back position. There is a wide variety of back cushions on the market, from small lumbar pillows to larger pieces that extend from the seat to the shoulders. Consult with the home medical supplier regarding cushion selection for the wheelchair. The goal is to use the most economical piece that helps the patient maintain the most upright position that his or her body structure will allow.

DOCUMENTATION GUIDELINES

Document the following on the visit report:
- The procedure and patient toleration
- The condition of the patient's skin
- Any patient/caregiver instructions and response to teaching, including the patient's adherence to seating recommendations
- Other pertinent findings

Update the plan of care.

Pulse

PURPOSE

- To assess pulse rate, rhythm, and volume
- To detect an irregular heart rate
- To assess a pulse deficit

EQUIPMENT

1. Stethoscope
2. Wrist watch, with second hand or digital display
3. Antiseptic wipes or home health agency disinfectant and an impermeable plastic trash bag (see *Infection Control*)

❖ Apical Pulse

PROCEDURE

1. Explain the procedure to the patient/caregiver.
2. Assemble the equipment at a convenient work area.
3. Assist the patient to a supine or sitting position.
4. Before and after patient use, clean the diaphragm of the stethoscope with antiseptic wipes or an approved home health agency disinfectant.
5. Expose the patient's chest area.
6. Palpate the point of maximal impulse (PMI) (also called Erb's point), which is located midchest and toward the patient's left side (over the apex of the heart, located in left fourth to fifth intercostal spaces).
7. Place the diaphragm over the PMI and auscultate for normal S_1 and S_2 (lub, dub) heart sounds.
8. Use a watch, and count the apical pulse for 1 minute.
9. Reclothe the patient.
10. Provide patient comfort measures.
11. Clean and replace equipment. Discard disposable items according to *Standard Precautions.*

❖ Apical-Radial Pulse

PROCEDURE

1. Follow steps *1* through *8* of the procedure for *Apical Pulse.*
2. With the other hand, palpate and assess the patient's radial pulse.
3. When the radial pulse can be felt, use a watch and count the apical and radial pulses simultaneously for 1 minute.
4. Assess any differences between the radial and apical pulses—the pulse deficit. Note the pattern or frequency of any irregularity.
5. Reclothe the patient.
6. Follow steps *10* and *11* of the procedure for *Apical Pulse.*

❖ Radial Pulse

PROCEDURE

1. Follow steps *1* through *4* of the procedure for *Apical Pulse.*

2. Gently bend the patient's elbow to a 90-degree angle, with the patient's wrist extended and palm up. Support the patient's lower arm with your arm as needed.
3. Palpate the radial pulse in the following manner:
   a. Exert slight pressure with the tips of your first two fingers on the patient's inner wrist and over the radial artery. Do not use your thumb.
   b. Apply pressure to the pulse initially, and then relax the pressure so that the pulse becomes easily palpable.
4. When the pulse can be felt, use a watch and count for a full minute.
5. Assess the rhythm, strength, and thrust of the radial pulse against your fingertips.
6. Follow steps *10* and *11* in the procedure for *Apical Pulse*.

NURSING CONSIDERATIONS

The radial pulse is commonly used during routine measurement of vital signs.

If the radial pulse is irregular or inaccessible because of dressings, follow the procedure for *Apical Pulse*.

DOCUMENTATION GUIDELINES

Document the following on the visit report:
- Characteristics of apical-radial pulse and heart sounds
- If a pulse deficit is detected, record the actual apical and radial pulses
- Correlate the apical-radial pulse characteristics with the prescribed medications, and notify the physician about any abnormal findings or deviations from the baseline status
- *Standard Precautions*
- Other pertinent findings

Update the plan of care.

Respirations

PURPOSE
• To assess the rate, depth, and quality of respirations

EQUIPMENT
1. A wrist watch with a second hand or digital display

PROCEDURE
1. Explain the procedure to the patient/caregiver.
2. Assist the patient to a position of comfort, preferably sitting.
3. Count respirations by watching the rise and fall of the chest, by placing your hand on the patient's chest to feel its rise and fall, or by listening to the patient's breathing (if it is audible).
4. Use a watch and count respirations for a full minute. One breath is made up of both 1 inspiration and 1 expiration.
5. While respirations are being counted, assess the depth and rhythm of the ventilatory movements.

DOCUMENTATION GUIDELINES
Document the following on the visit report:
• Respiratory rate
• Depth
• Rhythm
• Physician notification, if applicable
• Other pertinent findings
Update the plan of care.

Safety in the Community

PURPOSE

- To establish guidelines that maximize personal safety when working in the community and home setting

PROCEDURE

1. Take the following precautions before visits:
   a. *Appearance:*
      (1) Wear a name badge and uniform that clearly identifies you as a representative of the home health agency.
      (2) Call clients in advance and alert them to the approximate time of your visit. Confirm directions to their residence.
      (3) Request that unruly or overfriendly pets be properly secured before making visits. Back away, never run from a dog. Walk slowly around farm animals so as not to frighten them.
      (4) Keep change for a phone call in your shoe or pocket. Do *not* carry a purse. Before leaving the agency, lock your purse in the trunk of the car or cover your purse with a blanket if it will be visible.
   b. *Precautions when traveling:*
      Car
      (1) Keep your car in good working condition with plenty of gas. Obtain an automobile club membership for possible car problems.
      (2) Consider use of a personal cellular phone to maximize communication.
      (3) Store a blanket in the car in the winter and keep a thermos of cool water in the summer. Keep a snack in the glove compartment.
      (4) If your car fails, turn on emergency flashers, put a "CALL POLICE" sign in the window, and wait for the police. Do not accept rides from strangers.
      (5) Keep your car locked when parked or driving. Keep windows rolled up if possible.

    (6) Park in full view of the client's residence (avoid parking in alleys or deserted side streets).

On Foot

(1) Have nursing bag/equipment ready when exiting from the car. Keep one arm free.

(2) Walk in a professional, businesslike manner directly to the client's residence.

(3) When passing a group of strangers, cross to the other side of the street, as appropriate.

(4) When leaving the client's residence, carry car keys in your hand (pointed ends of the keys between fingers may make an effective weapon).

(5) Avoid subways or routes frequented by gangs.

(6) Use common walkways in buildings; avoid isolated stairs or darkened (unlit) areas.

  c. *Precautions during visits:*

In-the-Home Environment

(1) Always knock on the door before entering a client's home.

(2) If relatives or neighbors become a safety problem, consider the following:

    (a) Discuss the problem with the client and schedule a visit time when the relative is gone or the neighborhood is quiet.

    (b) Make joint visits with another home health nurse or arrange for escort service.

    (c) Close the case when the client, physician, and you are unable to resolve the problem.

(3) Request escort services, as appropriate for night visits.

Defense Techniques

(1) Run

(2) Scream or yell "fire" or "stranger"

(3) Kick the shins, instep, or groin

(4) Bite, scratch

(5) Use a whistle attached to your key ring, chemical sprays, or nursing bag or defense

> **NURSING CONSIDERATIONS**

Visit neighborhoods with questionable safety or gang-/drug-related problems in the morning. Some areas may have to be declared unsafe and, therefore, not serviced by your home health agency.

Regard uniforms and agency identification badges as an important part of identification to the public and an aid to your personal safety.

In the event of robbery, never resist to keep your nursing bag. It can easily be replaced.

When on duty, notify the home health agency clinical service manager for further instructions if there is any car trouble, auto accident, or incident in which personal safety is in question.

Never go into or stay in a home if you feel that your personal safety is in question. Always respect and listen to your "gut feelings."

Socioenvironmental Assessment

PURPOSE
- To obtain a data base to establish the plan of care
- To identify potential patient problems and needs on the patient care plan regarding resources, housing, finances, and support systems

GENERAL INFORMATION
The socioenvironmental assessment should be done when the patient is admitted to the home health agency. Data is both subjective and objective and is usually obtained from the patient. However, information may be supplemented from a secondary source, such as the caregiver or multidisciplinary team or from the referring institution's records.

PROCEDURE
1. Explain the purpose of the interview to the patient/caregiver.
2. Conduct the interview to include the following:

Personal data
Name, date of birth, age, Medicare or Medicaid number, nationality, religion, education, occupation, language barrier or cultural considerations, wishes regarding Advanced Directives

(durable power of attorney for health care or living will), interests, hobbies, and socialization

Household data

Address and directions to the patient's residence; telephone number; family members' names; inquire about conflict, substance abuse, weapons or pets, and farm animals

Support systems

Available caregivers (relationship to patient); caregiver's telephone number; local pharmacy; primary physician; physician's address and telephone number; patient, family members, or caregivers that are able to call the home health agency if problems arise; and church or other support group

Home

Size, condition, cleanliness, pests, water, heating, air-conditioning, smoke alarm, safety hazards, and accessibility from street or road

Neighborhood

Friendly or disruptive neighbors, bars, liquor stores, parks, gangs, crack houses, adequate street lighting, and urban versus rural setting

Food

How many meals are eaten each day, food preferences, special diet or food or fluid restrictions, Meals on Wheels, working refrigerator and stove, and an ability to prepare and obtain food

Economic data

Medical bills; ability to purchase medicine, heating, electric, gas, food, telephone, and housing

NURSING CONSIDERATIONS

Particular attention should be paid to the availability of support systems and to the extent that resources may be limited for health care needs.

Any problematic areas should be reported to the physician and reflected in the patient care plan. A referral to social services may be required.

DOCUMENTATION GUIDELINES

Use the data base to implement the plan of care and to develop the patient care plan.

Identified problems on the patient care plan then should be a focus on the visit report.

Update the plan of care to reflect the current patient status.

Temperature

PURPOSE
• To assess body temperature

RELATED PROCEDURES
• Radial Pulse
• Respirations

GENERAL INFORMATION

Most home health patients are issued an oral mercury thermometer by the home health agency. This thermometer is often kept in the patient's home record folder or with the patient's medical supplies. Because this is such a common practice, this procedure addresses usage of the standard mercury thermometer. The reader is referred to manufacturer guidelines for use of alternative thermometers.

EQUIPMENT
1. Oral or rectal mercury thermometer
2. Wrist watch
3. Water-soluble lubricant for rectal thermometer
4. Tissue
5. Disposable thermometer and plastic sleeves or protective coverings
6. Antiseptic wipes
7. Disposable nonsterile gloves and an impermeable plastic trash bag (see *Infection Control*)

❖ Axillary Temperature

PROCEDURE

1. Explain the procedure to the patient/caregiver.
2. Assemble the equipment at the bedside or a convenient work area.
3. Assist the patient to a sitting or a supine position.
4. Remove the thermometer from its container and wipe it with an antiseptic wipe from bulb end toward the fingers in a rotating manner. Rinse the thermometer with cold water. Place a protective cover on the thermometer if the patient does not have his or her own thermometer.
5. Shake the thermometer's mercury down to below 96° F.
6. Dry the area under the arm; place the bulb end of the thermometer into the center of the patient's axillae (Fig. 2-4, A).
7. Draw the patient's arm across his or her chest (Fig. 2-4, B).
8. Hold the thermometer in place for 5 minutes. Take the pulse and respiration measurements during this time.
9. Remove the thermometer from the axillae, and discard its protective covering.
10. Wipe any secretions off the thermometer with a tissue, cleaning in a rotating fashion from tip to bulb.
11. Read the thermometer at eye level to the nearest one-tenth degree.
12. Assist the patient to a comfortable position.
13. Clean the thermometer with lukewarm soapy water. Rinse it with cool water, and dry it.
14. Return the thermometer to its protective container.
15. Provide patient comfort measures.
16. Discard disposable items according to *Standard Precautions*.

NURSING CONSIDERATIONS

Perform the axillary procedure on adult patients who are not alert or who are combative.

❖ Oral Temperature

PROCEDURE

1. Follow steps *1* through *5* of the procedure for *Axillary Temperature*.

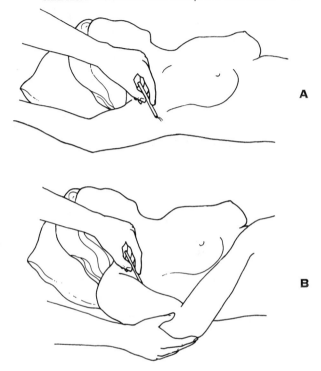

Fig. 2-4 Placement of thermometer for axillary temperature assessment.

2. Place the thermometer in the patient's mouth, well back under the tongue (Fig. 2-5). (Instruct the patient to keep his or her lips closed.)
3. Allow the thermometer to remain in the mouth at least 3 minutes.
4. Count the pulse and respirations while the temperature registers.
5. Remove the thermometer from the mouth and discard the protective cover.
6. Read the thermometer at eye level to the nearest one-tenth degree.
7. Wipe any secretions off the thermometer with a tissue, cleaning in a rotating fashion from tip to bulb.

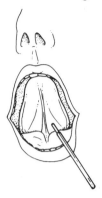

Fig. 2-5 Placement of thermometer for oral temperature assessment.

8. Clean the thermometer in warm soapy water. Rinse it in cool water, and dry it.
9. Shake down the mercury again.
10. Return the thermometer to its protective container.
11. Provide patient comfort measures.
12. Clean and replace equipment, and discard disposable items according to *Standard Precautions*.

NURSING CONSIDERATIONS

Consider issuing the patient his or her own thermometer when possible. (In this case, using a protective sleeve is not necessary.)

Do not take an oral temperature on patients who are disoriented, unconscious, on oxygen therapy, or on those who have had recent surgery of the mouth.

❖ **Rectal Temperature**

PROCEDURE

1. Follow steps *1* through *5* of the procedure for *Axillary Temperature*.
2. Apply a small amount of lubricant on the bulb of the thermometer.
3. Assist the patient onto his or her side, and drape the patient to expose the anal area only.

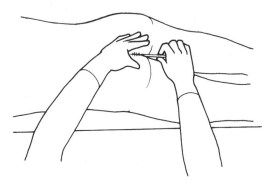

Fig. 2-6 Placement of thermometer for rectal temperature assessment.

4. Separate the buttocks, and insert the thermometer gently into the anus, about 1½ inches for an adult (Fig. 2-6). Leave the thermometer in place for 3 minutes. Stay with the patient.
5. Count the pulse and respiration while the thermometer is registering.
6. Remove the thermometer, and discard the protective cover.
7. Wipe any secretions off the thermometer with a tissue, cleaning in a rotating fashion from tip to bulb.
8. Read the thermometer at eye level to the nearest one-tenth degree.
9. Clean the patient's anal area to remove lubricant or feces.
10. Provide patient comfort measures.
11. Clean the thermometer with lukewarm, soapy water. Rinse it with cool water, and dry it.
12. Return the thermometer to its protective container, and place it in the nursing bag.
13. Discard disposable items according to *Standard Precautions.*

NURSING CONSIDERATIONS

Do not take rectal temperatures on patients with diarrhea, fecal impaction, or acute coronary artery disease; on those who have had surgery or disease of the rectum; or on any immunosuppressed patient.

Always hold the rectal thermometer while it is in place.

 DOCUMENTATION GUIDELINES

Document the following on the visit report:
- Temperature (indicate whether the patient's temperature was taken by oral, axillary, or rectal method)
- *Standard Precautions*
- Physician notification, if applicable
- Other pertinent findings

Update the plan of care.

Weight

PURPOSE

- To measure weight gain or loss
- To assess fluid status or edema
- To evaluate compliance with diet and medication regimen

RELATED PROCEDURES

- Edema
- Intake and Output (I/0)

EQUIPMENT

1. Scale (preferably patient's scale)

PROCEDURE

1. Explain the procedure to the patient/caregiver.
2. Use the same scale on the same flooring or rug each time the patient is weighed.
3. Weigh the patient as follows:
   a. Have the patient center his or her feet on the scale and stand erect.
   b. If it is possible, weigh the patient with the same

amount of clothing on and at the same time of day each visit.

4. Read the patient's weight indicated on the scale.
5. Provide patient comfort measures.

NURSING CONSIDERATIONS

Notify the patient's physician of a 3- to 4-pound weight gain in 1 week.

DOCUMENTATION GUIDELINES

Document the patient's weight, and evaluate his or her fluid status on the visit report in relation to the disease process, diet, medication regimen, and intake and output. Document physician notification of inappropriate weight gain or signs of respiratory distress, as appropriate.

Update the plan of care.

Wound Assessment and Documentation

PURPOSE

- To identify parameters of wound assessment
- To provide wound assessment documentation guidelines for Medicare reimbursement

RELATED PROCEDURES

- Wound Irrigation and Debridement (see Chapter 4)
- Wound Management (see Chapter 4)
- Wound Packing (see Chapter 4)

EQUIPMENT

1. Ruler or plastic measuring guide (all measurements should be given in centimeters)
2. Cotton-tip applicators or swabs
3. Disposable nonsterile and sterile gloves, protective apron, and an impermeable plastic trash bag (see *Infection Control*)

PROCEDURE

1. Explain the procedure to the patient/caregiver.
2. Be aware that Medicare views the following nursing skills as needed for wound care in the home health setting:
   a. Direct hands-on wound care treatment (procedural care)
   b. Skilled observation and assessment of the wound
   c. Patient and caregiver education regarding treatment and home management
3. Inspect and evaluate the condition of the wound in the following manner:
   a. Assess the wound location and its size; measure the length, width, and depth (use a sterile, cotton-tip applicator to measure the depth of the wound by inserting the applicator in the wound bed); compare the distance between the tip of the applicator and the surface of the wound to a tape measure (Fig. 2-7); probe the wound for evidence of undermining or tunneling. Measure the greatest length of the wound perpendicular to the greatest width. Describe the location of the undermining; picturing the face of a clock with the patient's head being at 12:00, measure/record the depth at the deepest point in relation to the markings on the face of a clock. (For ex-

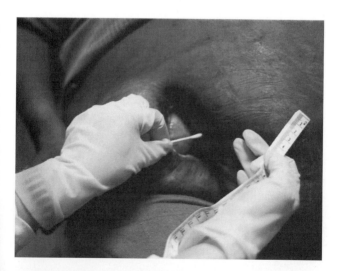

Fig. 2-7 Measuring a wound. (Photo courtesy Robyn Rice.)

ample, if undermining is deepest toward the patient's feet, document undermining 6 cm at 6 o'clock.)

b. Assess the color of the wound bed; a red or pink wound bed indicates healing, whereas a green, yellow, or black wound bed suggests infection or necrosis. Wounds tend to fill in and heal from the edges; the tissue is usually pink or red.

c. Assess wound drainage; clear or serosanguineous drainage is not unusual in a healing wound; green or yellow drainage is often referred to as *purulent* and suggests infection. Record the amount of drainage as none, slight, moderate, or heavy, and inspect the color and amount of drainage on old dressings when they are removed.

d. Assess wound odor; a sweet smell may indicate decay; a foul smell may indicate fecal contamination or a fistula. Occlusive and transparent adhesive dressings will cause a wound odor. When removing the dressing, always clean the wound before assessing it for odor. Document odor as "absent" or "present."

e. Stage the wound using the following descriptions (Fig. 2-8):

(1) *Stage 1:* Nonblanchable erythema of intact skin; can be reversible with proper treatment.

(2) *Stage 2:* Partial-thickness skin loss, involving epidermis and/or dermis; this may present clinically as an abrasion, blister, or shallow crater.

(3) *Stage 3:* Full-thickness skin loss, involving damage or necrosis of subcutaneous tissue that may extend down to, but not through, underlying fascia; undermining may or may not be present.

(4) *Stage 4:* Full-thickness skin loss with extensive destruction and tissue necrosis or damage to muscle, bone, or supporting structures (e.g., a tendon or joint capsule); undermining and sinus tracts may be present.

4. Assess the surrounding skin for redness, inflammation, or signs of breakdown.

5. Evaluate the response to treatment, as well as factors that may impede healing, such as inadequate diet, proximity of the wound to the perineum of incontinent patients, immobility, noncompliance with home dressing changes or skin care regimen, lack of patient's/caregiver's knowledge re-

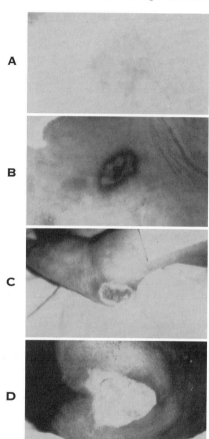

Fig. 2-8 Wound staging. **A,** Stage I. **B,** Stage II. **C,** Stage III. **D,** Stage IV. (From Perry AG, Potter PA: *Clinical nursing skills and techniques,* ed 3, St Louis, 1994, Mosby.)

garding home management of the wound, and lack of the patient's environmental resources.

6. Consult with the physician, and revise the plan of care as needed if the wound is not healing satisfactorily.

NURSING CONSIDERATIONS

Assessment of stage 1 pressure ulcers may be difficult in patients with darkly pigmented skin.

Irrigate the wound before measuring and staging. For consistent evaluation, it is advisable for the case manager to measure/stage the wound the first visit each week or PRN.

DOCUMENTATION GUIDELINES

Document the following on the visit report:

- The treatment and condition of the wound (each visit)
- Appearance of the wound bed (black, yellow, green, tan, red, or pink)
- Wound measurements (at least weekly), including the length, depth, and width of the wound in centimeters
- Depth and location of undermining in centimeters
- Inflammation or erythema of the skin around the wound
- Color, odor, and estimated amount of drainage
- Stage the wound weekly, and compare the progress with the goals of therapy
- Any patient/caregiver instructions on wound care and response to teaching, including ability to change dressings and manage the wound at home
- Physician notification, if applicable
- *Standard Precautions*
- Other pertinent findings

Describe the infected wound or the complex procedural requirements or signs of infection that require the services of a skilled nurse. Wound care is covered by Medicare as long as the need for skilled care and treatment is clearly and precisely documented on the visit report.

Update the plan of care.

CHAPTER 3

Cardiopulmonary Procedures

Administration of Oxygen Therapy

PURPOSE

- To review fundamental management of oxygen therapy in the home, including the following:
  a. Implementation and home safety guidelines
  b. Nasal cannula
  c. Oxygen face tent or shield
  d. Oxygen mask with a reservoir bag
  e. Simple face mask
  f. Venturi mask
  g. Tracheostomy collar
- To promote self-care in the home

RELATED PROCEDURES

- Administration of Medications: General Guidelines (see Chapter 9)
- Arterial Blood Gas Sampling (see Chapter 12)
- Home Ventilator Management
- Pulse Oximetry
- Suctioning

GENERAL INFORMATION

The respiratory therapist from the Home Medical Equipment (HME) vendor is usually responsible for the delivery, set up, patient education, and maintenance of home oxygen delivery systems (e.g., cylinders, concentrators, liquid oxygen).

The home health nurse is responsible for ensuring that oxygen is administered as prescribed and evaluating response to therapy. As advised by the respiratory therapist, follow manufacturer recommendations on the use of oxygen delivery systems at home.

EQUIPMENT

1. Source of oxygen supply (cylinder/liquid oxygen reservoirs/concentrator)
2. Regulator-flow meter (regulates gas flow in liters per minute [LPM])
3. Small-bore oxygen supply tubing for nasal cannula, simple mask, venturi mask, and rebreather mask; wide-bore corrugated supply tubing for tracheostomy collar and face tent
4. Humidifier
5. Sterile or distilled water, or tap water that has been boiled for 15 minutes
 6. Disposable nonsterile and sterile gloves, disinfectant and/or manufacturer-recommended solutions to clean respiratory equipment, and an impermeable plastic trash bag (see *Infection Control*)

❖ Oxygen Therapy: Implementation and Home Safety Precautions

PROCEDURE

1. Review the physician's prescription for type of therapy, source of oxygen supply, use of cannula or mask or tracheostomy collar, and desired liter flow.
2. Explain the procedure to the patient/caregiver.
3. Assess cognitive and cardiopulmonary status for signs/symptoms of hypoxia (Box 3-1).
4. Notify the physician when the patient's health changes or deviates from baseline status.
5. Evaluate patient/caregiver ability to administer oxygen. Assess the following:
   a. Correct liter flow
   b. Whether the patient knows when to use his or her oxygen
   c. Correct operation of the equipment (see manufacturer's recommendations, and review the procedure with the HME respiratory therapist)
   d. Whether the patient/caregiver knows what to do in case of power failure or equipment malfunction
   e. Home ventilator management, as applicable

  f. Suctioning, as applicable
  g. Cleaning and disinfection of reusable equipment
6. Implement home oxygen safety precautions with the following guidelines (oxygen is not flammable or explosive, but it does support combustion; anything that burns in an oxygen-rich environment burns faster and hotter):
  a. No open flames or smoking are allowed within 10 feet of the oxygen source.
  b. Do not use electrical equipment that may cause sparks from an electrical short, such as a space heater, near oxygen administration equipment.
  c. Care should be taken during use of gas/electric appliances with patients using oxygen.
  d. Oxygen is a drug and must be administered as ordered; use oxygen only at prescribed amounts because too little or too much is harmful and can cause death.
  e. Make sure that the oxygen tank is in an approved stand to prevent rolling or accidental fall. The oxygen in these tanks is under high pressure. If the tank falls over and the valve stem breaks, the pressure is released, causing the tank to be propelled like a projectile.

Box 3-1
SIGNS AND SYMPTOMS OF HYPOXIA

Early

Restlessness, headache, visual disturbances, slight confusion, hyperventilation, tachycardia, hypertension, and dyspnea

Chronic

Polycythemia, clubbing of the fingers, thrombosis, and pallor

Advanced

Hypotension, bradycardia, metabolic acidosis, cyanosis, and profound mental status changes (patient may be combative)

f. Store oxygen tanks away from direct sunlight or heat.

g. Keep oxygen concentrators away from walls to allow for adequate air return.

h. Oxygen concentrators should be plugged into a grounded electrical outlet.

7. Ensure that the patient/caregiver knows how to reach the HME vendor respiratory therapist 24 hours a day for supplies or problems with equipment.

8. Ensure that the patient/caregiver knows when to call the physician and when to go to the emergency room.

9. Evaluate caregiver ability to assist the patient and to comply with oxygen therapy recommendations.

❖ Nasal Cannula

GENERAL INFORMATION

This equipment is easily tolerated by most patients. It is simpler than a mask but provides less humidification (Fig. 3-1). The FIO_2 (fraction of inspired oxygen) level will vary depending on the liter flow and the rate/depth of patient breathing. The following provides a guideline regarding nasal cannula FIO_2 levels and corresponding oxygen liter flow for a patient breathing 12 breaths per minutes at a depth of 500 cc per breath:

a.	FIO_2	24%-28%	Flow: 1 to 2 LPM
b.	FIO_2	30%-35%	Flow: 3 to 4 LPM
c.	FIO_2	38%-44%	Flow: 5 to 6 LPM

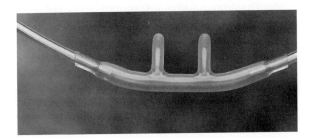

Fig. 3-1 Nasal cannula. (Courtesy Hudson Respiratory Care, Inc., Temecula, Calif.)

PROCEDURE

1. Follow the procedure for *Oxygen Therapy: Implementation and Home Safety Precautions.*
2. Connect the nasal cannula to the oxygen tubing and to the humidified oxygen source.
3. Adjust the oxygen flow meter to the prescribed liter flow.
4. Place the tips of the cannula no more than 1.25 cm into the patient's nares. Adjust the elastic headband or plastic slide guard for a snug and comfortable fit.
5. Secure the oxygen tubing to the clothing to prevent unnecessary pulling.
6. Clean and change equipment (tubing, cannula, humidifier) each visit or PRN.
7. Promote patient comfort by doing the following:
   a. Instruct the patient to place cotton balls over the ears or wrap moleskin around the tubing to prevent skin irritation. Foam curlers that have been split lengthwise and placed around the tubing may be used over the ears to reduce pressure from the tubing.
   b. Use a water-based lubricant on the nares to reduce irritation of the nose.
   c. If the oxygen delivery system does not have a humidifier jar, consider a room humidifier to prevent drying of mucosal membranes. Clean the humidifier daily to prevent nebulizing mold or bacteria.
   d. The patient may use 50-foot extension tubing to maximize independence and ambulation in the living area.
   e. Instruct the patient to wear his or her nasal cannula while eating, taking a shower, using the bathroom, during sexual activities, and as needed for shortness of breath.
8. Clean and replace the equipment. Discard disposable items according to *Standard Precautions.*

❖ Oxygen Face Tent or Shield

GENERAL INFORMATION

This device is rarely used in home care but may be seen in the treatment of a patient recovering from oromaxillofacial surgery. It is a shieldlike mask that fits under the patient's chin and sweeps around the patient's face (Fig. 3-2). An FIO_2 level of 21% to approximately 70% can be achieved in the home-care setting by having a high-output air compressor (50 psi) power

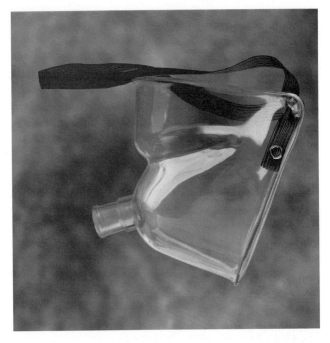

Fig. 3-2 Oxygen face tent or shield. (Courtesy Hudson Respiratory Care, Inc., Temecula, Calif.)

the nebulizer jar and by having oxygen bled-in from either an "H" cylinder, liquid reservoir, or an oxygen concentrator. The HME respiratory therapist adjusts the oxygen liter flow and analyzes the resulting FIO_2 level until that level matches the patient's prescription. The oxygen bleed-in liter flow should be clearly noted in the documentation.

PROCEDURE

1. Follow the procedure for *Oxygen Therapy: Implementation and Home Safety Precautions.*
2. Fill the nebulizer jar with either sterile, distilled, or boiled tap water.
3. Connect the face tent to the large-bore tubing of the high-humidity aerosol circuit. Mist should always be visible.
4. Adjust the oxygen bleed-in flow rate to the liter flow estab-

lished by the HME respiratory therapist as previously described.

5. Adjust the sides of the face tent to ensure a snug-yet-comfortable fit.

6. Water will condense in the circuit and must be drained into the drainage bag periodically. The condensate must be considered contaminated waste. Care must be taken to avoid contaminating the patient's airway or the water in the nebulizer jar with the condensate.

7. Keep tubing free of kinks.

8. If the patient is combative or confused, consider short-term use of restraints to keep the oxygen delivery device on. Combative behaviors or confusion often clear up once the patient is well-oxygenated. Arterial blood gas determinations may be indicated with combative behaviors.

9. Sit the patient up in bed. Support the patient with pillows, as needed.

10. Change face tent/tubing PRN. If the patient uses a face tent, obtain a physician's order for a nasal cannula for use during meals.

11. Provide patient comfort measures.

12. Clean and replace equipment. Discard of disposable items according to *Standard Precautions.*

❖ Oxygen Mask

GENERAL INFORMATION

Patients who require oxygen masks usually need more intensive management than home care permits. However, as sicker and sicker patients are being sent home, the use of oxygen masks are becoming more common. Limitations of oxygen masks include discomfort and frequent removal of the mask in order for the patient to eat, expectorate, or cough. If the patient uses a mask for oxygen delivery, obtain an order from the physician for a nasal cannula for use during meals.

Reservoir bag masks

Reservoir bag masks (Fig. 3-3, *A*) provide a high FIO_2 level, ranging from 40% to 90+%. Liter flow must be high enough to keep the reservoir bag inflated during inspiration; this prevents the risk of rebreathing carbon dioxide. Care must be taken to ensure that the oxygen-connecting tubing remains connected

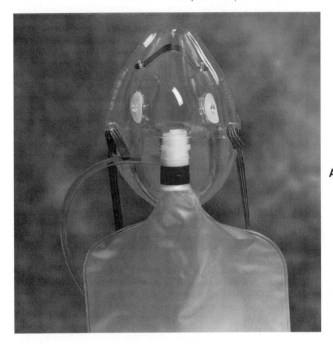

Fig. 3-3 Oxygen face masks. **A,** Reservoir bag mask. (Courtesy Hudson Respiratory Care, Inc., Temecula, Calif.)

Continued

to the oxygen source at all times to prevent suffocation. Two types of masks are available.

Non-rebreather mask

Oxygen from the oxygen source flows into the reservoir bag. When the patient inhales, a one-way valve between the bag and the mask opens to allow the patient to inhale oxygen. The one-way valve closes during expiration, and the exhaled air is forced out through one-way valves over the expiratory ports on the mask. This design allows for inhalation of oxygen yet prevents accumulation of expired CO_2. Because the one-way valves over the expiratory ports will not allow gas to flow into the mask from the room, it is extremely important to ensure that the reservoir remains inflated during inhalation. The reservoir bag is this patient's *only* source of oxygen. The FIO_2 level varies with the patient's ventilatory pattern.

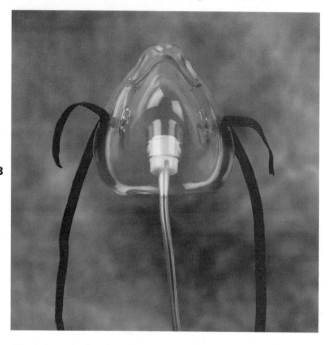

Fig. 3-3—cont'd B, Simple face mask. (Courtesy Hudson Respiratory Care, Inc., Temecula, Calif.)

Partial rebreather mask

Open ports are present on both sides of the partial rebreather mask. This mask provides a higher FIO_2 level than a simple mask by allowing patients to rebreathe some of their oxygen-enriched exhaled air from the attached reservoir bag. A minimum liter flow of 10 LPM is required to prevent deflation of the reservoir bag. Higher flows may be used if the reservoir bag deflates during inspiration. The FIO_2 level varies with the patient's ventilatory pattern.

Simple mask

This equipment requires a liter flow greater than 5 LPM to prevent rebreathing of carbon dioxide. The recommended liter flow is usually between 6 to 10 LPM (Fig. 3-3, *B*). An accurate FIO_2 level is difficult to estimate, and adequacy of

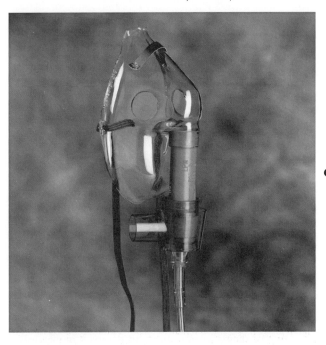

C

Fig. 3-3—cont'd   C, Venturi mask. (Courtesy Hudson Respiratory Care, Inc., Temecula, Calif.)

oxygenation may be assessed by pulse oximetry or arterial blood gases.

Venturi mask

This equipment allows the delivery of an accurate FIO_2 level (Fig. 3-3, C). The venturi mask kits come with a set of interchangeable or adjustable adapters. Each adaptor is calibrated by the manufacturer to provide a precise FIO_2 level when used with the recommended liter flow. The FIO_2 level and corresponding liter flow are determined by each manufacturer and will vary. Refer to the package insert for the flow rate settings and resulting FIO_2 level. Bubble humidifiers are *not* recommended for use with venturi masks. Venturi masks can provide a patient with chronic obstructive pulmonary disease (COPD) with a precise FIO_2 level that does not change with ventilatory pattern. These masks are especially efficacious for patients who are chronically hypercapnic and rely on their hypoxic drive to breathe. The venturi mask is used for patients when an accurate FIO_2 level is necessary for proper treatment.

PROCEDURE

1. Follow the procedure for *Oxygen Therapy: Implementation and Home Safety Precautions.*
2. Assist the patient to a comfortable position to wear the mask.
3. Attach the oxygen-supply tubing to the oxygen source.
4. Turn on the oxygen flow as prescribed by the physician.
5. Adjust the equipment specific to the type of mask being worn.
   a. Adjust the oxygen flow rate setting on the venturi mask
   b. As applicable, allow the reservoir bag to fill with oxygen before placing the venturi mask on the patient
6. Adjust the elastic strap behind the patient's head so that the mask fits snugly.
7. Gently pinch the metal strip located near the top of the mask to help ensure a tight mask fit across the bridge of the nose.
8. Observe the patient breathe with the mask in place. The patient should not show signs of respiratory distress or discomfort. If a mask with a reservoir bag is being used, the nurse should make sure that the bag remains inflated during the patient's inhalation. If the reservoir bag collapses, turn up the oxygen liter flow until the bag stays inflated during inhalation, and notify the physician and HME respiratory therapist of any changes in liter flow or problems with the equipment.
9. Provide patient comfort measures.
10. Clean and replace equipment. Discard disposable items according to *Standard Precautions.*

❖ Tracheostomy Collar

GENERAL INFORMATION

A tracheostomy collar is a curved device with an adjustable strap that fits around the patient's neck. The tracheostomy collar is designed to deliver high humidity and oxygen to patients with a tracheostomy (Fig. 3-4). The tracheostomy collar has an

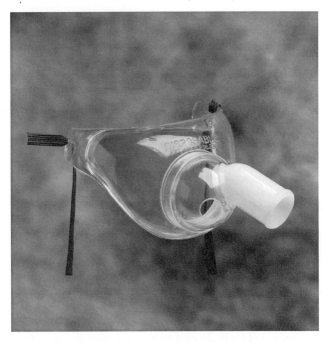

Fig. 3-4   Tracheostomy collar (Courtesy Hudson Respiratory Care, Inc., Temecula, Calif.)

exhalation port that must remain patent at all times and another port that connects to large-bore tubing.

An FIO_2 level of 21% to approximately 70% can be achieved in the home-care setting with the use of a high-output air compressor (50 psi) powering the nebulizer jar and by having oxygen bled-in from either an "H" cylinder, liquid reservoir, or oxygen concentrator. The HME respiratory therapist adjusts the oxygen liter flow and analyzes the resulting FIO_2 level until that level matches the patient's prescription. The oxygen bleed-in liter flow should be clearly noted in the documentation.

PROCEDURE

1. Follow the procedure for *Oxygen Therapy: Implementation and Home Safety Precautions.*

2. Fill nebulizer jar with sterile, distilled, or boiled tap water.
3. Connect the tracheostomy collar to the large-bore tubing of high-humidity aerosol circuit. Mist should always be visible.
4. Adjust the oxygen bleed-in flow rate to the liter flow established by the HME respiratory therapist as previously described.
5. Apply the tracheostomy collar so that it loosely covers the patient's tracheostomy.
6. Water will condense in the circuit and must be drained into the drainage bag periodically. The condensate must be considered contaminated waste. Care must be taken to prevent contaminating the patient's airway or the water in the nebulizer jar with the condensate.
7. Clean the collar with soap and water every day or more frequently, if needed, to remove secretions.
8. Instruct the patient/caregiver on suctioning.
9. Provide patient comfort measures.
10. Clean and replace the equipment according to *Standard Precautions.*

 NURSING CONSIDERATIONS

Consider obtaining physician's orders for pulse oximetry or arterial blood gas evaluation to measure adequacy of oxygenation and ventilation.

DOCUMENTATION GUIDELINES

Document the following on the visit report:
- The procedure and patient toleration
- Cardiopulmonary status
- Method of oxygen delivery
- Oxygen saturation via pulse oximetry or arterial blood gas analysis, as applicable
- Any patient/caregiver instructions and response to teaching, including the ability to operate oxygen equipment
- Physician notification, if applicable
- *Standard Precautions*
- Other pertinent findings

Oxygen is a medication. Oxygen liter flow and/or the FIO_2 level should be recorded on the medication record

Update the plan of care.

AUTHOR: Joan Vernitte-Kohorst, B.H.S., R.R.T.

Aerosol Therapy

PURPOSE
- To administer nebulizer medications
- To increase alveolar ventilation and improve cardiopulmonary status
- To promote self-care in the home

RELATED PROCEDURE
- Administration of Medications: General Guidelines (see Chapter 9)

GENERAL INFORMATION
The respiratory therapist from the HME vendor commonly delivers, assembles, and maintains the respiratory therapy equipment. The respiratory therapist usually initiates patient/caregiver training regarding the administration of prescribed respiratory treatments. The home health nurse is responsible for ensuring that the treatment is administered as prescribed and for evaluating the patient's response to therapy.

EQUIPMENT
1. Compressed air and/or oxygen source
2. Connective small-bore tubing
3. Nebulizer cup
4. Mouthpiece or flex tube and swivel adapter if the patient is tracheotomized
5. Sterile normal saline solution
6. Prescribed medication (bronchodilators, mucolytics, diluents)
 7. Face mask and an impermeable plastic trash bag (see *Infection Control*)

PROCEDURE
1. Explain the procedure to the patient/caregiver.
2. Assist the patient to a sitting or semi-reclining position.
3. Assess the patient's cardiopulmonary status before and after the treatment. Notify the physician if the findings are abnormal or if the patient's baseline status deviates.

4. Offer mouthwash to the patient or assist him or her with oral care as needed.

5. As appropriate, don a face mask.

6. Assemble the following equipment at a convenient work area:
   a. Fill the nebulizer with the prescribed medication
   b. Turn on the compressed air; a visible mist should flow out of the mouthpiece
   c. Occasionally, aerosol therapy may be given with oxygen; adjust the liter flow between 5 and 7 LPM per physician's orders to obtain a visible mist from the mouthpiece

7. Administer the following treatment:
   a. Instruct the patient to insert the mouthpiece and inspire slowly through his or her mouth to facilitate maximal ventilation of the lungs
   b. After each deep inhalation, instruct the patient to hold his or her breath for a few seconds to provide maximal absorption of the medication
   c. Stay with the patient; continue to provide reassurance and encourage slow, deep respirations

8. Turn the compressor off if the patient should have a coughing episode or if the treatment is interrupted for any reason.

9. Evaluate the patient's response to the treatment. Has the breathing improved? Does the patient feel relief? Note any signs of dyspnea, wheezing, agitation, tremors, tachycardia, or palpitations. If any adverse effects occur, stop the treatment and notify the physician for further orders.

10. Turn off the air compressor or oxygen and empty the nebulizer cup after treatment.

11. Rinse the nebulizer cup with hot running water, and allow it to air dry on a paper towel. Store the dry nebulizer cup in a sealed plastic bag at the patient's bedside.

12. Encourage the patient to cough once the treatment is completed. Provide a specimen cup for sputum, if needed. Instruct the patient in safe disposal of used tissues.

13. Perform postural drainage after aerosol therapy if ordered by the physician.

14. Provide patient comfort measures.

15. Clean and replace the equipment. Discard disposable items according to *Standard Precautions.*

NURSING CONSIDERATIONS

Make sure the nebulizer is kept in an upright position. (If the nebulizer is not level, the medication does not nebulize properly and may spill into the patient's mouth.)

If the patient is receiving supplemental oxygen by nasal cannula, leave the nasal cannula on and administer the treatment with compressed air.

Consult with the HME vendor's respiratory therapist regarding recommendations for applications and a model of the appropriate face mask.

DOCUMENTATION GUIDELINES

Document the following on the visit report:
- The procedure and patient toleration
- Cardiopulmonary status
- Any patient/caregiver instructions and response to teaching, including ability to administer treatment
- *Standard Precautions*
- Physician notification, if applicable

Document the length of the treatment and medications used on the medication record.

Update the plan of care.

Automatic Implantable Cardioverter Defibrillator

PURPOSE

- To provide guidelines for the home management of patients with an automatic implantable cardioverter defibrillator (AICD)
- To promote self-care in the home

GENERAL INFORMATION

The AICD is an implanted electrical device attached to the myocardium by sensing leads and two defibrillation patches. It is used to treat sudden onset ventricular tachycardia (VT) or ventricular fibrillation (VF) (Fig. 3-5). Patients who receive the

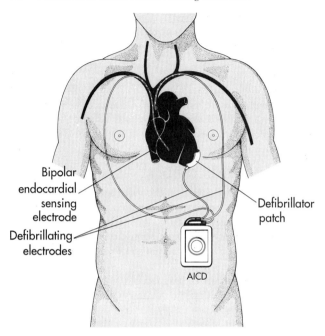

Bipolar endocardial sensing electrode

Defibrillating electrodes

Defibrillator patch

AICD

Fig. 3-5   The AICD pulse generator. (From Lewis SM, Collier IC, Heitkemper MM: *Medical-surgical nursing: assessment and management of clinical problems,* ed 4, St Louis, 1996, Mosby.)

AICD experience these lethal dysrhythmias despite medical management to control ventricular fibrillation and/or ventricular tachycardia.

The device is programmed to sense tachycardia and the width of QRS complexes to detect lethal dysrhythmias. Once an abnormal rhythm has been sensed, the AICD checks for rhythm verification and discharges 20 to 30 joules of energy in an attempt to convert the lethal dysrhythmias into a stable or normal sinus rhythm. A 5- to 10-second pause will occur. If the abnormal rhythm continues, the AICD will administer a series of shocks and pauses for a total of four shocks. The AICD is then programmed to reset, recharge, and be prepared to deliver a series of four more shocks after 35 seconds of a normal rhythm has been sensed. A magnet will activate and deactivate the AICD.

EQUIPMENT

1. Surgical wound care supplies
 2. Disposable nonsterile gloves and an impermeable plastic trash bag (see *Infection Control*)

PROCEDURE

1. Explain the procedure to the patient/caregiver.
2. Assess the patient's cardiopulmonary status and his or her compliance with the prescribed medications, diet, and activity restrictions.
3. Review the AICD manufacturer's instructional booklet with the patient/caregiver.
4. Provide the patient with reassurance that the AICD may deliver an occasional shock; however, the patient should be assured that the shock doesn't necessarily mean that he or she will have to go to the emergency room.
5. Instruct the patient that ordinary contact with another person will not activate the AICD. If someone is touching the patient when the AICD fires, that person may feel a slight-but-harmless shock.
6. Perform wound care; change the dressing as ordered. Observe for signs of redness, drainage, and/or swelling around the surgical incision site and report to the physician as appropriate.
7. Instruct the patient/caregiver in home management of AICD to include the following:
   a. Activities: no lifting for 4 to 6 weeks after surgery; avoid rough contact over the area of the power pack and the incision line; it is permissible to resume normal sexual relations; daily activities will not increase the risk of the AICD misfiring; driving is permitted unless the patient has neurologic problems or problems with syncope after AICD insertion.
   b. Clothing: wear loose-fitting clothes; avoid girdles or belts that may be constricting.
8. Instruct the patient/caregiver on the following safety precautions:
   a. Wear a Medic Alert bracelet at all times.
   b. Keep an information card about the AICD in the wallet.
   c. Avoid contact with magnetic fields (e.g., radio or television towers) because this contact may activate or de-activate the AICD; household appliances, such as a tele-

vision, microwave, and mixer, will not interfere with the AICD. Beeping from the AICD indicates exposure to electromagnetic interference—quickly move away from this area.

d. Post the local emergency room number or 911, the physician's number, and the home health agency number by your phone.

9. Instruct the patient/caregiver on the following actions to take if the AICD delivers a shock:

a. If a countershock occurs, the patient must stay calm, lie down, take the pulse, and wait. Shocks are not painful; however, they can be frightening. If the patient's pulse is regular and if he or she feels well, the day can be continued as normal.

b. If a second shock is consecutively delivered, the patient must take his or her pulse and notify the physician.

c. If a third shock is consecutively delivered, the patient must go to the emergency room or call emergency medical services.

d. The patient must keep a log of shocks (how many, time, and pulse aftershocks).

e. The patient should call the physician to report dizziness, chest pain, more than two shocks in the course of the day, or discomfort with shocks.

10. Instruct the patient on the importance of regular follow-up magnet testing to evaluate AICD function and predict the end of generator life.

11. Instruct the patient in the use of the transtelephonic phone system, if available.

12. Be prepared to follow cardiopulmonary resuscitation (CPR) protocols.

13. Provide patient comfort measures.

14. Clean and replace equipment. Discard disposable items according to *Standard Precautions*.

NURSING CONSIDERATIONS

Instruct the caregiver on CPR.

CPR should not be administered until the AICD fires unsuccessfully four times or fails to fire.

The AICD will not interfere with basic life support.

Provide emotional support to the patient/caregiver.

DOCUMENTATION GUIDELINES

Document the following on the visit report:

- The procedure and patient toleration
- Cardiopulmonary status
- Condition of the surgical wound
- Record of shocks and the patient's pulse afterwards
- Any patient/caregiver instructions and response to teaching, including knowledge of actions to take if the AICD should fire or if the patient should require CPR
- Physician notification, if applicable
- *Standard Precautions*

Update the plan of care.

BiPAP® Support Ventilator Management

PURPOSE

- To prevent nocturnal hypoxemia caused by sleep hypoventilation in patients with neuromuscular disorders
- To prevent respiratory fatigue in patients with COPD
- To improve ventilation and oxygen saturation in patients with obstructive apnea
- To promote self-care in the home

RELATED PROCEDURE

- Home Ventilator Management

GENERAL INFORMATION

The bi-positive airway pressure (BiPAP) ventilatory support system is a form of continuous positive airway pressure (CPAP) management. It is designed for mask-applied ventilation in the home. The BiPAP ventilatory support system delivers two different levels of positive airway pressure. The system cycles spontaneously between a preset level of inspiratory positive airway

---

SOURCE: Respironics Inc. Inclusion of this procedure does not imply endorsement of these products by either the author or Mosby, Inc.

pressure (IPAP) and expiratory positive airway pressure (EPAP). This system is used to control apnea (EPAP) and non-apneic events (IPAP) in hemodynamically stable patients. It may be used to offer ventilatory support without committing patients to the lifestyle associated with a tracheostomy. This ventilator is noncontinuous and is intended to augment the patient's breathing. It must not be used as a life-support ventilator; it is not intended to provide the total ventilatory requirements of the patient.

Under the direction of the physician, the respiratory therapist from the HME vendor is usually responsible for setting up the BiPAP ventilatory support system, readjusting settings, and instructing the patient/caregiver in the operation of equipment and in procedural care. Home health nurses should reinforce instructions, assess the patient's physiologic status, and evaluate the patient's compliance with the plan of care. It is important to refer to the manufacturer's recommendations to ensure safe and effective use of all equipment.

EQUIPMENT

1. BiPAP pressure support ventilator and patient circuit
2. Nasal mask and headstrap
3. Manufacturer-recommended disinfectant or equipment cleanser and an impermeable plastic trash bag (see *Infection Control*)

PROCEDURE

1. Explain the procedure to the patient/caregiver.
2. Assist the patient to a position of comfort.
3. Assess cardiopulmonary status, including vital signs, skin color, use of accessory muscles of ventilation, paradoxical movement of the chest wall (which may reflect impending muscle fatigue), auscultation of the lungs, oxygen saturation, and pertinent laboratory data.
4. Assemble the equipment at a convenient area. Place the BiPAP pressure support ventilator on a level surface close to where the patient will be resting or sleeping. Plug the machine into a standard three-prong home outlet.
5. Connect one end of the tubing to the airflow outlet port of the front of the BiPAP pressure support ventilator. Connect the other end of the tubing to the swivel end of the mask.

6. Place the mask over the patient's nose. The mask should extend from the end of the nasal bone to just below the nares. Ensure that the mask rests above the patient's upper lip to prevent air leaks or patient discomfort.

7. Turn on the BiPAP pressure support ventilator. The ON/OFF switch will light up.

8. Attach the headstrap to the mask. Adjust the straps until all significant air leaks are eliminated. Avoid making the headstrap too tight because this will cause patient discomfort and may cause air leaks because of distortion of the mask cushion. If possible, have the patient vary head positions to confirm mask seal during normal range of motion.

9. Check that all connections are secure.

10. Assess the prescribed BiPAP pressure support ventilator settings:
    a. IPAP control—sets prescribed pressure support level; range 4 to 20 cm H_2O; active in all modes except CPAP.
    b. EPAP control—sets prescribed positive end-expiratory pressure (PEEP) level; range 4 to 20 cm H_2O; active in all modes.
    c. Breaths per minute (BPM) control—sets the number of BPM; range 4 to 30 BPM; active in the S/T and T modes.
    d. BiPAP pressure support ventilator mode as clinically indicated:
       (1) Spontaneous (S) mode—the unit cycles between IPAP and EPAP in response to the patient rate
       (2) Spontaneous/timed (S/T) mode—the unit cycles as in the S mode; in addition, if the patient fails to initiate an inspiration, the unit will cycle based on the BPM control setting
       (3) Timed (T) mode—the unit cycles between IPAP and EPAP levels based solely on the set BPM and setting of IPAP time controls
       (4) CPAP mode—allows the system to be used for CPAP delivery
    e. FIO_2—match current administration

11. Ensure that the settings on the BiPAP pressure support ventilator match those on the plan of care. Obtain a physician's order for the current settings.

12. Assess the patient's comfort level. Observe the patient for

development of ear discomfort or conjunctivitis. Notify the physician as needed. Consult with the respiratory therapist and physician to add humidification if the patient complains of nasal dryness.

13. Clean and replace the equipment. Wipe off all surfaces of the ventilator with a clean, damp cloth. When the mask is not being used, store it in a plastic bag to keep it free from dust. Discard disposable items according to *Standard Precautions.*

NURSING CONSIDERATIONS

To make the mask and headgear fit more simply the next time, mark the straps with a permanent marker or safety pins.

To prevent abrasion from the mask, place a patch of hydrocolloid wound care dressing on the bridge of the patient's nose.

Instruct the patient to notify the physician of any unusual chest discomfort, shortness of breath, or severe headache on awakening or when using the BiPAP pressure support ventilator.

DOCUMENTATION GUIDELINES

Document the following on the visit report:
- The procedure and patient toleration
- Cardiopulmonary status
- BiPAP pressure support ventilator settings (BiPAP mode, FIO_2, IPAP/EPAP control, BPM control)
- Any patient/caregiver instructions and response to teaching, including the ability to operate the equipment
- Physician notification, if applicable
- *Standard Precautions*
- Other pertinent findings

Update the plan of care.

Breathing Exercises

PURPOSE
- To instruct the patient on how to strengthen respiratory muscles, clear mucus from the lungs, and improve ventilation
- To foster activity tolerance
- To promote self-care in the home

GENERAL INFORMATION

Diaphragmatic breathing and lateral-base expansion exercises strengthen respiratory muscles, promote mucous clearance, and improve ventilation. Pursed-lip breathing is used to control exhalation, help open the airways, and improve oxygenation. These exercises are typically prescribed for patients with lung disease and for postsurgical patients.

❖ Diaphragmatic Breathing

PROCEDURE

1. Explain the procedure to the patient/caregiver.
2. Offer mouthwash or assist with oral care as needed.
3. Instruct the patient to sit up as straight as possible with his or her head and shoulders relaxed to provide for maximal descent of the diaphragm. (Diaphragmatic breathing can be taught with the patient lying down and using books or hands over the abdomen to reinforce the proper technique.)
4. Instruct the patient to breathe out gently, feeling the lower ribs sink down and in toward the midline (Fig. 3-6).
5. Instruct the patient to breathe in while relaxing the upper abdominal muscles. The patient should feel air filling the lower part of the chest as the diaphragm descends (Fig. 3-7).
6. Instruct the patient to place one hand over the abdomen just below the breast bone. When the patient performs correct diaphragmatic breathing, the hand will move out as he or she inhales and will move in on exhalation.
7. Instruct the patient to use diaphragmatic breathing combined with forced expirations on the third or fourth breath to help cough up secretions.
8. Provide patient comfort measures.

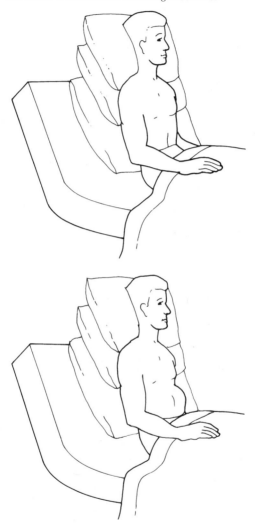

Fig. 3-6 Expiration during diaphragmatic breathing.

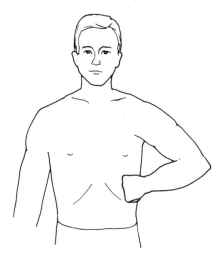

Fig. 3-7 Inspiration during diaphragmatic breathing.

❖ Lateral Base Expansion

PROCEDURE

1. Follow steps *1* through *3* of the procedure for *Diaphragmatic Breathing.*
2. Place your hands on the patient's lower ribs at the midaxillary line, and apply slight pressure to the ribs. (The pressure is used to fix the patient's attention on the part of the lung that is to be expanded and to note the direction in which expansion is required.)
3. Instruct the patient to breathe in through his or her nose and expand his or her ribs against the pressure of your hands as far as possible.
4. At the peak of inspiration, instruct the patient to relax and exhale while the ribs return to their original resting position.
5. Apply slight pressure at the end of expiration to make sure that the patient has fully exhaled.
6. Perform the exercise unilaterally or bilaterally as needed. (After a thoracotomy, emphasis must be given to the side of the incision, except when a pneumonectomy has been

performed. The patient is usually instructed to take six breaths at a time and then to rest.)

7. Provide patient comfort measures.

❖ Pursed-Lip Breathing

PROCEDURE

1. Explain the procedure to the patient/caregiver.
2. Offer oral care.
3. Have the patient sit in a comfortable position.
4. Instruct the patient to relax and breathe in slowly.
5. Instruct the patient to purse his or her lips in a whistling position and exhale slowly and evenly as long as he or she can tolerate it.
6. Exhalation is 2 to 3 times longer than inhalation. Count 1-2-3 for inhalation and 4-5-6-7-8-9 for exhalation.
7. Instruct the patient to use pursed-lip breathing when he or she is short of breath or performing strenuous activities, such as climbing stairs.
8. Provide patient comfort measures.

NURSING CONSIDERATIONS

Giving the patient a demonstration of energy-conservation techniques may enhance learning, reveal misunderstandings, and promote a utilization of breathing techniques by the patient.

Obtain physician's orders for rehabilitation services for a home exercise program to build the patient's strength and endurance.

Additionally, the services of a respiratory therapist from the HME vendor or pulmonary clinical nurse specialist may be useful when planning pulmonary rehabilitation and keeping staff up to date with available equipment.

DOCUMENTATION GUIDELINES

Document the following on the visit report:
- The procedure and patient toleration
- Cardiopulmonary status
- Any patient/caregiver instructions and response to teaching, including the ability to perform the breathing exercises
- Physician notification, if applicable
- Other pertinent findings

Update the plan of care.

Chest Physiotherapy

PURPOSE

- To assist in the removal of bronchial secretions
- To improve breathing
- To promote self-care in the home

RELATED PROCEDURE

- Breathing Exercises

GENERAL INFORMATION

Chest physiotherapy consists of procedures such as postural drainage, cupping, and vibration (Box 3-2, p. 85).

Postural drainage uses specific positions to let the force of gravity assist in removing lung secretions. Six basic positions are commonly used in home care. Each is specific for major areas of the bronchopulmonary segments (Fig. 3-8). Drainage positions should be maintained for 10 to 15 minutes each, as tolerated by the patient. During this time, alternate 2 to 5 minutes of percussion followed with 10 to 12 vibrations. These exercises should be performed before breakfast, before other meals, and at bedtime. Administer the inhaler or aerosol therapy before beginning.

EQUIPMENT

1. Foam wedge or pillows
 2. Cup, tissues, a towel, and an impermeable plastic trash bag (see *Infection Control*)

PROCEDURE

1. Explain the procedure to the patient/caregiver.
2. Position the patient to facilitate postural drainage. Elevate the hips and torso approximately 18 inches with pillows or a foam wedge to achieve best results.
3. Perform the following exercise to drain the lower bases first; then proceed to the apex of the lungs:
   a. To drain the base of the left lung (left lower lobe), place the patient in a right side-lying position; percuss and vibrate over the lower rib area
   b. To drain the base of the right lung (right lower lobe),

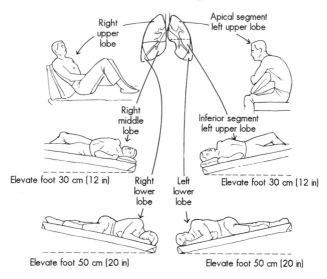

Fig. 3-8 Postural drainage positions commonly used in home care. (From Phipps WJ, Sands JK, Marek JF: *Medical-surgical nursing: concepts and clinical practice,* ed 6, St Louis, 1998, Mosby.)

place the patient in a left side-lying position; percuss and vibrate over the lower rib area

c. To drain the right middle lobe, place the patient in a left side-lying position, with the right side of body supported; percuss and vibrate over the midchest and nipple area

d. To drain the left upper lobe, place the patient as in step *c* but in the right side-lying position; percuss and vibrate over the midchest and nipple area

e. To drain the anterior upper lobes, instruct the patient to sit up and lean back; percuss and vibrate over the collarbone and shoulder area

f. To drain the posterior upper lobes, instruct the patient to sit up and then to lean forward over a pillow; percuss and vibrate over the shoulder area

4. When performing chest physiotherapy, have a cup or basin and paper tissue or towel available for draining mucus.

Box 3-2

MANEUVERS USED TO ASSIST IN THE REMOVAL OF PULMONARY SECRETIONS

1. *Percussion* is performed by clapping the cupped hand on the chest wall over the area of lung that is to be drained. Rhythmic clapping increases vibrations that stimulate the movement of secretions and helps to clear secretions that are sticking to the bronchial walls.

   The hands are cupped to create a cushion of air against the chest wall (Fig. 3-9). Raise the hands 3 to 4 inches above the chest wall, and alternately clap the lungs to vibrate secretions. Clapping should be vigorous but not painful and should not be done on the patient's bare skin. Remove rings before percussion.

2. *Vibration* is used to stimulate the flow of secretions into the larger airways, where they can be removed by coughing. To accomplish this technique, your hand should be pressed firmly over the area of the chest wall that is to be vibrated. The muscles of your upper arm and shoulder should be tensed (isometric contractions) to produce fine tremors on the chest wall as the patient exhales. Vibration is done with the flattened, not the cupped, hand. Perform vibration during exhalation. Encourage the patient to exhale as slow as possible.

3. *Deep breathing* by the patient assists in the movement of secretions and stimulates coughing. A deep, rapid inhalation followed by a slow, prolonged expiration moves secretions into the larger airways for expulsion by coughing. See the procedure for *Breathing Exercises* to strengthen respiratory muscles and to assist expectoration. Encourage deep breathing during chest physiotherapy. See the procedure for *Chest Physiotherapy.*

Continued

Box 3-2
MANEUVERS USED TO ASSIST IN THE REMOVAL OF PULMONARY SECRETIONS—CONT'D

4. *Productive coughing* is enhanced by placing the patient in a sitting position and having him or her lean forward. Encourage coughing after chest physiotherapy.
   a. *Cascade cough*—Have the patient take a deep, slow inhalation and then cough 2 to 3 times in a row at the end of the breath to move secretions to larger airways.
   b. *Huff cough*—Have the patient take a deep breath and make a *huff* sound when exhaling, instead of the usual cough.

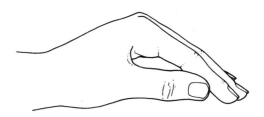

Fig. 3-9   Hand position for chest physiotherapy.

5. Offer mouthwash to the patient, and assist with oral care, as needed.
6. Encourage the patient to rest after the procedure.
7. Provide patient comfort measures.
8. Clean and replace equipment. Discard disposable items according to *Standard Precautions.*

NURSING CONSIDERATIONS

Observe for potential contraindications of the procedure, such as abdominal distention, an irregular heart rate, or a diagnosis of lung cancer. If any of these conditions exist, check with the physician before performing chest physiotherapy.

Vibrate as the patient exhales.

Use a manual resuscitation bag for patients who have a tracheostomy and are on a ventilator during the procedure. Bag breathing is carried out during percussion and vibration.

DOCUMENTATION GUIDELINES

Document the following on the visit report:
- The procedure and patient toleration
- Cardiopulmonary status (including lung sounds before and after the procedure and amount, color, and quantity of secretions)
- Any patient/caregiver instructions and response to teaching
- Physician notification, if applicable
- *Standard Precautions*
- Other pertinent findings

Update the plan of care.

Chest Tube Management

PURPOSE

- To evacuate air or fluid from the pleural space
- To allow full expansion of the lungs

GENERAL INFORMATION

Chest tubes are rarely seen in the home-care setting, with a few exceptions. Two situations that may require sending a patient home with a chest tube are spontaneous pneumothorax and empyema. Less often, a patient with a malignant pleural effusion is sent home with a standard chest tube and drainage system.

A spontaneous pneumothorax may occur in thin, healthy young males. If the patient has minimal symptoms, the physician may elect to insert a small pneumothorax catheter, which is connected to a Heimlich valve for air evacuation. Standard water-seal or drainage bottles are not used. The pneumothorax catheter is usually about the diameter of a large intravenous catheter; however, it may be larger. The catheter is placed percutaneously, with the patient under local anesthesia. A chest radiograph confirms placement. The home health nurse must maintain a secure connection between the pneumothorax catheter and the Heimlich valve, as well as maintain an airtight dressing.

An empyema is an infection in the pleural space. A chronic empyema requires long-term antibiotic therapy and an empyema chest tube for drainage of pus. The empyema chest tube usually has a large diameter—approximately 36 French. The chest tube is slowly pulled out—approximately 1 cm each week. This type of chest tube is not connected to a water-seal bottle or drainage system, since the area is not in contact with the lung parenchyma. An empyema is walled off from the lung, and there is minimal or no risk of pneumothorax The home health nurse must provide routine dressing changes, which sometimes include pleural space irrigations. The home health nurse may also be involved in the outward advancement of the chest tube.

A patient with cancer, involving the lung or breast, may develop a malignant pleural effusion, which compresses the lungs and impairs gas exchange. In this case the patient would require a standard chest tube and drainage system. The home health nurse is actively involved in both maintaining an airtight dressing and in maintaining a water-seal drainage system.

❖ Pneumothorax Catheter

EQUIPMENT

1. Sterile gauze
2. Petrolatum-impregnated gauze dressing
3. Tape (waterproof, adhesive, silk, or transparent—not paper)
4. Antiseptic wipes
5. Safety pin
6. Sterile bandage scissors
7. Chest tube catheter clamps
8. Disposable nonsterile and sterile gloves and an impermeable plastic trash bag (see *Infection Control*)

PROCEDURE

1. Explain the procedure to the patient/caregiver.
2. Assemble the equipment at a convenient work area.

3. Assess the cardiopulmonary status and patient toleration of the chest tube.

4. Notify the physician regarding abnormal findings or deviations from the patient's baseline status and concerns or problems with patient toleration of the chest tube.

5. Place the patient in a supine position, and uncover the chest to expose the catheter.

6. Assess the chest tube site for redness or signs of inflammation.

7. Aseptically open one or two packages of sterile gauze with a slit and one package (3 × 6 inches, or similar) of petrolatum-impregnated gauze.

8. Cut three or four (6 inches long × 2 inches wide) pieces of tape.

9. Don nonsterile gloves. Remove the old tape and the soiled dressing from the chest tube site; then discard everything, including the nonsterile gloves in a plastic trash bag.

10. Don sterile gloves.

11. Cleanse the chest tube site with an antiseptic wipe, moving from the center outward in a circular motion. Allow the area to dry; do not fan to dry. Some home health agencies remove iodine with alcohol.

12. Apply a new petrolatum-gauze dressing firmly around the chest tube insertion site to prevent air from entering the chest.

13. Cover with a dry gauze dressing.

14. Apply tape, overlapping the edges slightly to form an occlusive dressing. Completely encase the chest tube dressing and the chest tube with tape. Make sure there is no tunneling where the chest tube exits the dressing. A separate piece of tape may be needed to seal the tunnel from below.

15. Secure the connection between the chest tube and the Heimlich valve securely, using reverse spiral taping or a plastic band.

16. Tape the Heimlich valve to the patient's upper chest or wrap a piece of tape around the Heimlich valve, and use a safety pin to secure it to the patient's clothing. The distal tip of the valve must not be occluded by clothing or skin.

17. Provide patient comfort measures.

18. Clean and replace the equipment. Discard disposable items according to *Standard Precautions.*

❖ Empyema Chest Tube

EQUIPMENT

1. Sterile gauze dressings
2. Tape (waterproof, adhesive, silk, or transparent—not paper)
3. Liquid skin barrier or transparent adhesive dressing
4. Ostomy bag if required
5. Iodine swabs
6. Safety pin
7. Prescribed irrigation solution
8. Sterile cup
9. Emesis basin or bowl
10. Sterile catheter-tip syringe
11. Sterile bandage scissors
12. Chest tube catheter clamps
13. Disposable nonsterile and sterile gloves and an impermeable plastic trash bag (see *Infection Control*)

PROCEDURE

1. Follow steps *1* through *5* of the procedure for *Pneumothorax Catheter.*
2. Assemble the equipment at the bedside or a convenient work area.
3. Place the patient in a supine position, and uncover the chest.
4. Aseptically open one or two packages of sterile gauze.
5. Cut three or four (6 inches long × 2 inches wide) pieces of tape.
6. Don nonsterile gloves. Remove the old tape and soiled dressings from the chest tube site; then discard everything, including the nonsterile gloves, in a plastic trash bag.
7. Don sterile gloves.
8. Cleanse the site with an antiseptic wipe, moving from the center outward in a circular motion. Allow the area to dry; do not fan the area. Some home health agencies remove iodine with alcohol (refer to agency policy).
9. Apply a liquid skin barrier or hydrocolloid adhesive dressing to prevent skin breakdown and to secure the dressing when frequent dressing changes are required.
10. If irrigations are ordered by the physician, they are done

aseptically even though the area is already contaminated. Perform the chest tube irrigation as follows:

   a. Pour the prescribed irrigation solution into a sterile cup

   b. Draw the prescribed amount of irrigation fluid into the sterile catheter-tip syringe

   c. Insert the sterile catheter tip syringe directly into the chest tube

   d. Gently irrigate the chest tube; there may be a dwell time during which the chest tube is clamped and the syringe is left in place; after the dwell time, the clamp and syringe are removed, and the chest cavity is allowed to drain into a dressing or emesis basin

11. Apply an ostomy bag if drainage from the empyema or irrigation solution is excessive.

12. Apply a dry dressing over the tube exit, and tape it securely. (This chest tube is usually cut close to the patient's skin and secured with a safety pin that is inserted crosswise in the tube to prevent inward migration.)

13. Change the dressing when it is soiled or loose. This may occur several times a day or every several days.

14. Follow steps *17* and *18* of the procedure for *Pneumothorax Catheter*

❖ Chest Drainage System

EQUIPMENT

1. Sterile gauze
2. Petrolatum-impregnated gauze dressing
3. Tape (waterproof, adhesive, silk, or transparent—not paper)
4. Iodine swabs
5. Liquid skin barrier or transparent adhesive dressing
6. Chest tube drainage collection system and sterile normal saline solution
7. Chest tube clamp

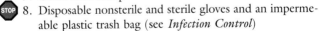

8. Disposable nonsterile and sterile gloves and an impermeable plastic trash bag (see *Infection Control*)

PROCEDURE

1. Follow steps *1* through *5* of the procedure for *Pneumothorax Catheter*.
2. Aseptically open one or two packages of sterile split gauze.

3. Cut three or four (6 inches long × 2 inches wide) pieces of tape.

4. Don nonsterile gloves. Remove the old tape and dressing from the chest tube site, and discard everything, including the nonsterile gloves, in a plastic trash bag.

5. Don sterile gloves.

6. Cleanse the site with an antiseptic wipe, moving it from the center outward in a circular fashion. Allow the area to dry; do not fan the area. Some home health agencies remove iodine with alcohol (refer to agency policy).

7. Apply a liquid skin barrier or hydrocolloid adhesive dressing to prevent skin breakdown and to secure the dressing when frequent dressing changes are required.

8. Apply new petrolatum gauze firmly around the chest tube insertion site to prevent air from entering the chest.

9. Apply a dry gauze dressing over the tube site.

10. Apply tape, overlapping the edges slightly, to form an occlusive dressing. Be sure to completely encase the chest tube dressing and the chest tube with tape. Make sure there is no tunneling where the chest tube exits the dressing. A separate piece of tape may be needed to seal the tunnel from below.

11. Firmly secure the connection between the chest tube and connecting tubing to the drainage system, using reverse spiral taping or a plastic band. You should be able to assess the 5-in-1 connector for clots.

12. Tape the chest tube to the patient's chest or abdomen to prevent pulling when the patient moves in the bed or gets up in a chair. (Pinch the tape together under the chest tube before taping it to the patient; this prevents the chest tube from slipping through the tape.)

13. Assess the drainage system for air leaks from the patient or from the system by systematically clamping the tubing below every connection. The leak or bubbling stops when the problematic connection is clamped. Use the following guidelines to assess for an air leak:

    a. If the leak stops when the chest tube itself is clamped, the leak is coming from the patient or from the chest tube insertion site.

    b. If changing the dressing or applying pressure on the dressing site does not change the bubbling, the leak is from the pleural space.

14. Evaluate the need to change the drainage bottle as it nears capacity. (This varies among systems. For a glass bottle, a volume of as little as 700 cc may indicate the need to change the bottle. For most commercial systems, a volume of about 2000 cc indicates the need for a new system.)

15. Use aseptic technique to change the drainage bottle when it is near capacity, as follows:
    a. Don sterile gloves to prevent self-contamination and contamination of the chest tube
    b. Open the new system and fill the water-seal chamber to the necessary height
    c. Remove the tape from the 5-in-1 connector
    d. Clamp the chest tube close to the patient and just proximal to the 5-in-1 connector
    e. Disconnect the chest tube from the 5-in-1 connector, and connect the new chest tube drainage system tubing
    f. Tighten the connection, and secure it with spiral wrapped tape
    g. Remove the clamps

16. Follow steps *17* and *18* of the procedure for *Pneumothorax Catheter.*

NURSING CONSIDERATIONS

It is imperative that the chest tube dressing remain occlusive to prevent the possible introduction of air or microorganisms into the pleural space.

The occlusive dressing is used in patients with empyema to contain contaminated material from aerosolization.

The only time a chest tube should be clamped is when the bottle or drainage system is changed.

If the tube accidentally becomes disconnected, quickly insert it in the bottle of sterile normal saline or water used to maintain a water seal.

Instruct the patient/caregiver to clamp an accidentally disconnected chest tube and immediately notify the home health agency.

DOCUMENTATION GUIDELINES

Document the following on the visit report:
- The procedure and patient toleration
- Patency of the chest tube (not empyema tube) or absence of bubbling in the water-seal chamber or air evacuation

from the Heimlich valve (sounds like flatus or a duck quack)
- Volume and characteristics of fluid drainage in the chest tube system or on the dressing
- Cardiopulmonary assessment, including the rate, depth, and pattern of breathing; percussion notes; and auscultation findings
- Safety measures, such as clamps or saline at the bedside; intactness of dressing and taped or banded connections; and any adverse events, such as accidental disconnection
- Any patient/caregiver instructions and response to teaching
- Physician notification, if applicable
- *Standard Precautions*
- Other pertinent findings

Update the plan of care.

Controlled Cough Exercise

PURPOSE
- To instruct the patient how to clear his or her lungs of secretions and improve ventilation
- To foster activity tolerance
- To promote self-care in the home

RELATED PROCEDURE
- Breathing Exercises

GENERAL INFORMATION
Breathing techniques such as the controlled cough exercise strengthen respiratory muscles, promote mucus clearance, and improve patient ventilation. The controlled cough technique is typically prescribed for patients with chronic lung disease.

EQUIPMENT

1. Tissues
 2. Impermeable plastic bag for disposal of tissues (see *Infection Control*)

PROCEDURE

1. Explain the procedure to the patient/caregiver.
2. Review the principles of diaphragmatic and pursed-lip breathing with the patient/caregiver (see the procedure for *Breathing Exercises*).
3. Instruct the patient to sit forward in a leaning position with his or her feet on the floor and tissues in hand.
4. To promote a controlled cough, instruct the patient to do the following:
   a. Slowly inhale and take a deep breath
   b. Hold the deep breath for 4 seconds
   c. Cough twice with the mouth open; use tissues to dispose of mucus
   d. Pause
   e. Inhale by sniffing gently
   f. Rest and repeat
5. Provide patient comfort measures.

NURSING CONSIDERATIONS

Instruct the patient/caregiver to place used tissues in a waste basket with a plastic lining for disposal (e.g., family should avoid directly handling tissues).

Consider a referral to rehabilitation services for a home exercise program to build the patient's strength and endurance.

DOCUMENTATION GUIDELINES

Document the following on the visit report:
- The procedure and patient toleration
- The color, amount, odor, and viscosity of sputum
- Any patient/caregiver instructions and response to teaching, including patient's ability to perform the controlled cough technique
- Physician notification, if applicable
- *Standard Precautions*
- Other pertinent findings

Update the plan of care.

Coronary Precautions in the Home

PURPOSE

- To decrease the cardiac workload by reducing stress from physical activity
- To return the patient to an optimum level of health with regard to limitations
- To instruct the patient/caregiver in home coronary precautions
- To promote self-care in the home

RELATED PROCEDURES

- Temperature (see Chapter 2)
- Weight (see Chapter 2)

EQUIPMENT

1. Bedside commode
2. Oral thermometer

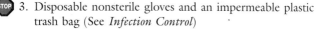

3. Disposable nonsterile gloves and an impermeable plastic trash bag (See *Infection Control*)

PROCEDURE

1. Explain the procedure to the patient/caregiver.
2. Assess cardiopulmonary status, focusing on the symptomology of chest pain or heart failure. Ask the patient whether he or she has any problems with chest pain, indigestion, palpitations, dizziness, or shortness of breath.
3. Report abnormal findings or deviations from baseline status to the physician.
4. Evaluate adherence with prescribed medications, diet, and activity regimen each visit. Weigh the patient weekly.
5. Review the physician's orders for progressive increases in the patient's physical activities, and instruct the patient/caregiver regarding the following:
   a. Bed rest with commode privileges, provided that no postural hypotension or dysrhythmia exists
   b. May feed self
   c. Rest after meals; delay all activities, such as bathing or sitting up in a chair, for at least 30 minutes

    d. Change position by self (encourage active rather than passive movement and assist the patient as needed)

    e. May have back rubs but not a vigorous massage

    f. Bed bath with assistance

    g. Temperature taken orally

    h. May sit up in chair with assistance *three times a day* provided no postural hypotension or dysrhythmia exists

    i. No smoking

    j. Sexual activity may be resumed when determined by the physician

6. Instruct the patient/caregiver in the following prescribed nutritional and fluid recommendations:

    a. Eat small, frequent meals

    b. Drink cool or warm liquids; avoid extreme cold or hot temperatures

    c. Coffee and tea must be decaffeinated

    d. Follow prescribed diet and nutritional modifications

7. Instruct the patient/caregiver about the following elimination needs:

    a. Take stool softeners as prescribed

    b. Avoid straining or bearing down

8. Instruct the patient/caregiver about the following chest pain management:

    a. Symptom identification (often occurs with activity); sit quietly for a few minutes

    b. Take up to 3 nitroglycerin tablets as prescribed by the physician 5 minutes apart for continued pain

    c. If chest pain is not resolved after third nitroglycerin tablet, go to the emergency room for evaluation

    d. Contact the physician if nausea, vomiting, or dizziness exists and with other concern

NURSING CONSIDERATIONS

Teach patient/caregiver how to measure pulse, respirations, and weight and to contact the physician with abnormal findings.
Instruct the caregiver/family on CPR.

DOCUMENTATION GUIDELINES

Document the following on the visit report:

- The procedure and patient toleration
- Cardiopulmonary status, including complaints of chest pain, indigestion, or syncope

- Any patient/caregiver instructions and response to teaching
- Physician notification, if applicable
- *Standard Precautions*
- Other pertinent findings

Update the plan of care.

Home Dysrhythmia Monitoring

PURPOSE

- To record an electrocardiogram (ECG) tracing
- To assess cardiopulmonary status

GENERAL INFORMATION

Home dysrhythmia monitoring provides the tools necessary to document cardiac events that are not captured by alternative monitoring methods. It is a tool to document symptomatic cardiac dysrhythmias. Home dysrhythmia monitoring can be used to document the absence or the presence of an irregular cardiac dysrhythmia. The telephone ECG is used with patients who complain of a pounding heart or dizziness.

There are a number of home dysrhythmia monitors available on the market. The author has chosen to describe a basic procedure for home dysrhythmia monitoring.

Carefully review and follow the manufacturer's recommendations regarding operation of home dysrhythmia monitors and ECG transmitter systems. Follow the manufacturer's recommendations regarding maintenance and battery replacement of the monitor. Most home dysrhythmia monitors have either a skin, chest plate, or wrist electrode(s). The physician will prescribe the electrode type.

EQUIPMENT

1. Home dysrhythmia monitor
2. Telephone

PROCEDURE

1. Explain the procedure to the patient/caregiver.
2. Assist the patient to a sitting or a semi-reclining position near the telephone.
3. Assess the patient's cardiopulmonary status.
4. Evaluate the patient for signs and symptoms of cardiac failure, such as dizziness, fainting spells, shortness of breath, blurred vision, changes in heart rate from baseline status, chest pain, and sudden weight gain or edema.
5. Assemble the equipment at a convenient work area. Open the dysrhythmia monitoring kit. The monitor has two buttons. The ON/OFF switch turns the monitor on and off. The RECORD/PLAY button is used to record and transmit the ECG.
6. To turn on the dysrhythmia monitor and to record the ECG, do the following:
   a. Move the ON/OFF switch to the ON position; you will hear two distinct tones that last about 4 seconds; this indicates that the monitor is ready to record the ECG; if you do not hear two distinct tones when the ON/OFF switch is in the ON position, turn the monitor off and then on again; if you still do not hear the tones, install a new battery; contact the physician and manufacturer if the equipment does not work properly.
   b. Press and release the RECORD/PLAY button; you will hear a high-pitched tone that will last 45 to 60 seconds; instruct the patient not to move during this recording period; unnecessary movement will distort the recording of the ECG; the recording of the ECG is completed when the high-pitched tone stops; the memory of the monitor is capable of storing only one recording; therefore, do not attempt to make a second recording until you have transmitted the first recording; do not unplug the lead(s) while recording the patient's ECG.
   c. Leave the ON/OFF switch in the ON position until the stored ECG has been transmitted; if the monitor is turned off, the ECG will be lost.
7. To record the ECG use one of the following methods:
   a. *Recording with wrist electrodes*
      (1) Insert the wrist electrode plug into the holes labeled Channel 1 (+) (−); insert the plug with the (+) side on top

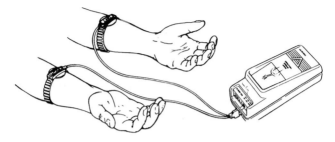

Fig. 3-10 Placement of wrist electrodes. (From Medtronic, Inc., Minneapolis, Minn.)

- (2) Turn on the dysrhythmia monitor
- (3) Slide the wrist electrode marked LEFT onto the left wrist and move it up the patient's forearm for a snug fit (3 to 4 inches below the elbow); the marked areas of the electrodes should be on the hairless portion of the inside arm
- (4) In a similar manner, apply the RIGHT wrist electrode to the right forearm (Fig. 3-10)
- (5) Press and release the RECORD/PLAY button; record the ECG
- (6) Remove the wrist electrodes
- b. *Recording with the chest electrode*
  - (1) Using the chest electrode, insert the electrode plug into the monitor and turn on the monitor, as described previously
  - (2) Place the hand-held chest electrode in the center of the bare chest at the level of the armpit; make sure all four of the metal buttons on the chest electrode touch the skin (Fig. 3-11)
  - (3) Press and release the RECORD/PLAY button; record the ECG
  - (4) Remove the chest electrode
- c. *Recording with skin electrodes*
  - (1) Remove or shave body hair from the electrode placement areas, if necessary; scrub the area with alcohol; allow the skin to dry
  - (2) Remove the electrode from the package, and gently peel the skin electrode off the protective cover;

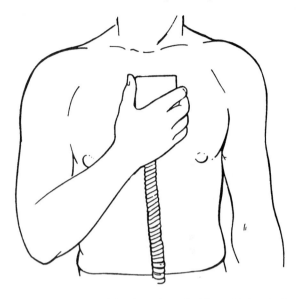

Fig. 3-11 Placement of the chest electrode. (From Medtronic, Inc., Minneapolis, Minn.)

Fig. 3-12 shows the standard placement of the skin electrodes; place the electrode securely onto the prepared skin area or as instructed by the physician; attach the appropriate color-coded clip to the snap of the skin electrode by gently squeezing the clip (Fig. 3-13)

(3) Insert the white plug into the Channel 1 hole, with the (+) side on top; insert the black plug into the Channel 2 hole with the (+) side on top

(4) Turn on the dysrhythmia monitor

(5) Press and release the RECORD/PLAY button; record the ECG

(6) Replace the skin electrodes every 3 to 4 days or when they become loose

8. To transmit the ECG tracing use the following steps:

a. Place the dysrhythmia monitor on a flat surface

b. Call the telephone number to send the ECG

c. When instructed, place the mouthpiece of the tele-

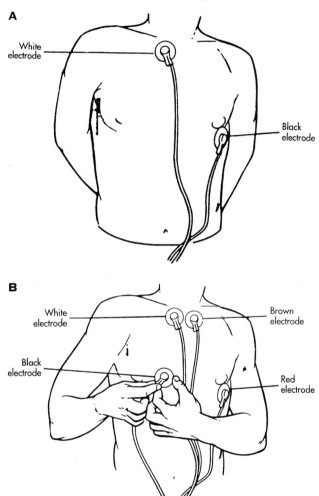

Fig. 3-12 Placement of skin electrodes. **A,** Single-channel recording. **B,** Dual-channel recording. (From Medtronic, Inc., Minneapolis, Minn.)

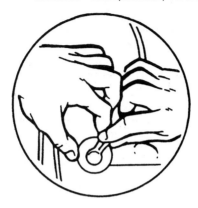

Fig. 3-13 Attaching the skin electrode. (From Medtronic, Inc., Minneapolis, Minn.)

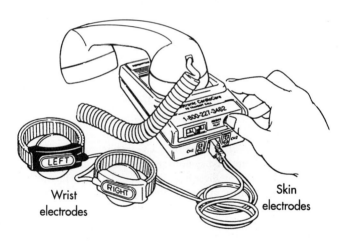

Fig. 3-14 Telephone placement of the dysrhythmia monitor. (From Medtronic, Inc., Minneapolis, Minn.)

phone on the dysrhythmia monitor's speaker hole; follow the markings on the dysrhythmia monitor for correct telephone placement (Fig. 3-14)
d. Press and release the RECORD/PLAY button
e. Wait for the tone to stop

    f. Pick up the telephone and follow any additional instructions given to you

    g. When instructed to do so, slide the ON/OFF switch to the OFF position; this will erase the ECG recording

    h. Turn the dysrhythmia monitor off only after you are instructed to do so

9. Assist the patient to a position of comfort.

10. Clean and replace the equipment. Clean the exterior of the home dysrhythmia monitor with a damp cloth moistened with water, mild detergent, or alcohol. Discard disposable items according to *Standard Precautions.*

 NURSING CONSIDERATIONS

Instruct the patient/caregiver how and when to transmit the home telephone ECG.

The ECG may be transmitted by the home health nurse during planned home visits and by the patient or caregiver whenever the patient experiences dizziness, palpitations, or signs of cardiac failure.

Do not place the home dysrhythmia monitor in water.

Instruct the patient/caregiver not to wear the monitor while bathing, showering, or swimming.

 DOCUMENTATION GUIDELINES

Document the following on the visit report.
- The procedure and patient toleration
- The time and to whom the ECG tracing was sent
- Signs and reported symptoms of cardiac failure
- Any patient/caregiver instructions, including ability to operate equipment and response to teaching
- Physician notification, if applicable
- *Standard Precautions*
- Other pertinent findings

Update the plan of care.

Home Ventilator Management

PURPOSE
- To define the responsibilities of the home health nurse caring for the ventilator-dependent patient
- To provide guidelines for home ventilator management
- To maximize high-tech, quality patient care in the home setting
- To promote self-care in the home

RELATED PROCEDURES
- Administration of Oxygen Therapy
- Arterial Blood Gas Sampling (see Chapter 12)
- Chest Physiotherapy
- Manual Ventilation with a Hand-Held Resuscitator or Ambu-Bag
- Pulse Oximetry
- Suctioning
- Tracheostomy Care

GENERAL INFORMATION
Defining the roles of the HME vendor respiratory therapist and the home health nurse regarding care of the ventilator patient in the home is the responsibility of the discharge planning team. Weeks before the patient's discharge, the patient's home care team, including the caregiver, should be given instructions about actual and potential patient care needs. Caregivers who are *willing* and *able* to assist with the patient's needs are necessary for home discharge.

The home health nurse is advised to review the HME vendor's patient care manual, which should outline ventilator management in the home and also serves as an additional instructional guide for the patient/caregiver. It is important to refer to individual manufacturer's recommendations to ensure safe and effective use of all equipment.

Although the respiratory therapists from the HME vendor are responsible for instructing the patient/caregiver in the procedural aspects of care, home health nurses should reinforce instructions and evaluate compliance with the plan of care during visits. The patient and caregiver should be familiar with ventilator alarms, know what they mean, and know how to take appropriate action. An important role of the home health nurse in patient/caregiver education regarding home ventilator management is to provide a basis for sound decision making and to foster a sense of competency and good judgment.

EQUIPMENT

1. Ventilator
   a. Ventilator circuits and filters
   b. Heated humidifier or cascade
      (1) Sterile or distilled water, or tap water if boiled 15 minutes
      (2) Condensation drainage bags
      (3) Heat and moisture exchanger (optional)
   c. External 12-volt battery with power cord
   d. Volume bag (optional)
   e. Manual self-inflating resuscitation bag
   f. Disinfectant (see *Infection Control*)
2. Oxygen and related supplies
   a. Oxygen source (optional): oxygen concentrator with backup compressed-gas cylinder (tank)
   b. Oxygen-connecting tubing: pressure-compensated flow meters are recommended with the use of 50 feet of connecting tubing
   c. Air compressor and tubing for aerosol treatments (optional) (see the procedure for *Aerosol Therapy*)
3. Tracheostomy equipment and related supplies
4. Durable medical equipment
   a. Hospital bed (optional)
   b. Patient communication aids
   c. As needed: equipment to assist with patient bowel and bladder management and personal care
   d. As needed: cane, walker, and wheelchair

PROCEDURE

1. Explain the procedure to the patient/caregiver.
2. Maintain a copy of the most recent plan of care to ensure that all orders are being implemented correctly.
   a. When faced with questions that fall outside of the established care plan, contact the HME respiratory therapist *and* the physician for answers; if available, consult with the pulmonary clinical nurse specialist or dis-

charge planning coordinator from the referring hospital

3. Perform a physical assessment to include the following:
   a. Subjective assessment based on, but not limited to, patient/caregiver comments on shortness of breath, color change, mucus production, fever, and machine or equipment concerns
   b. Objective assessment of physiologic data, such as blood pressure, pulse, respiratory rate, breath sounds, and oxygen saturation
      (1) Assess for complications of ventilator dependence, such as skin breakdown, infection, fluid and electrolyte imbalance, malnutrition, and depression

4. Assess patient/caregiver ability to manage ventilator dependence at home; assess his or her concerns regarding equipment, resources, psychosocial, spiritual, and teaching needs, etc.

5. Perform a safety check of all equipment to include the following:
   a. Patient circuit
      (1) Drain all tubing of water; excess water should be considered contaminated and disposed of accordingly
      (2) Inspect the circuit for wear and cracks
      (3) Check all connections for tightness
      (4) Make sure tubing is routed to prevent excess water from draining into the patient's airway or back into the humidifier or ventilator
   b. Inspect all equipment for proper function and wear, including battery level and operational hours of the ventilator
   c. Confirm that the equipment is being cleaned and changed as ordered or per manufacturer's recommendations

6. Assess the *mode* of delivery:
   a. Control mode—delivers a preset tidal volume at a fixed rate; the patient cannot initiate breaths or change the ventilatory pattern
   b. Assist control volume or rate (ACV)—allows patients to initiate breaths so that they can breathe at a faster rate than the preset number of breaths per minute generated by the ventilator; each breath is delivered at the same preset tidal volume

    c. Intermittent mandatory ventilation (IMV)—delivers a preset number of mechanical breaths at a preset tidal volume, but it also allows the patient to breathe with no assistance (positive pressure) from the ventilator at his or her own tidal volume

    d. Synchronized intermittent mandatory ventilation (SIMV)—the ventilator senses the patient's spontaneous breath and synchronizes the timed breath with the patient's breather; this syncopation reduces competition between machine-delivered breaths and patient-spontaneous breaths

7. Assess the breath rate (ventilator plus patient); approximate normal range up to 38 breaths each minute.

8. Assess the tidal volume (VT) that the ventilator is giving the patient. Normal VT is 10 to 15 ml/kg. The dial setting of the tidal volume may be compared with results obtained from the use of a volume bag.

    a. The HME vendor provides a clear, plastic sleeve called a volume bag that is used to measure the VT. Attach the volume bag to the exhalation valve or gas collection head on the tubing. Count the number of breaths it takes to completely fill the bag. On the back of the volume bag, a diagram shows total number of breaths taken to fill the volume bag with the corresponding tidal volume.

    b. Dial settings from the tidal volume *should* be similar to those obtained from the volume bag measurement. If discrepancies are noted, inform the HME vendor's respiratory therapist for follow-up

9. Assess the low-pressure alarm setting. When the pressure falls below the set rate, the alarm will sound. For example, if the patient becomes disconnected from the ventilator, the low-pressure alarm with be triggered; approximate normal range is 2 to 32 cm H_2O.

10. Assess the high-pressure alarm limit setting. When the pressure rises above the set rate, the alarm will sound. For example, mucous plugs, excessive secretions, coughing, and lying on the ventilator circuit tubing will increase pressure, inhibiting the ventilator effort to deliver oxygen, and will trigger the high-pressure alarm. Approximate normal range is 15 to 90 cam H_2O.

11. Assess patient pressures by observing low and high limits as the patient breathes.

12. Assess the FIO$_2$ level (room air is 21%) or the amount of prescribed oxygen being delivered. Approximate normal range 24% to 40%. An FIO$_2$ level greater than 40% is rarely used in home care.

13. Assess PEEP, if used. High levels of PEEP (more than 5 cm H$_2$O) may use barotrauma. PEEP is rarely used in home care.

14. Instruct the patient/caregiver to post the following phone numbers by the telephone: the HME vendor, the physician, the home health agency, local power/electricity service, and local emergency service for emergencies or problems with equipment. Assist the patient/caregiver to identify circumstances when emergency numbers should be called.

15. Notify the local power and emergency services of the patient's home address, and arrange for priority service.

16. Provide patient comfort measures.

17. Clean and replace equipment. Discard disposable items according to *Standard Precautions.*

NURSING CONSIDERATIONS

Instruct the patient/caregiver in the use of alternative ventilatory support systems.

Have the patient/caregiver demonstrate the use of the manual self-inflating resuscitation bag.

The ventilator-dependent patient is at risk for respiratory failure, and care should be planned accordingly. Make the initial visits with the respiratory therapist from the HME vendor to review equipment and to mutually assess the needs of the patient/caregiver.

For the first week, daily visits are advised. The frequency of visits after this period depends on the progress of the patient/caregiver with procedural aspects of care. During the first week, 24-hour private duty care may be required because this is an anxious time for the patient and caregiver, who are developing independence from the hospital setting.

DOCUMENTATION GUIDELINES

Document the following on the visit report:
- The procedure and patient toleration of ventilator dependence
- Cardiopulmonary status

- Teaching, intervention, or procedures implemented (e.g., suctioning) and response to teaching
- Ventilator settings or any changes or pertinent findings, such as mode, breath rate, high- and low-pressure alarm limit settings, the patient's high- and low-pressure reading, VT, FIO_2 level, and PEEP (if used)
- Multidisciplinary services and care coordination (physical therapy, occupation therapy, speech therapy, social worker or home health aide may be involved)
- Any patient/caregiver concerns regarding the home environment, equipment, resources, or psychosocial needs
- Physician notification, if applicable
- *Standard Precautions*
- Other pertinent findings

Update the plan of care.

Incentive Spirometer

PURPOSE

- To increase tidal volume
- To maximize inspiration to prevent postoperative atelectasis
- To improve cough effectiveness
- To promote self-care in the home

EQUIPMENT

1. Incentive spirometer
2. Tissue
3. Basin
4. Disposable nonsterile gloves and an impermeable plastic trash bag (see *Infection Control*)

PROCEDURE

1. Review physician's orders for volume and frequency of treatments.
2. Explain the procedure to the patient/caregiver.
3. Assemble the equipment at a convenient work area.

4. Assist the patient to an upright sitting or semi-reclining position.
5. Offer mouthwash, or assist with oral care as needed.
6. Instruct the patient to exhale to a resting exhalation level and then to seal his or her mouth around the flow tube or mouthpiece (Fig. 3-15).
7. Instruct the patient to inspire slowly and hold the inspired breath for 5 to 10 seconds, as tolerated.
8. Instruct the patient to exhale normally.
9. Assess the volume achieved. Encourage the patient to reach a higher volume each day, until the volume ordered by the physician is reached or exceeded.
10. Encourage the patient to cough (abdominal splinting with a pillow may be necessary to control pain from a surgery). Offer the patient a basin and tissue.
11. Instruct the patient to repeat the procedure 5 to 10 times each hour or according to physician orders.
12. Provide patient comfort measures.
13. Clean and replace equipment. Discard disposable items according to *Standard Precautions.*

NURSING CONSIDERATIONS

Hyperventilation may occur with associated symptoms of light-headedness and paresthesia. Instruct the patient to breathe slower to avoid such symptoms.

DOCUMENTATION GUIDELINES

Document the following on the visit report:
- The procedure and patient toleration
- Volume achieved
- Frequency
- Cardiopulmonary status
- Description of cough and color, amount, and consistency of mucus
- Any patient/caregiver instructions and response to teaching, including the ability to use the spirometer
- Physician notification, if applicable
- *Standard Precautions*
- Other pertinent findings

Update the plan of care.

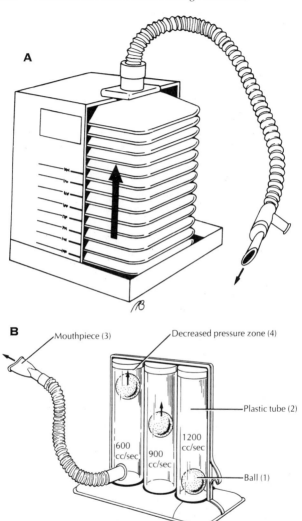

Fig. 3-15 A, Volume-incentive breathing exerciser. **B,** Flow-oriented incentive spirometer. (From Eubanks DH, Bone RC: *Comprehensive respiratory care,* ed 2, St Louis, 1990, Mosby.)

Inhalation (Steam) Therapy

PURPOSE

- To introduce moist vapor into the respiratory tract
- To relieve congestion and drying of the mucosal membranes of the respiratory tract
- To improve breathing
- To promote self-care in the home

EQUIPMENT

1. Steam humidifier
 2. Distilled water and an impermeable plastic trash bag (see *Infection Control*)

PROCEDURE

1. Explain the procedure to the patient/caregiver.
2. Assemble the equipment at the bedside or a convenient work area.
3. Assess the cardiopulmonary status before and after steam therapy.
4. Fill the steamer with distilled water to the level indicated.
5. Place the steamer by the patient's bedside on a night stand, dresser, or safe place where it will not be accidentally overturned.
6. Check the cord and apparatus for defects to prevent injury to the patient.
7. Plug in and turn on the steamer.
8. Direct the stream of mist toward the patient.
9. Be sure that the steamer is refilled with distilled water as needed and that the steamer is not on when the available water supply is depleted. Follow the manufacturer's recommendations regarding operation of the steamer.
10. Close the windows and doors as necessary to prevent drafts and to accumulate the desired amount of moisture in the air.
11. Provide patient comfort measures.
12. Evaluate steam therapy. Does the patient feel relief? Has the patient's breathing improved?

13. Clean and replace the equipment. Discard disposable items according to *Standard Precautions.*

NURSING CONSIDERATIONS

Instruct the caregiver to keep the patient's door closed during the treatment in order for the steamer to effectively humidify the room.

Keep children away from the steamer.

The steamer should be cleaned daily to prevent the growth of harmful bacteria or molds. Wash it in soap and water; rinse and air dry.

DOCUMENTATION GUIDELINES

Document the following on the visit report:
- The procedure and patient toleration or response to the treatment
- Cardiopulmonary status
- Any patient/caregiver instructions, including the patient's/caregiver's ability to safely use the steamer and response to teaching
- Physician notification, if applicable
- *Standard Precautions*
- Other pertinent findings

Update the plan of care.

Manual Ventilation with a Hand-Held Resuscitator or Ambu-Bag

PURPOSE

- To manually ventilate the patient when the patient is unable independently ventilate himself or herself
- To promote the patient's oxygenation status

RELATED PROCEDURES

- Administration of Oxygen Therapy
- Home Ventilator Management
- Suctioning
- Tracheostomy Care

GENERAL INFORMATION

Manual ventilation can be used during a respiratory emergency, during temporary disconnection from a mechanical ventilator, during failure of the mechanical ventilator, or before suctioning to prevent patient hypoxia. If used independently of oxygen, the resuscitator will supply room air (21% oxygen).

EQUIPMENT

1. Hand-held resuscitator or Ambu-bag
2. Cuffed face mask
3. Oxygen source if appropriate
4. Oxygen tubing
5. Nipple adaptor attached to oxygen flow meter
 6. Disposable nonsterile gloves and an impermeable plastic trash bag (see *Infection Control*)

PROCEDURE

1. Explain the procedure to the patient/caregiver.
2. Assemble the equipment in a convenient work area.
3. Position patient for comfort (if conscious, many patients prefer to sit upright during this procedure).
4. If the patient experiences an emergency situation, call 911. If the patient should lose consciousness, check his or her pulse. If the patient becomes pulseless, initiate CPR. Stay with the patient until emergency medical services (EMS) arrives.
5. If the resuscitator is to be used with oxygen, connect the resuscitation bag to the oxygen by attaching one end of the oxygen tubing to the bottom of the bag and the other end of the tubing to the nipple adaptor on the flow meter of the oxygen tank.
6. Check the patient's airway for obstruction. Remove any foreign matter that could impair resuscitation. If the patient has a tracheostomy tube in place, suction the tube to remove any secretions that may block the airway.
7. Use the nondominant hand to tightly seal the mask against the patient's face (the mask should be applied under the chin and up and over the patient's mouth and nose—if the patient has a tracheostomy tube, attach the resuscitation bag directly to the tube).
8. Use the dominant hand to ventilate the patient by compressing the bag (allow time between inspirations for the patient's passive exhalation and bag re-expansion).

9. Slowly compress the bag every 5 seconds to deliver about 1 L of air.
10. Observe the patient's chest rise and fall to ensure that air is inspired and exhaled with each compression.
11. Observe the patient's comfort level and color; to assess ventilation, ask the patient to nod his or her head if he or she feels like he or she is getting enough air.
12. Provide patient comfort measures.
13. Clean and replace equipment. Discard disposable items according to *Standard Precautions*.

NURSING CONSIDERATIONS

If the patient is experiencing respiratory distress, *stay with him or her* until he or she is stable or EMS arrives.

Notify the respiratory therapist and HME company with any problems regarding the operation or function of any respiratory therapy equipment, including the home mechanical ventilator.

When using a hand-held resuscitator, observe for vomiting because gastric distention may be caused by forcing air into the patient's stomach. If the patient vomits, remove the face mask and turn the patient on his or her side to assist in clearing the airway. As soon as possible, reapply the face mask and manually resuscitate until the patient is stable or EMS arrives.

Keep the resuscitator at the patient's side, visible at all times, and ready to use for those patients whose disease state or condition may require the use of a hand-held resuscitator.

Instruct the caregiver/family how to use the hand-held resuscitator (for home mechanical ventilator patients, this teaching should be done *before* patient discharge from the hospital and reinforced during the home health admission visit).

DOCUMENTATION GUIDELINES

Document the following on the visit report:
- The procedure and patient toleration
- Any patient/caregiver instructions and response to teaching, including the caregiver's ability to use the hand-held resuscitator
- *Standard Precautions*
- Other pertinent findings

Update the plan of care.

Metered Dose Inhaler Use

PURPOSE
- To deliver aerosolized medication
- To improve oxygenation
- To instruct the patient how to administer the metered dose inhaler
- To promote self-care in the home

RELATED PROCEDURE
- Administration of Medications (see Chapter 9)

GENERAL INFORMATION
Metered dose inhalers are hand-held, pocket-sized nebulizers. Each inhaler contains approximately 200 puffs. An empty cartridge will float, whereas one that is half-full will partially submerge in water (Fig. 3-16).

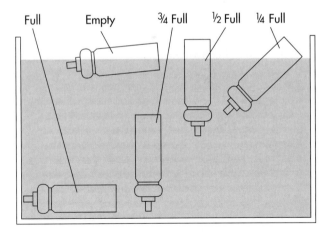

Fig. 3-16 Method to determine the amount of medication left in an MDI. (From Beare PG, Myers IL: *Adult health nursing,* ed 2, St Louis, 1994, Mosby.)

EQUIPMENT

1. Inhaler
2. Prescribed medication (bronchodilator)

❖ Open Mouth Technique

PROCEDURE

1. Explain the procedure to the patient/caregiver.
2. Assemble the equipment at a convenient work area.
3. Assist the patient to a sitting or semi-reclining position.
4. Instruct the patient/caregiver in the following procedure:
   a. Shake the inhaler canister 15 to 20 times
   b. Take a slow, deep breath in, and exhale completely
   c. Open your mouth wide (Fig. 3-17)
   d. Hold the inhaler canister 1 to 1½ inches from your lips
   e. Press down the canister while deeply inhaling a puff of medication
   f. Hold your breath as long as comfortable
   g. Exhale slowly through pursed lips
   h. Wait 1 minute between puffs, and then repeat steps *a* through *g;* recommended dosage is one or two puffs every 3 to 4 hours
5. Provide patient comfort measures.

❖ InspirEase Technique

PROCEDURE

1. Follow steps *1* through *3* of the procedure for *Open Mouth Technique.*
2. Instruct the patient/caregiver in the following procedure:
   a. Insert the inhaler canister in the mouthpiece
   b. Make sure the bag is connected to the mouthpiece
   c. Shake the inhaler canister 15 to 20 times
   d. Take a slow breath in, and then exhale completely
   e. Insert the mouthpiece between the teeth, and close the lips (Fig. 3-18)
   f. Gently compress the inhaler canister
   g. Take 3 to 4 deep, slow breaths from the bag: *do not* make the InspirEase whistle; hold your breath as long as it is comfortable between breaths to allow the medicine to

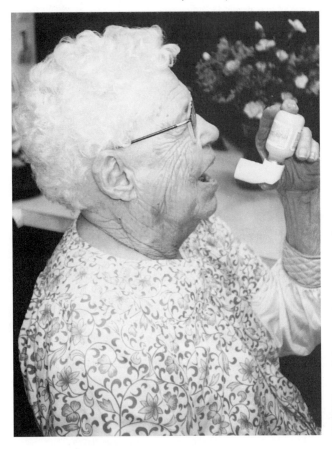

Fig. 3-17 Using a metered dose inhaler—open mouth technique. (Photo courtesy Robyn Rice.)

deposit in the lungs; recommended dosage is one or two breaths every 3 to 4 hours
3. Provide patient comfort measures.

NURSING CONSIDERATIONS

If the patient experiences palpitations or muscle tremors, discontinue using the medication and immediately notify the physician.

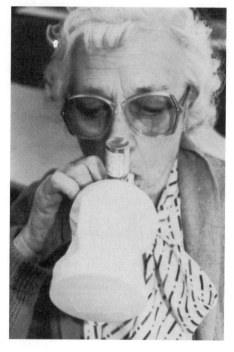

Fig. 3-18 Using a metered dose inhaler—InspirEase technique. (From Dettenmeier PA: *Pulmonary nursing care,* St Louis, 1992, Mosby.)

DOCUMENTATION GUIDELINES

Document the following on the visit report:
- The procedure and patient toleration
- Cardiopulmonary status (e.g., improved respiratory status with the use of inhaler)
- Any patient/caregiver instructions and response to teaching, including the ability to correctly administer the inhaler and response to teaching
- Physician notification, if applicable
- *Standard Precautions*
- Other pertinent findings

Document medications on the medication record.

Update the plan of care.

Pulse Oximetry

PURPOSE

- To provide a noninvasive measurement of the arterial oxygen saturation (SAO_2)

RELATED PROCEDURE

- Arterial Blood Gas Sampling (see Chapter 12)

GENERAL INFORMATION

Pulse oximetry is used in the home-care setting to spot and trend arterial oxygen saturation. Pulse oximetry measures the amount of saturation for hemoglobin bound with oxygen as a percentage of the hemoglobin available to combine with oxygen. It is important to know the patient's actual hemoglobin level because the oxygen saturation alone may be misleading and the patient may not be adequately oxygenated. Pulse oximetry does not measure carbon dioxide. An arterial blood gas measurement is recommended if the patient retains or is suspected of retaining carbon dioxide.

The pulse oximeter works by sending lights through the vascular bed of the digit (finger or toe) and measuring the amount of hemoglobin that is bound with oxygen. The sensor has both an infrared light and red light–emitting diodes (LEDs). When the sensor is placed around the digit, the LEDs shine through the area and are received by the photodetector on the other side. Oxyhemoglobin (oxygenated hemoglobin) absorbs more infrared light than the reduced hemoglobin (unoxygenated hemoglobin), which absorbs more red light. The information is registered by the photodetector and transmitted to the microprocessor in the oximeter, where it is converted into a meaningful number.

EQUIPMENT

1. Portable pulse oximeter
2. Oximeter probe

PROCEDURE

1. Explain the procedure to the patient/caregiver.
2. Assemble the equipment and prepare the oximeter in the following manner:
   a. Ensure that the batteries work
   b. Check the paper supply
   c. Complete the calibration of the oximeter
3. Select the appropriate sensor.
4. Assess the patient's digits to select the one with the best blood flow.
5. Attach the sensor to the patient's digit. Be careful not to attach the sensor too tightly.
6. Connect the sensor to the pulse oximeter.
7. Turn on the pulse oximeter (Nellcor N-10), then do the following:
   a. Press the button once for a single reading
   b. Press and hold the button for a continuous reading; the pulse oximeter will take a reading every 30 seconds for 20 minutes and record the data on the printout
8. Obtain a saturation reading.
9. Check patient pulse and compare with the measured heart rate on the oximeter.
10. Record the results.
11. Remove the probe, and turn off the oximeter.
12. Provide patient comfort measures.
13. Clean and replace equipment. Discard disposable items according to *Standard Precautions.*

NURSING CONSIDERATIONS

If the patient's blood pressure is less than 90 mm Hg systolic, question the reliability of the arterial blood saturation. Inadequate blood flow will result in an erroneous reading.

Be aware that the saturation reported by the pulse oximeter is usually 2% to 4% higher than the actual measured arterial oxygen saturation.

Do not use cold digits because the reading will be inaccurate.

If oxygen saturation levels with exercise are ordered be sure to have the patient ambulate in the home—having the patient sit quietly for the pulse oximeter reading will not give a true picture of the patient's oxygen requirements.

DOCUMENTATION GUIDELINES

Document the following on the visit report:
- The procedure and patient toleration
- Cardiopulmonary status, including the patient's heart rate
- Arterial oxygen saturation by pulse oximeter (SAO_2)
- FIO_2 level
- The oxygen delivery system (e.g., nasal cannula, face mask)
- The digit used to obtain the reading
- The patient's activity at the time the reading was obtained
- Any patient/caregiver instructions and response to teaching
- Physician notification, if applicable
- *Standard Precautions*
- Other pertinent findings

Update the plan of care.

AUTHOR: Pamela Becker Weilitz, M.S.N.-R., R.N., C.S., A.W.P.

Suctioning

PURPOSE

- To relieve airway obstruction
- To prevent respiratory infection
- To improve breathing
- To promote self-care in the home

EQUIPMENT

1. Number 14 or 16 French catheter
2. Suction machine
3. Specimen container, as required
4. Distilled water or tap water
5. Disposable nonsterile and sterile gloves and an impermeable plastic trash bag (see *Infection Control*)

PROCEDURE

1. Explain the procedure to the patient/caregiver.
2. Assemble the equipment at a convenient work area. A portable suction machine should be at the bedside.
3. Place the conscious patient in a semi-reclining position and the unconscious patient in a supine position, unless contraindicated. Turn the patient's head to face you.
4. Check and regulate the suction machine. Set the gauge between 5 and 10 inches of mercury.
5. Open the sterile catheter and follow sterile technique if the patient is on a ventilator, requires deep suctioning, or is immunosuppressed. Otherwise, clean catheter technique is acceptable in the home.
6. Prepare the irrigation solution. Tap water may be placed in a clean cup. Afterwards, rinse out the cup, and air dry. Instruct the caregiver to use a clean cup each day.
7. Don disposable gloves.
8. Attach the catheter to the suction machine.
9. Open the finger adapter, and insert the catheter:
   a. For a patient with a nasopharynx or oronasopharynx: measure the length of the suction catheter from the top of the patient's nose to his or her earlobe, and gently insert the catheter
   b. For a patient with a tracheostomy: insert the catheter until resistance is felt (4 to 6 inches) or until patient tolerance level is met
10. Begin suctioning when the catheter is at the required depth. Apply suction as the catheter is pulled out. Suction 10 to 12 seconds only.
11. Close the finger adaptor to withdraw the catheter, using a gentle rotation motion while withdrawing.
12. If the catheter gets clogged, apply suction and rinse.
13. Stop suction a few seconds between respirations. The patient's color should return to normal before you suction again.
14. Obtain a sputum specimen if ordered.
15. Provide patient comfort measures, and assist with oral care.
16. Clean and replace the equipment. Discard disposable items according to *Standard Precautions.*

NURSING CONSIDERATIONS

Instruct caregivers to irrigate suction catheters with distilled or tap water and store them in a paper towel after use.

Suction catheters must be discarded after 24 hours, or they must be cleaned with a 50% hydrogen peroxide solution and then boiled in water for 10 minutes, air dried, and stored in a new plastic bag for reuse.

The suction collection bottle should be emptied and cleaned with soap and hot water every 24 hours.

Suction tubing also may be routinely cleaned with soap and hot water and air dried. Hang tubing in the bathroom shower to dry.

A Yankauer catheter is useful for suctioning excessive oral secretions. This catheter is plastic, rod-shaped, and has holes at the end. Suction pressure is constant because there may be no finger adaptor for regulation. Clean a Yankauer catheter with soap and water daily, rinse, and air dry.

DOCUMENTATION GUIDELINES

Document the following on the visit report:
- The procedure and patient toleration
- Amount and color of mucus suctioned (normal mucus is white, thin, and watery)
- Cardiopulmonary status, including auscultatory findings
- Any patient/caregiver instructions and response to teaching, including ability to suction
- Physician notification, if applicable
- *Standard Precautions*
- Other pertinent findings

Update the plan of care.

Tracheostomy Button or Plug: Changing, Cleaning, and Care

PURPOSE
- To prevent infection
- To maintain patent airway
- To instruct the patient/caregiver on how to manage a tracheostomy button or plug in the home
- To promote self-care in the home

EQUIPMENT
1. Tracheostomy button or plug
2. Water-soluble lubricant
3. Hydrogen peroxide
4. 4- × 4-inch gauze pad
5. Pipe cleaners or small brush
6. Sterile disposable gloves and an impermeable plastic trash bag (see *Infection Control*)

PROCEDURE
1. Explain the procedure to the patient/caregiver.
2. Assemble equipment in a convenient work area.
3. Place the patient in a sitting or a semi-reclining position, with the neck slightly hyperextended. Instruct the patient/caregiver on the following:
   a. Clean the soma per physician's orders. Soap and warm water work well. If possible, avoid hydrogen peroxide or povidone iodine (Betadine) because these solutions can irritate the skin.
   b. Remove the tracheostomy button or plug by using an outward and downward movement.
   c. Inspect the stoma for redness or signs of infection; report to the physician as necessary.
   d. Apply a thin layer of water-soluble lubricant to the cannula portion of the tracheostomy button or plug.
   e. Using an upward and slightly downward motion, gently insert the tracheostomy button or plug until it rests snugly against the patient's neck.

4. Ask the patient to nod his or her head if the tracheostomy button or plug is a comfortable fit; reinsert as necessary.
5. Provide patient comfort measures.
6. Clean and replace equipment. Discard disposable items according to *Standard Precautions.*

NURSING CONSIDERATIONS

Do *not* use bleach to clean and disinfect the tracheostomy button or plug. Consider the following practices:

a. Discard old or worn-looking tracheostomy buttons or plugs and reinsert a new one.
b. Consult with the HME vendor respiratory therapist regarding preferences for cleaning the tracheostomy button or plug.
c. Clean the tracheostomy button or plug with soap and water, rinse with tap water, and reinsert; a hydrogen peroxide solution followed by a tap water rinse may help remove crusted material; pipe cleaners or small brushes can be used to clean the inside of the tracheostomy button or plug; do not use hydrogen peroxide with metal tracheostomy buttons or plugs or tubes because it will corrode metal.

Instruct the patient/caregiver on how to manage a tracheostomy button in the home; provide time for return demonstrations of the technique.

DOCUMENTATION GUIDELINES

Document the following on the visit report:
• The procedure and patient toleration
• Cardiopulmonary status before and after the procedure
• Condition of the patient's stoma
• Any patient/caregiver instructions and response to teaching, including the ability to change, clean, and care for the tracheostomy button or plug
• Physician notification, if applicable
• *Standard Precautions*
• Other pertinent findings
Update the plan of care.

Tracheostomy Care: Inner Cannula Change and Nondisposable Cannula Care

PURPOSE
- To prevent infection
- To instruct the patient/caregiver how to manage a tracheostomy in the home
- To promote self-care in the home

RELATED PROCEDURES
- Tracheostomy Care: Outer Cannula Tube Change for the Ventilator-Dependent Patient
- Suctioning
- Administration of Medications (see Chapter 9)

GENERAL INFORMATION
Inner cannula changes should be routinely performed by the patient or caregiver daily. Implement clean technique unless the patient is immunosuppressed or has an infected stoma. Inner cannulas may be disposable or nondisposable.

EQUIPMENT
1. 25% hydrogen peroxide solution
2. Tap water
3. Pipe cleaners
4. Sterile or clean tracheostomy sponge
5. Clean bowls
6. Inner and outer cannulas (may be clean or sterile, as necessary)
7. Antibiotic ointment, if prescribed by the physician
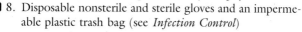 8. Disposable nonsterile and sterile gloves and an impermeable plastic trash bag (see *Infection Control*)

PROCEDURE
1. Explain the procedure to the patient/caregiver.
2. Assemble the equipment at a convenient work area.
3. Place the patient in a sitting or a semi-reclining position, with the neck slightly hyperextended.
4. Remove the soiled tracheostomy sponge.

5. Inspect the stoma for redness and drainage, and report to the physician as necessary.

6. Clean the stoma per physician's orders. Soap and water work well. Avoid hydrogen peroxide or Betadine because these solutions can cause skin breakdown. Apply antibacterial ointment if ordered.

7. Remove the inner cannula from the tracheostomy tube. (Some inner cannulas are directly pulled out of the tracheostomy tube, whereas others must be rotated and *unlocked* for removal. Review specific manufacturer recommendations for cannula removal.)

8. Suction as needed.

9. Insert a new inner cannula, using the manufacturer's recommendations. Many slide into the outer cannula and lock into place.

10. Apply clean tracheostomy tape before removing the soiled tape to prevent the outer cannula from coming out. Tie securely with two knots at the lateral aspect of the neck, rotating the sides. Allow room for one finger between the patient's neck and the tape.

11. Apply a clean tracheostomy sponge.

12. Provide patient comfort measures.

13. Do not use bleach to clean and disinfect disposable cannulas. Consider the following practices:
    a. Discard disposable inner cannulas
    b. Consult with the HME vendor respiratory therapist regarding preferences for cleaning inner and outer cannulas; not all tracheostomy tubes have inner cannulas
    c. Clean nondisposable cannulas daily; clean cannulas with soap and water, rinse with tap water, air dry, and store in plastic bags for future use; a 25% hydrogen peroxide solution followed by a tap water rinse may help remove crusted material; pipe cleaners or small brushes can be used to clean the inside of the cannulas
    d. Clean reusable metal tracheostomy tubes with soap and water, boil for 5 minutes, and then air dry for storage; store dry metal tracheostomy tubes in a plastic bag for future use; *do not* use hydrogen peroxide with metal tracheostomy tubes because it will corrode metal

14. Clean and replace the equipment. Discard disposable items according to *Standard Precautions.*

NURSING CONSIDERATIONS

Instruct the patient/caregiver in the procedure; provide time for return demonstrations.

DOCUMENTATION GUIDELINES

Document the following on the visit report.
- The procedure and patient toleration
- Cardiopulmonary status
- Condition of the stoma
- Any patient/caregiver instructions and response to teaching, including the ability to manage the tracheostomy at home
- Physician notification, if applicable
- *Standard Precautions*
- Other pertinent findings

Document medications on the medication record.

Update the plan of care.

Tracheostomy Care: Outer Cannula Tube Change for the Ventilator-Dependent Patient

---

PURPOSE

- To provide guidelines for outer cannula tracheostomy tube change in the home
- To prevent infection
- To prevent tissue adhesions to the tracheostomy tube
- To promote self-care in the home

RELATED PROCEDURES

- Suctioning
- Tracheostomy Care: Inner Cannula Change and Non-Disposable Cannula Care

GENERAL INFORMATION

This is a sterile procedure because patients on ventilators are at high risk for pulmonary infections. For these patients, reuse of cleaned outer cannulas is not routinely recommended.

A clean technique is permissible for most patients **not on a ventilator.** Follow the manufacturer's recommendations for cleaning and reusing outer cannulas. Many can be boiled, air-dried, and stored in a plastic bag.

Outer cannula tube changes are usually done on a monthly basis according to the physician's order regarding the frequency of change and the type and size of tracheostomy tube. It is recommended that two persons assist with the outer cannula changes.

Never force insertion of the tracheostomy tube. If insertion of the tube cannot be achieved, attempt to place a tube that is one-size smaller. If a smaller tube is not available, seal the patient's stoma, and assist the patient's ventilation with a self-inflating resuscitation bag until assistance arrives. Some patients may require that this procedure be performed in the doctor's office or in the emergency room.

❖ Cuffed Tracheostomy Tube Change

EQUIPMENT

1. Tracheostomy tube (Fig. 3-19)
2. Tracheostomy set (ordered by the patient/caregiver in accordance with the HME vendor's recommendations; it is recommended that extra tracheostomy tubes be kept on hand [styles vary according to patient need])
   a. Tracheostomy tube
   b. Obturator
   c. Inner cannula
   d. Tracheostomy ties or tape
3. Sterile tracheostomy sponge and pad
4. Sterile 4- × 4-inch gauze pads
5. Water-soluble lubricant
6. 10-ml syringe
7. Goggles and/or mask, as needed
8. Sterile gloves and an impermeable plastic trash bag (see *Infection Control*)

PROCEDURE

1. Explain the procedure to the patient/caregiver. Trained caregivers may serve as assistants in this procedure.
2. Assemble the equipment at a convenient work area.
3. Perform cardiopulmonary assessment to include the fol-

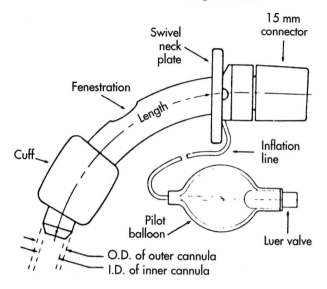

Fig. 3-19   Fenestrated cuffed tracheostomy tube. (Courtesy of Pfizer/Shiley, San Francisco.)

lowing: vital signs, lung sounds, and heart sounds; check for edema.

4. Perform home ventilator assessment.
5. Suction the patient's airway before the procedure. Then, suction above the tracheostomy cuff before deflating it.
6. Position the patient for the procedure in a sitting position or with the head of the bed raised. (Assess the position that is more comfortable for the patient. The patient may be placed in a supine position, with a towel between his or her shoulder blades; however, many patients tolerate this particular procedure best when they are sitting in an upright position. Consult with the physician regarding positioning of the patient.)
7. Prepare the tracheostomy tube, using an assistant's help and in as sterile manner as possible. *Avoid touching the cannula.* Hold the cannula at the connector by the neck plate.
   a. Test the cuff for leaks; always test the cuff and inflation system for leakage before inserting the tube by inflating the cuff and observing it for leaks; the cuff of the tube

       may also be submerged in a sterile cup of sterile water to check for bubbles.

   b. Remove the inner cannula, and insert the obturator into the outer cannula.

   c. Put ties and tape onto the neck plate of the new tracheostomy tube.

   d. Apply a thin film of water-soluble lubricant to the outer cannula and cuff and to the protruding portion of the obturator to facilitate insertion.

   e. Place the prepared tracheostomy tube in the original sterile container tray, keeping the tube's ties away from the cannula until it is needed for insertion.

8. Inspect the stoma site for redness and swelling or for signs of bleeding.

9. Clean the stoma according to the physician's orders. Soap and water work well. Avoid using hydrogen peroxide or Betadine because they may enhance skin breakdown.

10. Instruct an assistant to remove the ties and tape from the old tracheostomy tube neck plate; then turn down or turn off the ventilator alarms.

11. Hyperoxygenate the patient for a minimum of 30 seconds before extubation with an FIO_2 level of 100%.

12. Deflate the old cuff by evacuating air from the Luer valve of the inflation line, using a 5- to 10-ml syringe.

13. Instruct an assistant to disconnect the patient from the ventilator. Place the end of the ventilator tubing on sterile 4- × 4-inch gauze pads; protect the tubing from contamination.

14. Quickly remove the old tracheostomy tube (grasp the neck plate and remove the tube in a downward and outward motion). Suction the airway if necessary.

15. Immediately insert the lubricated tube into the patient's tracheostomy using an upward and then downward curved motion that follows the anatomic position of the patient's neck. Consider asking the patient to look up at the ceiling and to swallow to ease insertion of the tracheostomy tube.

16. Remove the obturator.

17. Insert the inner cannula, and secure.

18. Instruct an assistant to immediately reconnect the patient to the ventilator. Turn the ventilator alarms back on.

19. Inflate the cuff at 1 ml/mm tube size. Usually 4 to 7 cc of air is used to inflate the cuff.

20. Follow the manufacturer's recommendations to assess cuff pressure. Cuff pressure should not exceed 18 mm/Hg or 22 cm H_2O pressure. Evaluate the patient's comfort level.
21. Apply a new sponge and pad to the stoma. Suction the airway as needed.
22. Assess cardiopulmonary status. Ask the patient to nod head if he or she is getting enough air and feels all right. Administer a few breaths of 100% oxygen from the ventilator if needed. Return the FIO_2 level to the prescribed setting.
23. Instruct the caregiver that if the tracheostomy tube accidentally comes out and the caregiver cannot reinsert it, he or she must make a tight seal over the patient's stoma and ventilate the patient with a self-inflating resuscitation bag via a face mask until assistance arrives.
24. Provide patient comfort measures
25. Clean and replace the equipment. Discard disposable items according to *Standard Precautions.*

NURSING CONSIDERATIONS

This procedure may need to be individualized according to specific patient needs; use essentially the same procedure for uncuffed tracheostomy tube changes.

Clean technique is permissible for most patients who are not on a ventilator. In this case it is permissible to reuse a clean outer cannula.

Many patients tolerate this procedure best sitting up in a chair with side arms for support. Instruct the patient to look up at the ceiling and to swallow while the tracheostomy tube is being inserted. This accomplishes the following:

1. It positions the neck to facilitate tracheostomy tube insertion
2. It gives the patient a "job" to do, which therefore may be distracting and lessen patient anxiety

See the procedures for *Inner Cannula Change* and *Nondisposable Cannula Care.*

DOCUMENTATION GUIDELINES

Document the following on the visit report.
- The procedure and patient toleration
- Size and lot number of tracheostomy tube inserted
- Volume and pressure millimeters of air used to inflate the cuff

- Cardiopulmonary status before and after the procedure
- Ventilator settings (make sure to include high- and low-pressure patient readings before and after the procedure)
- Any patient/caregiver instructions and response to teaching
- Physician notification, if applicable
- *Standard Precautions*
- Other pertinent findings

Update the plan of care.

❖ FOME-Cuf Tracheostomy Tube Change*

EQUIPMENT

1. FOME-Cuf tracheostomy tube kit and spare (Fig. 3-20)
2. Sterile tracheostomy sponge and pad dressing
3. Water-soluble lubricant
4. Sterile Cuff Maintenance Device (CMD); 60-ml syringe and attached to three-way stopcock
5. AutoControl connector (sideport adaptor) included in the FOME-Cuf

 6. Sterile gloves and an impermeable plastic trash bag (see *Infection Control*)

PROCEDURE

1. Follow steps *1* through *6* of the procedure for *Cuffed Tracheostomy Tube Change*. Hyperoxygenate the patient before and after the procedure, suction as needed, and return the FIO_2 level to the prescribed setting.
2. Prepare the tube using an assistant's help in as sterile a manner as possible. *Avoid touching the cannula*. Hold the cannula by the connector at the neck plate, and do the following:
   a. Insert the CMD with the three-way stopcock into a red-wing pilot port and evacuate all the air from the FOME-Cuf
   b. Firmly pinch the red-wing pilot port with your fingers, and remove the pilot port from the syringe while maintaining the collapsed state of the cuff; never clamp or place excessive traction on the pilot port tubing

---

*Inclusion of the FOME-Cuf (Bivona-Gary, Ind.) procedure does not indicate an endorsement by the author or Mosby, Inc.

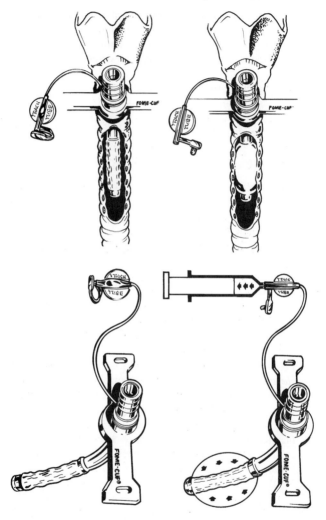

Fig. 3-20   The Bivona FOME-Cuf. (Courtesy Bivona, Inc., Gary, Ind.)

   c. Plug the red-wing pilot port with the attached red stopper; this procedure ensures the smallest possible cuff diameter for ease of tube insertion and for maximum patient comfort

   d. Insert the obturator

    e. Put ties and tape onto the neck plate of a new tracheostomy tube

    f. Apply a thin film of water-soluble lubricant to the outer surface of the tracheostomy tube, cuff, and protruding portion of the obturator to facilitate insertion

    g. Place the tube in the original sterile container tray, keeping ties away from the cannula until it ready for use

3. Instruct an assistant to remove the ties and tape from the old tracheostomy tube neck plate.

4. Inspect the stoma site for redness and swelling or for signs of bleeding.

5. Clean the stoma according to the physician's orders. Soap and water work well. Avoid using hydrogen peroxide or Betadine because they may enhance skin breakdown.

6. Instruct the assistant to use the CMD to evacuate all the air from the old cuff. Repeat steps *2a* through *2c* to evacuate all the air from the old cuff. Collapse of the red-wing pilot port indicates complete evacuation of the cuff volume.

7. Instruct the assistant to disconnect the patient from the ventilator. Place the end of the ventilator tubing on sterile 4- × 4-inch gauze pads; protect the tubing from contamination.

8. Quickly remove the old tracheostomy tube (grasp the neck plate and remove the tube in a downward and outward motion).

9. *Immediately* insert the lubricated FOME-Cuf tracheostomy tube into the patient's tracheostomy in an upward and then downward curved motion that follows the anatomic position of the patient's throat. Consider asking the patient to look up at the ceiling and to swallow to ease insertion of the tracheostomy tube.

10. Remove the obturator.

11. Instruct the assistant to reconnect the patient to the ventilator. Turn the ventilator alarms back on.

12. Disconnect the red stopper from the red pilot port to allow the cuff to passively inflate, gently and naturally sealing the patient's trachea.

13. Ensure the integrity and fit of the newly intubated FOME-Cuf by evacuating all the air from the cuff with the CMD in the following manner:

    a. Pull the syringe plunger to evacuate all the air from the cuff (note the dimple on the red pilot port that indicates complete and proper evacuation of the cuff)

b. While maintaining a forceful pull on the plunger, turn the stopcock selector to isolate the syringe (the dimple created on the red-wing pilot port tells you that the integrity of the cuff has been maintained)

c. Measure the residual cuff volume to ensure proper tracheostomy tube size (when at least 6-ml residual volume can be evacuated from the cuff, you are assured of a safe resting-cuff-to-tracheal-wall pressure and that the tube size is appropriate for the patient)

d. Remove the CDM from the red pilot port, and allow the cuff to passively inflate

14. Attach the Sideport AutoControl connector to the self-inflating resuscitation bag for maintaining a positive seal during manual resuscitation.

15. Instruct the caregiver to totally evacuate the cuff at least every 8 hours as described in steps *2a* through *2c*.

16. Follow steps *24* and *25* of the procedure for *Cuffed Tracheostomy Tube Change.*

NURSING CONSIDERATIONS

Never plug the pilot port or add air to the FOME-Cuf while it is in the patient.

Many patients tolerate this procedure best sitting up in a chair with side arms for support. Instruct the patient to look up at the ceiling and to swallow while the tracheostomy tube is being inserted. Then, do the following:

1. Position the neck to facilitate tracheostomy tube insertion
2. During this procedure, give the patient a "job" to do, which therefore may be distracting and lessen patient anxiety

Review the manufacturer's guidelines for FOME-Cuf insertion and maintenance.

DOCUMENTATION GUIDELINES

See the procedure for Cuffed Tracheostomy Tube Change.

Dermatologic and Wound Care Procedures

Butterfly or Steri-Strips

PURPOSE
- To close a small wound
- To reinforce a staple or suture line

GENERAL INFORMATION
Butterfly or steri-strips may be used on a small wound where the tissue is closed and there is not a great deal of movement in the surrounding area. For primary skin closure to occur, allow the butterfly strips to remain on for 5 to 7 days.

RELATED PROCEDURES
- Wound Assessment and Documentation (see Chapter 2)
- Wound Management

EQUIPMENT
1. Butterfly or steri-strips (available commercially or can be made from tape)
2. Hypoallergenic tape
3. Scissors
4. Disposable nonsterile gloves and an impermeable plastic trash bag (see *Infection Control*)

PROCEDURE
1. Explain the procedure to the patient/caregiver.
2. Assemble the equipment at a convenient work area.

3. Assist the patient to a comfortable position and expose the wound. Drape the patient for privacy.
4. Inspect the wound, and evaluate it for signs of healing versus infection.
5. Apply butterfly or steri-strips by the following method:
   a. To make a butterfly strip: Fold a 3- to 4-inch long strip of ½-inch wide tape back on itself and cut off the corners at the folded ends to make nicks; butterfly and steri-strips are also commercially available
   b. Apply the strips across the wound, being careful to approximate wound edges. Space the strips evenly along the wound.
6. Provide patient comfort measures.
7. Cleanse and replace equipment. Discard disposable items according to *Standard Precautions*.

 NURSING CONSIDERATIONS

Patient may report itching.

Report signs and symptoms of wound infection to the physician.

Allow the strips to remain in place as ordered by physician. Replace as necessary.

 DOCUMENTATION GUIDELINES

Review documentation guidelines of the procedures for *Wound Assessment and Documentation* and *Wound Management*.

Update the plan of care.

Dressing Changes: Biobrane

PURPOSE
- To promote wound healing
- To control fluid loss
- To minimize infection and discomfort

RELATED PROCEDURES
- Dressing Changes: Sterile Technique
- Wound Assessment and Documentation (see Chapter 2)
- Wound Irrigation and Debridement
- Wound Management

GENERAL INFORMATION
Biobrane is an adherent, flexible, biosynthetic wound dressing. It is a nontoxic, hypoallergenic mixture of purified porcine peptide bonded to an elastic silicone membrane. The impermeable membrane functions to (1) control water-vapor loss at rates comparable to normal skin, (2) provide a flexible covering for the wound surface, and (3) allow joint movement and early ambulation.

Biobrane dressings are commonly applied over partial-thickness wounds or burns (Fig. 4-1). It may be necessary to immobilize the affected area of joint for 48 hours after application; review the manufacturer's recommendations.

EQUIPMENT
1. Biobrane dressing(s) as prescribed by the physician
2. Cleansing or irrigation solution as prescribed by the physician
3. Sterile gauze roll dressing
4. Cotton-tip applicators
5. Hypoallergenic tape, bandage scissors
6. Plastic sheet or towels
7. Disposable nonsterile and sterile gloves, protective apron, and an impermeable plastic trash bag (see *Infection Control*)

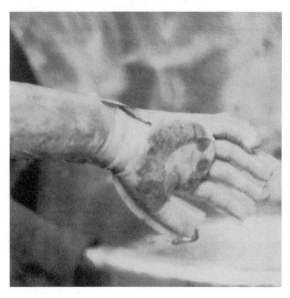

Fig. 4-1 Biobrane dressing over partial-thickness burn. (From Wong DL: *Whaley and Wong's essentials of pediatric nursing,* ed 4, St Louis, 1993, Mosby.)

PROCEDURE

1. Explain the procedure to the patient/caregiver.
2. Assemble the equipment at a convenient work area.
3. Assist the patient to a comfortable position, and expose the wound. Place a plastic sheet or towel under the patient to prevent soiling of linen. Drape the patient for privacy.
4. Cleanse and irrigate the wound as ordered by the physician. Clean from the least contaminated area to the most contaminated area.
5. Evaluate the wound for signs of healing versus infection.
6. Apply the Biobrane dressing in the following manner:
   a. Cover more area than necessary; apply the Biobrane wrinkle-free with a slight stretch
   b. Wrap and cover the Biobrane with a snug, bulky, or absorbent dressing; then secure the dressing with tape (do not get the dressing wet, and do not remove the dressing for the first 24 hours)

7. Remove the gauze dressing 24 to 36 hours after applying the Biobrane. Inspect the condition of the dressing site and take the following actions:
   a. If the Biobrane is adherent and no fluid has accumulated, rewrap the area with gauze, then secure it with tape.
   b. If the Biobrane is loose but the underlying tissue is pink, remove any nonpurulent fluid with a sterile cotton-tip swab, rewrap the area with a gauze dressing, and secure it with tape. Inspect the dressing 24 and 48 hours after application for adherence and for condition of the wound.
   c. If the Biobrane is loose and there is purulent drainage underneath, notify the patient's physician for further orders; assess for other signs of infection; instruct the patient/caregiver to observe the wound area daily for drainage, edema, inflammation, blistering, or separation—notify the physician if any of these occur.
8. Continue to inspect the Biobrane dressing for bubbles, drainage, or purulence; treat as previously advised.
9. Remove the Biobrane dressing when the wound has healed or adherence to the surgical suture line is achieved.
10. Provide patient comfort measures.
11. Clean and replace the equipment. Discard disposable items according to *Standard Precautions*.

NURSING CONSIDERATIONS

Perform burn wound care using sterile technique.

There may be some drainage on the gauze because Biobrane is porous and small amounts of fluid may escape.

Secure Biobrane with a clean gauze dressing.

After 7 to 14 days the Biobrane may appear dry and loose in spots. Patients may report itching.

Patient reports of fever within the first 48 hours after application of the dressing may indicate an allergic reaction; notify the physician.

DOCUMENTATION GUIDELINES

Review documentation guidelines of the procedures for *Wound Assessment and Documentation* and *Wound Management*.

Update the plan of care.

Dressing Changes: Calcium Alginate

PURPOSE
- To promote wound healing
- To control drainage
- To minimize discomfort and infection

RELATED PROCEDURES
- Dressing Changes: Sterile Technique
- Wound Assessment and Documentation (see Chapter 2)
- Wound Irrigation and Debridement
- Wound Management

GENERAL INFORMATION

Calcium alginate dressings are commonly used on full-thickness wounds. They are commonly used to control wound drainage. Secondary dressings should be nonocclusive because oxygen interacts with the calcium alginate dressing to promote wound healing.

EQUIPMENT
1. Calcium alginate dressing, as prescribed by the physician (see Table 4-1, *Dermal Wound Care Products,* on pp. 183-190)
2. Sterile normal saline solution, as prescribed by the physician
3. Sterile 4- × 4-inch gauze dressings and pads
4. Hypoallergenic tape, bandage scissors
5. Plastic sheet or towel
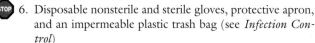 6. Disposable nonsterile and sterile gloves, protective apron, and an impermeable plastic trash bag (see *Infection Control*)

PROCEDURE
1. Explain the procedure to the patient/caregiver.
2. Assemble the equipment at a convenient work area.
3. Assist the patient to a comfortable position to expose the wound. Place a plastic sheet or towel under the patient to prevent soiling the linen. Drape the patient for privacy.

4. Gently remove the old tape and dressing. Assess the drainage on the old dressing, then discard it in a plastic trash bag.

5. Clean and irrigate the wound with sterile normal saline solution. Clean the wound from the least contaminated area to the most contaminated area; then blot the surrounding area dry with 4- × 4-inch gauze pads.

6. Inspect the wound, and evaluate it for healing versus signs of infection.

7. Apply a calcium alginate dressing to the moist wound bed, and gently pat the dressing to conform to the wound bed. (If packing is required, gently layer the calcium alginate dressings by folding them back on the previous layer.)

8. Cover the wound with a secondary porous or gas-permeable dressing, such as gauze; then secure it with tape.

9. Change the calcium alginate dressing daily (more frequently if the secondary gauze dressing becomes moist), using the following methods:

   a. Gently lift the secondary gauze dressing from the wound

   b. Remove and discard any nongelled calcium alginate dressing from the wound bed

   c. Flush away any remaining gelled calcium alginate dressing with normal saline solution irrigation

   d. Dry the surrounding tissue surface with 4- × 4-inch gauze pads

   e. Reapply new calcium alginate dressings to the moist wound bed; secure with a secondary gauze dressing and tape

10. Provide patient comfort measures.

11. Clean and replace the equipment. Discard disposable items according to *Standard Precautions.*

NURSING CONSIDERATIONS

Perform wound care using sterile technique, unless ordered otherwise by the physician.

Instruct the patient/caregiver in clean technique as approved by the physician.

Calcium alginate dressings may appear to crystallize and not gel in wounds that have minimal drainage. If this should occur, it may be necessary to dampen the dressing with normal saline solution before dressing removal. Use calcium alginate dressings **only** on moderate to copious draining wounds.

DOCUMENTATION GUIDELINES

Review documentation guidelines of the procedures for *Wound Assessment and Documentation* and *Wound Management*.

Update the plan of care.

Dressing Changes: Dry to Dry

PURPOSE
- To protect the wound from injury or trauma
- To minimize pain and infection
- To promote wound healing

RELATED PROCEDURES
- Administration of Medications: General Guidelines (see Chapter 9)
- Dressing Changes: Sterile Technique
- Montgomery Straps
- Wound Assessment and Documentation (see Chapter 2)
- Wound Irrigation and Debridement
- Wound Management
- Wound Packing

GENERAL INFORMATION

Dry dressings are commonly used for abrasions and non-draining postoperative incisions. A dry dressing does not debride the wound and should not be used for wounds requiring debridement.

EQUIPMENT
1. Sterile gauze dressing (as required for the wound) as prescribed by the physician
2. Sterile normal saline or irrigant/topical medication as prescribed by the physician
3. Hypoallergenic tape, bandage scissors
4. Plastic sheet or towel
5. Disposable nonsterile and sterile gloves, protective apron,

and an impermeable plastic trash bag (see *Infection Control*)

PROCEDURE

1. Explain the procedure to the patient/caregiver.
2. Assemble the equipment at a convenient work area.
3. Assist the patient to a comfortable position to expose the wound. Place a plastic sheet or towel under the patient to prevent soiling the linen. Drape the patient for privacy.
4. Gently remove the old tape and dressing. Assess the drainage on the old dressing, then discard it in a plastic trash bag.
5. Irrigate the wound with sterile normal saline (or other irrigant solution) as ordered by the physician.
6. Inspect the wound; evaluate it for signs of healing versus signs of infection.
7. Apply topical medication if ordered by the physician.
8. Apply dry dressing over the wound, then secure with tape (for frequent dressing changes, it is advised to use Montgomery straps).
9. Provide patient comfort measures.
10. Clean and replace equipment. Discard disposable items according to *Standard Precautions.*

NURSING CONSIDERATIONS

Perform wound care using sterile technique, unless ordered otherwise by the physician. Be aware that sterile technique is recommended for deep or infected wounds.

Generally, a chronic wound can be managed with a clean glove.

Instruct the patient/caregiver in clean technique as approved by the physician.

The dressing may be reinforced with an abdominal dressing (ABD) or absorbent cotton pad for wounds with large amounts of drainage.

Tape located over body hair should be removed in the direction of the hair growth to reduce irritation and discomfort.

If a catheter or drain is present, remove dressings one layer at a time to avoid accidental removal of the drain/catheter.

Report signs and symptoms of wound infection to the physician.

DOCUMENTATION GUIDELINES

Review documentation guidelines of the procedures for *Wound Assessment and Documentation* and *Wound Management*.

Update the plan of care.

Dressing Changes: Foam Dressing

PURPOSE

- To promote wound healing
- To debride the wound
- To minimize pain and infection

RELATED PROCEDURES

- Dressing Changes: Sterile Technique
- Wound Assessment and Documentation (see Chapter 2)
- Wound Irrigation and Debridement
- Wound Management

GENERAL INFORMATION

Foam dressings are nonadhesive, hydrophilic dressings used to treat partial- and full-thickness wounds with minimal to moderate drainage. Be aware that a secondary dressing may be required to secure the foam in place.

EQUIPMENT

1. Foam dressing (e.g., Epi-Lock, Lyofoam, Allevyn) as prescribed by the physician (see Table 4-1, *Dermal Wound Care Products,* on pp. 183-190)
2. Sterile normal saline (or other irrigant) as prescribed by the physician
3. Sterile 4- × 4-inch gauze dressings
4. Plastic sheet or towel
5. Disposable nonsterile and sterile gloves, protective apron, and an impermeable plastic trash bag (see *Infection Control*)

PROCEDURE

1. Explain the procedure to the patient/caregiver.
2. Assemble equipment in a convenient work area.
3. Position the patient to expose the wound. Place a plastic sheet or towel under the patient to prevent soiling the linen. Drape the patient for privacy.
4. Gently remove the old dressing.
5. Irrigate and cleanse the wound as ordered by the physician.
6. Inspect the wound, and evaluate for signs and symptoms of infection versus signs of healing.
7. Using gauze dressings, blot excess moisture from the wound surface, and dry intact skin around the wound.
8. Apply foam dressing according to the manufacturer's instructions.
9. Provide patient comfort measures.
10. Clean and replace equipment. Discard disposable items according to *Standard Precautions.*

NURSING CONSIDERATIONS

Perform wound care using sterile technique, unless ordered otherwise by the physician. Be aware that sterile technique is recommended for deep or infected wounds.

Generally, a chronic wound can be managed with a clean glove.

Instruct the patient/caregiver in clean technique as approved by the physician.

Foam dressings may be left in place 5 to 7 days; if adherent, they may be allowed to fall off on their own.

Foam dressing may be secured with roll gauze, tape, adhesive dressings, or a dressing sheet (e.g., Mefix or Hypafix).

Report signs and symptoms of wound infection to the physician.

DOCUMENTATION GUIDELINES

Review documentation guidelines of the procedures for *Wound Assessment and Documentation* and *Wound Management.*

Dressing Changes: Hydrocolloid Dressings and Transparent Adhesive Films

PURPOSE
- To promote wound healing
- To minimize pain and infection
- To protect the skin

RELATED PROCEDURES
- Dressing Changes: Sterile Technique
- Wound Assessment and Documentation (see Chapter 2)
- Wound Irrigation and Debridement
- Wound Management

GENERAL INFORMATION

Hydrocolloid dressings and transparent adhesive films are useful to protect excoriated, reddened, or blistered areas of skin (Fig. 4-2). They are used on partial-thickness wounds. Transparent adhesive films are semipermeable dressings that are also commonly used to protect skin against friction.

EQUIPMENT

1. Hydrocolloid dressing and transparent adhesive film as prescribed by the physician (see Table 4-1, *Dermal Wound Care Products*, on pp. 183-190)
2. Hypoallergenic tape, bandage scissors
3. Plastic sheet or towel
4. Disposable nonsterile and sterile gloves, protective apron, and an impermeable plastic trash bag (see *Infection Control*)

PROCEDURE

1. Explain the procedure to the patient/caregiver.
2. Assemble the equipment at a convenient work area.
3. Assist the patient to a comfortable position to expose the wound. Place a plastic sheet or towel under the patient to prevent soiling the linen. Drape the patient for privacy.
4. Gently remove the old tape and dressing. Assess the drain-

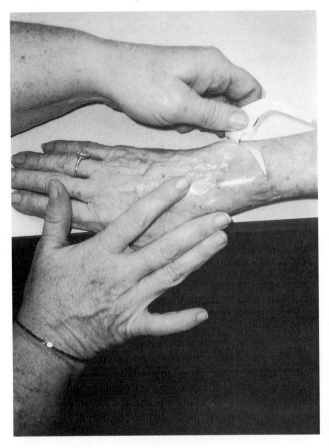

Fig. 4-2 Applying a hydrocolloid dressing as a protective dressing. (Gloves are not worn because the skin is intact.) (Photo courtesy Robyn Rice.)

age on the old dressing, then discard the dressing in a plastic trash bag and secure.

5. Clean and irrigate the wound as prescribed by the physician. Clean from the least contaminated area of the wound to the most contaminated area.

6. Inspect the wound, and evaluate it for signs of healing versus signs of infection.

7. Pat the wound edges dry with a gauze pad, making sure that the surrounding skin is free of oily or greasy substances. Consider using a skin preparation to anchor the dressing.
8. Prepare the dressing (hydrocolloid dressings and adhesive films are sterile and should be handled appropriately) in the following manner:
   a. Cut and prepare the dressing so that it covers a 1.5-inch margin of healthy skin
   b. Carefully remove the paper backing from the dressing to prevent contamination of the sterile adhesive side
9. Apply the hydrocolloid dressing and adhesive film in the following manner:
   a. Gently *roll* the dressing over the wound (avoid stretching)
   b. Shape and mold the dressing into place, securing it around the wound edges; shape, mold, cut, and taper the dressing for hard-to-fit areas.
10. Secure the hydrocolloid dressing and adhesive film with hypoallergenic tape, as needed.
11. Change the hydrocolloid dressing and transparent adhesive film about every 3 to 7 days or as required for leakage. (The hydrocolloid dressing may leave a gel residue in the wound bed; irrigate the wound bed with a normal saline solution, then apply a new dressing.)
12. Provide patient comfort measures.
13. Clean and replace the equipment. Discard disposable items according to *Standard Precautions.*

NURSING CONSIDERATIONS

Perform wound care using sterile technique, unless ordered otherwise by the physician.

Instruct the patient/caregiver in clean technique as approved by the physician.

DOCUMENTATION GUIDELINES

Review documentation guidelines of the procedures for *Wound Assessment and Documentation* and *Wound Management.*

Update the plan of care.

Dressing Changes: Hydrogel

PURPOSE
- To promote wound healing
- To debride the wound
- To minimize pain and infection

RELATED PROCEDURES
- Dressing Changes: Sterile Technique
- Wound Assessment and Documentation (see Chapter 2)
- Wound Irrigation and Debridement
- Wound Management

GENERAL INFORMATION
Hydrogel dressings expand in water but do not dissolve in it. The gel is available in a sheet form or as a viscous fluid.

Hydrogels debride the wound by rehydration; they absorb exudate and encourage healing by maintaining a moist wound environment conducive to healing. The gel dressings are nonadherent and must be covered by a secondary dressing.

Hydrogels are best suited for the treatment of leg ulcers, pressure ulcers, and minor burns. Hydrogels are not recommended for infected wounds with large amounts of drainage.

EQUIPMENT
1. Hydrogel (e.g., Carrington Gel, Intrasite Gel) as prescribed by the physician (see Table 4-1, *Dermal Wound Care Products,* on pp. 183-190)
2. Sterile normal saline solution or other irrigant as prescribed by the physician
3. Sterile 4- × 4-inch gauze dressings
4. Cotton-tip applicators
5. Hypoallergenic tape, bandage scissors
6. Plastic sheet or towel
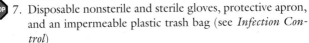 7. Disposable nonsterile and sterile gloves, protective apron, and an impermeable plastic trash bag (see *Infection Control*)

PROCEDURE

1. Explain the procedure to the patient/caregiver.
2. Assemble equipment in a convenient work area.
3. Assist the patient to a comfortable position to expose the wound. Place a plastic sheet or towel under the patient to prevent soiling the linen. Drape the patient for privacy.
4. Gently remove the old dressing.
5. Assess the drainage on the old dressing, then discard in a plastic trash bag.
6. Irrigate and clean the wound as ordered by the physician.
7. Inspect the wound, and evaluate it for signs and symptoms of infection versus signs of healing.
8. Using a cotton-tip applicator, apply the gel approximately ¼- to ½-inch thick across the wound surface.
9. Cover the wound with a secondary dressing: gauze, hydrocolloid, or foam. As needed, secure the dressing with tape.
10. Provide patient comfort measures.
11. Clean and replace equipment. Discard disposable items according to *Standard Precautions.*

NURSING CONSIDERATIONS

Perform wound care using sterile technique, unless ordered otherwise by the physician. Be aware that sterile technique is recommended for deep or infected wounds.

Generally, a chronic wound can be managed with a clean glove.

Instruct the patient/caregiver in clean technique as approved by the physician.

Hydrogel dressings should be changed daily.

Report signs and symptoms of wound infection to the physician.

DOCUMENTATION GUIDELINES

Review documentation guidelines of the procedures for *Wound Assessment and Documentation* and *Wound Management.*

Dressing Changes: Sterile Technique

PURPOSE
- To minimize infection
- To enhance wound healing

RELATED PROCEDURES
- Wound Assessment and Documentation (see Chapter 2)
- Wound Irrigation and Debridement
- Wound Management

GENERAL INFORMATION

It is recommended that the nurse use sterile technique whenever possible when performing wound care, unless otherwise ordered by the physician. Patients, however, are unlikely to infect themselves in their own environment and may be taught clean technique as approved by the physician.

EQUIPMENT

1. Sterile dressing as prescribed by the physician (see Table 4-1, *Dermal Wound Care Products,* on pp. 183-190)
2. Wound irrigation solution as prescribed by the physician
3. Plastic sheet or towel
 4. Disposable nonsterile and sterile gloves, protective apron, and an impermeable plastic trash bag (see *Infection Control*)

PROCEDURE

1. Explain the procedure to the patient/caregiver.
2. Assemble the equipment at a convenient work area.
3. Assist the patient to a comfortable position to expose the wound. Place a plastic sheet under the patient to prevent soiling the linen. Drape the patient for privacy.
4. Place a clean towel underneath the working area to minimize contamination.
5. Open the sterile dressings, the irrigation and cleaning solution, and the instrument set to provide a sterile field.

6. Wear a protective apron when caring for a patient with a draining wound. Don nonsterile gloves.
7. Gently remove and discard the old tape and soiled dressings in a plastic trash bag. If the dressing sticks to the wound, moisten the dressing with a sterile normal saline solution, and then remove.
8. Remove and discard the nonsterile gloves. Don sterile gloves.
9. Cleanse and irrigate the wound as prescribed by the physician. Clean from the least contaminated area to the most contaminated area.
10. Inspect the wound, and evaluate it for signs of healing versus signs of infection.
11. Apply a dressing, and secure it with hypoallergenic tape.
12. Provide patient comfort measures.
13. Clean and replace the equipment. Discard disposable items according to *Standard Precautions.*

DOCUMENTATION GUIDELINES

Review documentation guidelines of the procedures for *Wound Assessment and Documentation* and *Wound Management.*

Update the plan of care.

Dressing Changes: Unna Boot

PURPOSE

- To promote healing of venous stasis ulcers and to minimize cellulitis
- To minimize pain and infection

RELATED PROCEDURES

- Dressing Changes: Sterile Technique
- Wound Assessment and Documentation (see Chapter 2)
- Wound Irrigation and Debridement
- Wound Management

GENERAL INFORMATION

An Unna boot wrap or medicated dressing is used to control edema and to promote healing of poorly vascularized areas of the leg and foot. The Unna boot is often used to treat venous stasis ulcers.

EQUIPMENT

1. Unna boot or medicated compression dressing as prescribed by the physician (see Table 4-1, *Dermal Wound Care Products,* on pp. 183-190)
2. Irrigation or cleansing solution as prescribed by the physician
3. Gauze or elastic bandage
4. Hypoallergenic tape, bandage scissors
5. Plastic sheet or towel

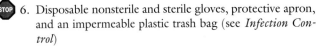

6. Disposable nonsterile and sterile gloves, protective apron, and an impermeable plastic trash bag (see *Infection Control*)

PROCEDURE

1. Explain the procedure to the patient/caregiver.
2. Assemble the equipment at a convenient work area.
3. Assist the patient to a comfortable position to expose the lower leg. Place a plastic sheet or towel underneath the leg to prevent soiling the linen or the floor. Drape the patient for privacy.
4. Gently remove the old tape and dressing. Assess the drainage on the old dressing, then discard the dressing in a plastic trash bag. Clean and irrigate the wound as ordered by the physician. Clean from the least contaminated area to the most contaminated area.
5. Inspect the wound, and evaluate it for signs of healing versus signs of infection.
6. Apply the Unna boot by wrapping the dressing from above the toes to below the knee to control edema (Fig. 4-3).
7. Cover the heel with oblique turns.
8. Make circular, figure-of-eight turns around the leg, overlapping each turn by half the width of the medicated dressing.
9. Cover the entire area 2 to 3 times. Do not make reverse turns, because such turns cause unnecessary creases and pressure.
10. Cut and smooth the dressing to avoid creases or pleats.

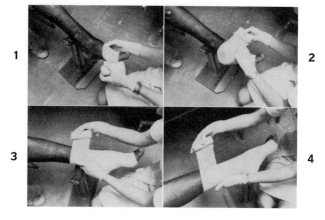

Fig. 4-3 Application of Unna boot. (From Phipps WJ, Long BC, Woods NF, Cassmeyer VL: *Medical-surgical nursing: concepts and clinical practice,* ed 4, St Louis, 1991, Mosby.)

11. Apply a clean gauze or elastic bandage over the medicated dressing for support and to absorb copious drainage, then secure the gauze or elastic bandage with hypoallergenic tape.

12. Change the dressing 1 or 2 times a week. Remove the Unna boot in the following manner:
    a. Remove the elastic bandage or gauze wrap
    b. Carefully cut and remove the dressing from the leg (soaking the dressing loose decreases the debriding effect)

13. Provide patient comfort measures.

14. Clean and replace the equipment. Discard disposable items according to *Standard Precautions.*

NURSING CONSIDERATIONS

Perform wound care using sterile technique, unless ordered otherwise by the physician.

Clean technique is often used with leg ulcers.

DOCUMENTATION GUIDELINES

Review documentation guidelines of the procedures for *Wound Assessment and Documentation* and *Wound Management.*

Update the plan of care.

Dressing Changes: Wet-to-Dry

PURPOSE
- To promote wound healing
- To debride the wound
- To prevent infection

RELATED PROCEDURES
- Dressing Changes: Sterile Technique
- Wound Assessment and Documentation (see Chapter 2)
- Wound Irrigation and Debridement
- Wound Management

GENERAL INFORMATION
A wet-to-dry dressing change is helpful for wounds that require debridement. The wet portion of the dressing absorbs exudate from the wound bed and cleans the infected wound. The dry-wound covering pulls moisture and wound drainage into the dressing by capillary action.

EQUIPMENT
1. Sterile normal saline solution as prescribed by the physician
2. Sterile 4- × 4-inch gauze dressings
3. Hypoallergenic tape, bandage scissors
4. Plastic sheet or towel
 5. Disposable nonsterile and sterile gloves, protective apron, and an impermeable plastic trash bag (see *Infection Control*)

PROCEDURE
1. Explain the procedure to the patient/caregiver.
2. Assemble the equipment at a convenient work area.
3. Assist the patient to a comfortable position to expose the wound. Place a plastic sheet or towel under the patient to prevent soiling the linen. Drape the patient for privacy.
4. Gently remove the tape and older dressing. Assess the drainage on the old dressing, then discard it in a plastic trash bag, and secure.
5. Clean and irrigate the wound as ordered by the physician.

Clean from the least contaminated area to the most contaminated area.

6. Inspect the wound, and evaluate it for signs of healing versus signs of infection.
7. Apply moist gauze directly on the surface of the wound (Fig. 4-4). (Gently feed moist gauze into the wound with

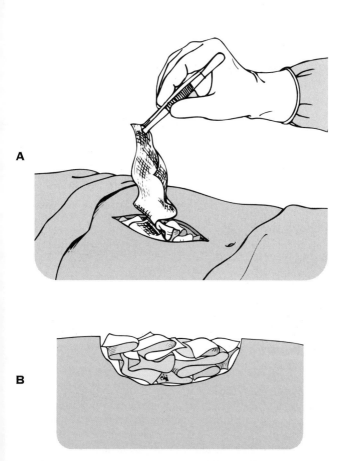

Fig. 4-4 Wet-to-dry dressing. **A,** Applying dressing. **B,** Lightly packing wound. (From Potter PA, Perry AG: *Fundamentals of nursing: concepts, process and practice,* ed 4, St Louis, 1997, Mosby.)

forceps or cotton-tip applicators if packing is required; do not stuff packing into the wound.)

8. Place dry gauze over wet gauze. Then cover with a gauze dressing, surgi-pad, or ABD pad. Secure the dressing with tape, Montgomery ties, or a binder.
9. Provide patient comfort measures.
10. Clean and replace the equipment. Discard disposable items according to *Standard Precautions*.

NURSING CONSIDERATIONS

Perform wound care using sterile technique, unless ordered otherwise by the physician.

Instruct patient/caregiver to use clean technique as approved by the physician.

DOCUMENTATION GUIDELINES

Review documentation guidelines of the procedures for *Wound Assessment and Documentation* and *Wound Management*.

Update the plan of care.

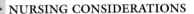

Moist Compress

PURPOSE

• To reduce inflammation of the skin

RELATED PROCEDURE

• Skin Care

GENERAL INFORMATION

A moist compress is effective in the treatment of cellulitis, furunculosis, and oozing dermatitis. The cooling effect of the compress may relieve itching and burning of the skin.

EQUIPMENT

1. Gauze dressings for compress
2. Wetting solution (room temperature: tap water, normal

saline, aluminum acetate solution [e.g., Burrow's solution]) as prescribed by the physician
3. Clean bowl
STOP 4. Disposable nonsterile gloves and an impermeable plastic trash bag (see *Infection Control*)

PROCEDURE

1. Explain the procedure to the patient/caregiver.
2. Assemble the equipment at a convenient work area.
3. Assist the patient to a comfortable position to expose the affected area. As necessary, drape the patient for privacy.
4. Place gauze dressings in a bowl and moisten with the wetting solution to the point of slightly dripping.
5. Apply a moist compress to the affected area and leave in place for 20 to 30 minutes.
6. Remove and discard gauze dressings.
7. Provide patient comfort measures.
8. Clean and replace equipment. Discard disposable items according to *Standard Precautions.*

NURSING CONSIDERATIONS

Instruct the patient/caregiver in skin care (see the procedure for *Skin Care* in this chapter).

DOCUMENTATION GUIDELINES

Document the following on the visit report:
• The procedure and patient toleration
• Condition of the patient's skin
• Physician notification, if applicable
• *Standard Precautions*
• Any other pertinent findings
Update the plan of care.

Montgomery Straps

PURPOSE

- To prevent skin irritation from tape during repeated dressing changes

RELATED PROCEDURES

- Dressing Changes: Hydrocolloid Dressings and Transparent Adhesive Films
- Dressing Changes: Sterile Technique
- Wound Assessment and Documentation (see Chapter 2)
- Wound Management

GENERAL INFORMATION

Montgomery straps should be used for patients who receive frequent dressing changes. The straps with ties essentially hold the dressing in place and prevent skin irritation caused by repeated use of tape. Montgomery straps are commercially available.

EQUIPMENT

1. Montgomery straps
2. Adhesive dressing
3. Cotton-twill tape for ties
4. Skin-protectant wipes
5. Soap and water, washcloth
6. Plastic sheet or towel
 7. Disposable nonsterile and sterile gloves, protective apron, and an impermeable plastic trash bag (see *Infection Control*)

PROCEDURE

1. Explain the procedure to the patient/caregiver.
2. Assemble the equipment at a convenient work area.
3. Assist the patient to a comfortable position to expose the wound. Place a plastic sheet or towel under the patient to prevent soiling the linen. Drape the patient for privacy.
4. Gently remove the old dressing.

5. Inspect the wound, and evaluate it for signs of healing versus signs of infection.
6. Perform wound care as ordered by the physician.
7. Wash the patient's skin surrounding the wound with soap and water to prevent irritation.
8. Apply the skin protectant to the area around the wound where the Montgomery straps with adhesive dressing will adhere. Allow the skin protectant to air dry.
9. Apply the adhesive dressing for the Montgomery ties to the skin along the side of the wound.
10. To apply the Montgomery ties, do the following:
    a. Apply the Montgomery ties with the hole ends placed on opposite sides of the dressing (the tie edges have an adhesive backing and should stick to the adhesive dressing).
    b. Thread the holes with cotton tape. Draw the opposing straps together and tie.
11. Provide patient comfort measures.
12. Clean and replace the equipment. Discard disposable items according to *Standard Precautions.*

NURSING CONSIDERATIONS

Instead of cotton-twill tape, safety pins can be placed through the holes on each side of the straps. Rubber bands are then hooked into the safety pins to hold the dressing in place. The dressing is changed by unsnapping the safety pins on one side.

Replace Montgomery straps whenever they become soiled (usually every 4 to 7 days).

Use a hydrocolloid adhesive dressing under the straps if the skin becomes irritated.

Report signs and symptoms of wound infection to the physician.

DOCUMENTATION GUIDELINES

Review documentation guidelines of the procedures for *Wound Assessment and Documentation* and *Wound Management.*

Update the plan of care.

Pediculosis

PURPOSE
- To eliminate head lice (pediculosis)
- To prevent spread of the infestation

RELATED PROCEDURE
- Administration of Medications: General Guidelines (see Chapter 9)

GENERAL INFORMATION

The louse is a small (about one-sixteenth of an inch), blood-sucking insect. It is spread through direct contact with an infected person or, less commonly, through contact with an infected person's belongings (e.g., combs, hats, clothing, bedding). Head lice attach themselves to the hair shaft so they have ready availability to their food source—the blood of the human scalp. Itching is the main symptom of head lice. The female louse lays eggs (nits) that firmly attach to the hair and, unlike dandruff, cannot be shaken off.

Be aware that some preparations are not recommended for infants, young children, and pregnant or lactating women; follow manufacturer's recommendations regarding usage.

EQUIPMENT
1. Delousing shampoo or crème rinse (prescription or over-the-counter because regular shampoos will not work)
2. Fine-tooth comb
3. Towels
 4. Disposable nonsterile gloves and an impermeable plastic trash bag (see *Infection Control*)

PROCEDURE
1. Explain the procedure to the patient/caregiver.
2. Assemble the equipment in a convenient work area.
3. Apply delousing shampoo or crème rinse. Follow manufacturer's instructions for the shampoo, **exactly.** Do not allow the shampoo to get into the patient's eyes.
4. Remove nits with a fine-tooth comb. A solution of 50%

vinegar and 50% water, used as a rinse, will help loosen the nits. Although most treatments kill both the adult lice and the nits, many schools will not allow children back in school until the nits are removed.

5. Instruct the household in environmental management of head lice to include the following:
   a. Wash articles that have come into contact with the patient's head in the last 48 hours in hot (at least 130° F) water. Dry in a hot dryer.
   b. Vacuum all carpeting, furniture, and mattresses. Car seats and headrests should also be vacuumed.
   c. Put articles that cannot be washed or vacuumed (such as stuffed animals) in a plastic bag and seal for 10 days.
   d. Disinfect combs and brushes by washing them in hot water or soak them in a louse shampoo. Rinse and air dry.
6. Provide patient comfort measures.
7. Clean and replace equipment. Discard disposable items, including the vacuum cleaner bag, according to *Standard Precautions.*

NURSING CONSIDERATIONS

Instruct the patient/caregiver in shampoo application and nit removal. All members of the household and close contacts should be checked for head lice.

As appropriate, treat everyone in the household infected with head lice at the same time.

Body lice and pubic lice (crabs) are slightly different but are treated in the same basic manner. Lice or nits in the eyelashes can be treated by applying petroleum jelly twice a day for 1 week.

Spraying the house with insecticide or fumigation is not necessary.

Inspect the patient's and, as appropriate, each household member's hair for 1 week to ensure that all lice and nits are gone. If eggs survive after 7 to 10 days, retreatment may be necessary.

There is no prophylactic treatment for head lice; do not treat people without seeing the lice or nits.

Be aware that there have been reported cases of head lice resistant to commonly used treatments. When resistance is reported, consult with the physician or local public health department and consider the following alternatives: (1) apply a heavy layer of petroleum jelly, regular mayonnaise (not non- or low-fat), or olive oil to the scalp; cover with a shower cap overnight or for several hours; wash out, using first a dishwashing liquid and then regular shampoo (combing with a fine-tooth comb is essential) or (2) daily combing of wet hair with a fine-tooth metal comb (this needs to be done on a continuous basis for 1 to 2 weeks).

DOCUMENTATION GUIDELINES

Document the following on the visit report:
- The procedure and patient/caregiver toleration
- The response to treatment
- Any patient/caregiver instructions and response to teaching, including adherence with recommendations
- Physician notification, if applicable
- *Standard Precautions*
- Other pertinent findings

Document medications on the medication record.

Update the plan of care.

AUTHOR: Anne Cahill Schappe, Ph.D., R.N.

Scabies

PURPOSE
- To eliminate scabies
- To prevent spread of the infestation

RELATED PROCEDURE
- Administration of Medications: General Guidelines (see Chapter 9)

GENERAL INFORMATION

Scabies is a parasitic disease of the skin caused by a mite *(Sarcoptes scabiei)*. The mite burrows into the cracked and folded regions of the skin and forms tunnels in the stratum corneum. Eggs are laid and hatched in the burrows. Resulting larvae form their own burrows and grow into adulthood within 2 months. Scabies is usually contracted after close personal contact with an infested individual.

EQUIPMENT

1. Medication to treat scabies (e.g., Kwell or Eurax) as prescribed by the physician; use with caution with infants and pregnant women as recommended by the physician
2. Soap and water
3. Towel and washcloth
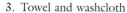 4. Disposable nonsterile gloves, protective apron, and an impermeable plastic trash bag (see *Infection Control*)

PROCEDURE

1. Explain the procedure to the patient/caregiver and family household members.
2. Assemble the equipment at a convenient work area.
3. Apply Kwell or Eurax from neck to toes. Follow the manufacturer's recommendations for the product **exactly.** One application is usually sufficient.
4. Wash, rinse, and dry the entire body according to manufacturer's instructions.
5. Provide patient comfort measures.
6. Clean and replace the equipment. Discard disposable items according to *Standard Precautions.*

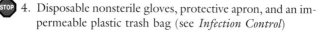

NURSING CONSIDERATIONS

Instruct the patient/caregiver that itching may persist for 1 to 2 weeks after the treatment.

Treat prophylactically those who have had skin-to-skin contact (this includes family members, caregivers, and home-care staff).

Overtreatment is common and should be avoided because of neurotoxicities associated with the medication.

Wash all items that come into contact with the patient's skin.

Store any item that cannot be washed in a sealed plastic bag for 10 days. Items may then be removed and reused.

It is not necessary to treat furniture, etc.

DOCUMENTATION GUIDELINES

Document the following on the visit report:
- The procedure and patient/caregiver toleration
- Any caregiver instructions, including adherence with recommendations
- Physician notification, if applicable
- *Standard Precautions*
- Any other pertinent findings

Document medications on the medication record.
Update the plan of care.

Skin Care

PURPOSE
- To prevent skin breakdown
- To instruct the patient/caregiver in skin-care precautions
- To promote self-care in the home

RELATED PROCEDURES
- Dressing Changes: Hydrocolloid Dressings and Transparent Adhesive Films
- Wound Assessment and Documentation (see Chapter 2)
- Wound Management

GENERAL INFORMATION
When patients who are at risk for skin breakdown and decubitus ulcer formation are admitted to the home health agency, they should be placed on a regimen of skin care that controls exposure to forces of friction, shearing, and pressure. Risk factors for skin breakdown and decubitus ulcer formation include being bed- and chair-bound, immobile, and incontinent; consuming an inadequate dietary intake; and having an altered level of consciousness. A skin-care program should be instituted by the home health agency and implemented by staff, patients, and caregivers.

EQUIPMENT
1. Lanolin-based moisturizer
2. Elbow and heel protectors or socks and sheepskin
3. Pressure-reduction devices (e.g., water mattresses, gel pads, and foam mattresses or pads)
4. Pressure-relief devices (consider air-fluidized therapy)
5. Hydrocolloid dressing and transparent adhesive film as prescribed by the physician
6. Disposable nonsterile gloves and an impermeable plastic trash bag (see *Infection Control*)

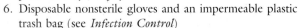

PROCEDURE

1. Explain the procedure to the patient/caregiver.
2. Assemble the equipment at a convenient work area.
3. Explain to the patient/caregiver that bedsores are likely to occur over weight-bearing areas; bony prominences; or where the body is exposed to a firm, unyielding surface.
4. Implement the following skin-care precautions with the patient/caregiver:
   a. Inspect the skin for redness; protect reddened areas from further damage. All patients at risk for skin breakdown should inspect the skin daily, paying particular attention to bony prominences.
   b. Wash the skin with a mild soap and soft washcloth; avoid hot water. During the cleansing process, be careful to minimize the force and friction applied to skin. Skin should be cleansed at the time of soiling and at routine intervals.
   c. Rinse thoroughly with clear water, and blot dry with a towel.
   d. Apply lotion; massage and stroke lightly around the bony prominence; avoid massaging over a bony prominence.
   e. Change the bed linen daily and whenever it is soiled by urine or feces; minimize skin exposure to moisture caused by incontinence, perspiration, or wound drainage; topical agents that act as barriers to moisture may also be used.
   f. Keep sheets and linens wrinkle free.
   g. Place the bed-bound patient in a 30-degree oblique position when he or she is at rest to prevent pressure over bony prominences (this can be accomplished by using pillows).
   h. Plan a simple schedule of turning the immobile patient every 2 hours from side, to back, to side to reduce the effects of prolonged pressure; minimize skin injury caused by friction and shear forces through proper positioning, transferring, and turning techniques.
   i. Instruct patients who are able to do so to shift their weight every 15 minutes.
   j. Use elbow and heel protectors, socks, or a sheepskin to relieve friction and excessive pressure on areas that are vulnerable to skin breakdown.
   k. Consider using pressure-reduction and relief devices with the immobile or chair-bound patient. Follow the

manufacturer's recommendations for use; do not use "doughnut-type" devices.

   l. Use lifting devices, such as a trapeze or bed linen, to move (rather than drag) individuals who are in bed and who cannot assist with transfers or position changes.

5. Apply transparent adhesive film or hydrocolloid dressing over areas at risk for skin breakdown. Use lubricants (e.g., cornstarch or creams), pads, and protective dressings to prevent friction.

6. Encourage adequate hydration and a diet high in protein and vitamin C to prevent skin breakdown and to enhance wound healing.

7. Obtain a physician's order for protein supplements if the patient's intake is not adequate. If dietary intake remains poor, more aggressive nutritional interventions, such as enteral or parenteral feedings, should be considered.

8. Provide patient comfort measures.

9. Clean and replace equipment. Discard disposable items according to *Standard Precautions.*

NURSING CONSIDERATIONS

A written schedule for systematically turning and repositioning the patient should be used.

A systematic risk assessment can be accomplished by using a validated risk assessment tool, such as the Braden Scale or Norton Scale. Update the risk assessment periodically.

Consider a physical therapy referral if the potential exists for improving the patient's mobility and activity status; obtain physician's orders.

Consider a home health aide referral for assistance with activities of daily living (ADLs); obtain physician's orders.

DOCUMENTATION GUIDELINES

Document the following on the visit report:
- The procedure and patient toleration
- Condition of the patient's skin
- Any patient/caregiver instructions and response to teaching, including adherence to recommendations
- Physician notification, if applicable
- *Standard Precautions*
- Other pertinent findings

Update the plan of care.

Skin Suture and Staple Removal

PURPOSE
- To remove cutaneous sutures or staples, using principles of asepsis

RELATED PROCEDURES
- Dressing Changes: Sterile Technique
- Wound Assessment and Documentation (see Chapter 2)

EQUIPMENT
1. Basic suture or staple removal set
2. Sterile dressing supplies if needed
3. Steri-strips
4. Towels
5. Antiseptic wipes
6. Disposable sterile gloves and an impermeable plastic trash bag (see *Infection Control*)

❖ Skin Suture Removal

PROCEDURE
1. Explain the procedure to the patient/caregiver.
2. Assemble the equipment at a convenient work area.
3. Position the patient to expose the suture. Drape the patient for privacy.
4. Place a clean towel underneath the suture kit and dressing supplies to minimize contamination.
5. Open the suture kit and supplies.
6. Cleanse the suture or staple line with antiseptic wipes.
7. Hold the thumb forceps in one hand and the scissors in the other hand. Gently grasp the suture with thumb forceps.
8. Gently pull on the suture to permit the insertion of the scissor's blade between the suture and the skin.
9. Cut the exposed portion of the suture, and remove it with a smooth, pulling motion of the thumb forceps.
10. Repeat steps 7 through 9, until all the sutures are removed.
11. Gently wipe the incision line with antiseptic wipes.
12. Apply a gauze dressing or steri-strips as necessary.

13. Provide patient comfort measures.
14. Clean and replace the equipment. Discard disposable items according to *Standard Precautions.*

❖ Skin Staple Removal

PROCEDURE

1. Repeat steps *1* through *6* of the procedure for *Skin Suture Removal.*
2. Place the staple remover's lower jaws beneath the span of the first staple.
3. Squeeze the handles until they are completely closed; lift the staple away from the skin, and discard the staple by releasing the handle.
4. Repeat steps *2* and *3* until all the staples are removed.
5. Repeat steps *11* through *14* of the procedure for *Skin Suture Removal.*

NURSING CONSIDERATIONS

Assess the wound for signs of healing. Do not remove suture or staples if the wound edges may separate.

It may be necessary to soak the scabs off with a warm washcloth before suture or staple removal on wounds that have a heavy or moderate scab formation.

DOCUMENTATION GUIDELINES

Document the following on the visit report:
- The procedure and patient toleration
- Appearance of the incision
- Amount and description of the drainage if present
- Physician notification, if applicable
- *Standard Precautions*
- Other pertinent findings

Review documentation guidelines of the procedure for *Wound Assessment and Documentation.*

Update the plan of care.

Wound Irrigation and Debridement

PURPOSE
- To cleanse and debride the wound
- To promote healing

RELATED PROCEDURES
- Dressing Changes: Sterile Technique
- Wound Assessment and Documentation (see Chapter 2)
- Wound Care: Scoring of Eschar

EQUIPMENT
1. Dressing as prescribed by the physician (see Table 4-1, *Dermal Wound Care Products,* on pp. 183-190)
2. Irrigation solution as prescribed by the physician
3. Hypoallergenic tape, bandage scissors
4. Sterile dressing tray, container, and syringe; or sterile 60-ml syringe attached to an 18-gauge needle, spray bottle, dental water pick, or home whirlpool
5. Emesis basin or clean bowl
6. Plastic sheet or towel
7. Disposable nonsterile and sterile gloves, protective apron, and an impermeable plastic trash bag (see *Infection Control*)

PROCEDURE
1. Explain the procedure to the patient/caregiver.
2. Assemble the equipment at a convenient work area. Open the sterile supplies and irrigation solution. Place a clean towel underneath the work area to minimize contamination.
3. Position the patient so that the irrigation solution will drain from the upper part of the wound into the basin or bowl held below the wound. Place a plastic sheet under the patient to avoid soiling the linens. Drape the patient for privacy.
4. Gently remove the old tape and dressing, and discard them in a plastic trash bag.

5. Irrigate and debride the wound in the following manner:
   a. Use sterile technique when irrigating and cleansing the wounds of patients who are immunocompromised, who have diabetes, or who have active infections.
      (1) Pour the irrigation solution into a sterile container
      (2) Place a bowl or emesis basin under area of wound to be irrigated
      (3) Fill a sterile syringe with irrigation solution
      (4) Irrigate all areas of the wound; irrigate the pockets or sinus tracts in the wound. Do not touch the wound or surrounding tissue with the tip of the irrigation syringe; irrigate from the center of the wound outward
      (5) Continue irrigating until the solution drains clear from the wound or until the solution is used up
   b. Use a home whirlpool, wet-to-dry normal saline dressing changes, or enzymatic topical debriders to cleanse and debride yellow, green, or black wound beds (carefully follow the product's instructions when applying enzymatic topical debriders to prevent damaging healthy tissue).
   c. Irrigate pink, healthy tissue with a physiologic solution, such as normal saline solution, via a spray bottle, a dental water pick, or a syringe attached to an 18-gauge needle when clean technique is acceptable.
   d. Wash the wound with soap and water to remove necrotic tissue when clean technique is not acceptable.
6. Inspect and evaluate the wound for healing versus signs of infection.
7. Dry the skin around the wound. Apply the dressing and secure it with hypoallergenic tape.
8. Consult with the physician for surgical debridement.
9. Provide patient comfort measures.
10. Clean and replace the equipment. Discard disposable items according to *Standard Precautions.*

NURSING CONSIDERATIONS

Perform wound care using sterile technique, unless ordered otherwise by the physician.

Instruct the patient/caregiver in wound irrigation, using a clean technique as approved by the physician.

DOCUMENTATION GUIDELINES

Document the following on the visit report:

- The procedure and patient toleration
- Irrigation solution used and amount
- Any patient/caregiver instructions on wound irrigation, including response to teaching and ability to irrigate and manage the wound
- Physician notification, if applicable
- *Standard Precautions*
- Other pertinent findings

Review documentation guidelines of the procedures for *Wound Assessment and Documentation* and *Wound Management*.

Update the plan of care.

Wound Care: Scoring of Eschar

PURPOSE

- To break down and remove hard, black eschar on pressure ulcers to allow chemical agents to debride the wound
- To minimize pain and infection
- To promote wound healing

RELATED PROCEDURES

- Dressing Changes: Sterile Technique
- Dressing Changes: Wet-to-Dry
- Wound Assessment and Documentation (see Chapter 2)
- Wound Management

GENERAL INFORMATION

Hard, black tissue in the wound is called eschar. Until wound eschar is removed, healing will not take place. Scoring of eschar should be done by a certified enterostomal therapist or registered nurse who has had formal training in the procedure.

EQUIPMENT

1. Sterile normal saline or irrigation solution as prescribed by the physician
2. Enzymatic debriding agent (e.g., Elase, Santyl, Travase) as prescribed by the physician (see Table 4-1, *Dermal Wound Care Products,* on pp. 183-190)
3. Gauze sponges
4. Cotton-tip applicators
5. Hypoallergenic tape, bandage scissors
6. Antiseptic wipes
7. Sterile scalpel
8. Plastic sheet or towel

9. Disposable nonsterile and sterile gloves, protective apron, and an impermeable plastic trash bag (see *Infection Control*)

PROCEDURE

1. Explain the procedure to the patient/caregiver.
2. Assemble the equipment at a convenient work area.
3. Assist the patient to a comfortable position to expose the wound. Place a plastic sheet or towel under the patient to prevent soiling the linen. Drape the patient for privacy.
4. Gently remove the old dressing.
5. Cleanse the eschar with antiseptic wipes, working in a circular motion from inside out to remove necrotic material from the wound. Use a new wipe for each circular stroke.
6. Irrigate the wound with normal saline to remove all traces of antiseptic wipe so that there is no interaction with the chemical agent.
7. Inspect the wound, and evaluate it for signs and symptoms of infection versus signs of healing.
8. Make parallel, vertical, or horizontal incisions about every one-fourth inch (.5 cm) into the black eschar. Make a criss-cross pattern. Make the incision into the eschar until a pink color is observed in the cut. It may be necessary to go over the incisions more than once to achieve an effective depth.
9. Using a cotton-tip applicator, apply a thin layer of enzymatic debriding agent *only on the eschar.*
10. Cover with a wet-to-dry dressing, as ordered by the physician.
11. Provide patient comfort measures.

12. Clean and replace equipment. Discard disposable items according to *Standard Precautions*.

NURSING CONSIDERATIONS

Perform wound care using sterile technique, unless ordered otherwise by the physician. Be aware that sterile technique is recommended for deep or infected wounds.

Generally, a chronic wound can be managed with a clean glove.

Consider surrounding or covering the wound edges with an adhesive dressing to protect healthy tissues from the enzymatic debriding agent.

Do not score wounds larger than 2 to 5 cm.

Do not score wounds that are in close proximity to the bone, where the danger of debriding to the bone exists.

Report signs and symptoms of wound infection to the physician.

DOCUMENTATION GUIDELINES

Review documentation guidelines of the procedures for *Wound Assessment and Documentation* and *Wound Management*.

Update the plan of care.

Wound Management

PURPOSE

- To provide guidelines for wound management in the home based on the degree of tissue destruction
- To apply current trends and products useful in wound management
- To promote self-care in the home

RELATED PROCEDURES

- Skin Care
- Wound Assessment and Documentation (see Chapter 2)
- Wound Irrigation and Debridement

GENERAL INFORMATION

Current trends in wound management and treatment suggest that wound repair is enhanced by (1) a moist environment; (2) a wound bed free of necrotic tissue, eschar, and environmental contamination or infection; (3) an adequate blood supply to meet metabolic demands for tissue generation; and (4) sufficient oxygen and nutrition for cellular metabolism and tissue generation.

EQUIPMENT

1. Review Table 4-1, *Dermal Wound Care Products,* on pp. 183-190

🛑 2. Disposable nonsterile or sterile gloves as needed and an impermeable trash bag (see *Infection Control*)

PROCEDURE

1. Explain the procedure to the patient/caregiver.
2. Apply current principles of wound management in the following manner:

   Stage 1: Erythema (redness, swelling, warmth over affected area) and pain are present but no damage is found to the dermis or epidermis; the condition is reversible with prompt interventions.

   Interventions: Prevention—use pressure-reduction techniques along with the application of hydrocolloid and transparent adhesive dressings to protect *reddened* areas of skin that are at risk for breakdown.

   Stage 2: Loss of epidermal, and possibly dermal, tissue may present as excoriation or blistering; shallow, superficial wound with pink wound bed, painful (referred to as partial-thickness wounds).

   Interventions: Cleanse and Protect—gently cleanse and irrigate the pink wound bed with physiologic solution, such as normal saline solution. Application of a hydrocolloid dressing, transparent adhesive film, foam, topical moisturizer, or impregnated gauze dressing will maintain a moist environment for healing and will protect the wound from environmental contamination.

   Stage 3: Loss of dermal and possibly subcutaneous tissue; undermining, eschar, copious drainage and exudates, and infection may be present; painless; referred to as a shallow, full-thickness wound.

Interventions: Disinfect, Debride, Absorb, and Protect—use an antiseptic solution to cleanse and irrigate; consult with the physician because antibiotic therapy, either systemic or topical (silver sulfadiazine cream), may be useful; eliminate dead space; fill the wound with an absorber (foam, granules, or gel) and cover with a protective dressing; calcium alginate dressings are helpful to control drainage.

Stage 4: Loss of subcutaneous tissue may expose the muscle, bone, or joint; these are typically deep wounds, with eschar, copious drainage, undermining, and sinus tract formation; usually painless; referred to as deep, full-thickness wounds.

Interventions: Essentially the same as for stage 3; avoid solitary use of transparent adhesive films or hydrocolloid dressings because these will not fill dead space.

3. Institute a skin-care regimen for stages 1 through 4.
4. Evaluate for short-term urinary catheterization or evaluate the fecal incontinence pouch for bladder or bowel contamination of the wound.
5. Instruct the patient/caregiver on home wound management. Evaluate for patient/caregiver compliance.
6. Evaluate the response to treatment. Consult with the physician, and revise the plan of care accordingly.

NURSING CONSIDERATIONS

Obtain the physician's orders for wound care supplies.

Review the fiscal intermediary guidelines for reimbursement of wound care supplies.

A number of wound care products are available. Become familiar with what products work well with which type of wound.

Three to four weeks may be needed before improvement is evident.

DOCUMENTATION GUIDELINES

Document the following on the visit report:

- The procedure and patient toleration
- The wound's response to treatment (signs of healing versus infection)
- Any patient/caregiver instructions and response to teaching, including the ability to perform dressing changes and manage the wound at home
- Physician notification, if applicable

- *Standard Precautions*
- Other pertinent findings

Review documentation guidelines of the procedure for *Wound Assessment and Documentation*.

Update the plan of care.

Wound Packing

PURPOSE

- To keep a wound open and allow it to heal from the inside out
- To minimize pain and infection

RELATED PROCEDURES

- Administration of Medications: General Guidelines (see Chapter 9)
- Dressing Changes: Sterile Technique
- Montgomery Straps
- Wound Assessment and Documentation (see Chapter 2)
- Wound Management

GENERAL INFORMATION

Moist-wound packing eliminates dead space and promotes wound healing. It is particularly useful for wounds with large tissue loss.

EQUIPMENT

1. Dressing (as required for the wound) prescribed by the physician
2. Sterile normal saline or irrigation solution and topical medication as prescribed by the physician
3. Sterile forceps and scissors
4. Hypoallergenic tape, bandage scissors
5. Plastic sheet or towel
6. Disposable nonsterile and sterile gloves, protective apron, and an impermeable plastic trash bag (see *Infection Control*)

PROCEDURE

1. Explain the procedure to the patient/caregiver.
2. Assemble the equipment at a convenient work area.
3. Assist the patient to a comfortable position to expose the wound. Place a plastic sheet or towel under the patient to prevent soiling the linen. Drape the patient for privacy.
4. Gently remove the old dressing. Assess the drainage on the old dressing, then discard in a plastic trash bag.
5. Irrigate the wound with sterile normal saline (or other irrigant solution) as ordered by the physician.
6. Inspect the wound, and evaluate it for signs and symptoms of infection versus signs of healing.
7. Apply topical medication if ordered by the physician.
8. Using sterile forceps gently pack the wound with loose layers of gauze dressings; make sure to cover all areas of the wound with dressings. Place enough dressings over the wound to absorb drainage until the next scheduled change (it may be necessary to use an ABD pad or absorbent cotton pad over the outer layer of the dressing for wounds with large amounts of drainage). Do **not** stuff dressing into the wound because overpacking will slow healing (see Fig. 4-4, *B*).
9. Secure dressing with tape.
10. Provide patient comfort measures.
11. Clean and replace equipment. Discard disposable items according to *Standard Precautions.*

> **NURSING CONSIDERATIONS**

Perform wound care using sterile technique, unless ordered otherwise by the physician. Be aware that sterile technique is recommended for deep or infected wounds.

Generally, a chronic wound can be managed with a clean glove.

Do not pack the wound too tightly because this will impair healing.

Table 4-1 Dermal wound care products

Product	Manufacturer	Comments
PHYSIOLOGIC SOLUTIONS		
Normal saline	Generic	Isotonic solutions used in wound irrigation and mechanical debride-
Ringer's lactate	Generic	ment; no chemical or antiseptic action
ANTISEPTIC SOLUTIONS		
Acetic acid	Generic	Known to inhibit growth of *Pseudomonas aeruginosa, Trichomonas vaginalis,* and *Candida albicans;* strong concentrations may destroy fibroblasts; dilute to 0.25%
Alcohol/ethanol	Generic	Use only on iodine-sensitive patients
Povidone iodine	Generic	Can be absorbed through any body surface except adult intake skin; dries skin; may destroy fibroblasts unless properly diluted to <1%
Dakin's (diluted sodium hypochlorite)	Generic	Controls odor; may interfere with coagulation; solution unstable; replace every day
Hydrogen peroxide	Generic	Use only on wounds with necrotic debris; can separate new epithe- lium from underlying tissue; do not use in abdominal cavity because gas may invade capillaries and lymphatics; slightly warms wound, enhancing vasodilation and decreasing inflammation; in strong concentrations, shown to destroy fibroblasts; dilute to <3%

Continued

Table 4-1   Dermal wound care products—cont'd

Product	Manufacturer	Comments
ANTISEPTIC SOLUTIONS—CONT'D		
Zephiran chloride (benzalkonium)	Generic	Inactivated by soaps; rinse wound thoroughly with normal saline solution before use; reported to enhance growth of some *Pseudomonas* species; do not cover with occlusive dressings
DETERGENT SOLUTIONS		
Cara Klenz	Carrington Labs	Isotonic solutions used in wound irrigation and mechanical debridement; no antiseptic action
Saflens	Calgon-Vestal-Merck	
Constant-Clens	Sherwood Medical	
COTTON DRESSINGS (GAUZE)		
Fine-mesh gauze	Generic	Approximately 41-47 thread count in a 4- × 4-inch pad; capillary beds rarely grow into the interstices of fine mesh and are not damaged when dressing is removed
Wide-mesh gauze	Generic	Approximately 30-39 thread count in a 4- × 4-inch pad; used in mechanical debridement because coarse weave allows necrotic debris to adhere to dressing for removal

COTTON DRESSINGS (IMPREGNATED)		Drying out adversely affects wound healing
Adaptic	Johnson & Johnson	
Melolite	Smith-Nephew	
Mesalt	Scott Health Care	
Scarlet-Red	Cheesbrough-Ponds	
Zeroform	Sherwood Medical	
Vaseline gauze	Cheesbrough-Ponds	
COMBINATION DRESSINGS		Provide nonadherent, absorbent layer within a transparent membrane
Viasorb	Cheesbrough-Ponds	
Polymen	Ferris	
Nu-Derm	Johnson & Johnson	
COTTON DRESSINGS (PASTE BANDAGE)		Cotton mesh, impregnated with zinc oxide, calamine (Unna boot), and gelatin; dries to provide extremity with compression and support; no gaps should be left in bandage, otherwise edema will accumulate
Unna boot	Miles Pharmaceuticals	
Viscopaste	Smith-Nephew	

Continued

Table 4-1 Dermal wound care products—cont'd

EXUDATE ABSORPTIVE DRESSINGS		Absorb and wick up bacteria and exudates
Bard Absorption	Bard Home Health	
Debrisan	Johnson & Johnson	
DuoDerm Granules	ConvaTec	
DuoDerm Paste	ConvaTec	
Hydra-Gran	Baxter	
Hydron	Bioderm Sciences	
Algosteril	Johnson & Johnson	
Kaltostat	Calgon-Vestal-Merck	May be used in conjunction with prescribed solution for copious-draining wounds; is not the treatment of choice for wound management because gauze may leave particles and fibers in the wound
Sorbsan	Dow Hickman	
Wound Exudate Absorber	Hollister	
Gauze	Generic	
FOAM DRESSINGS		Avoid using in wounds with dry eschar
Allevyn	Smith-Nephew	
Epi-Lock	Calgon-Vestal-Merck	
Lyofoam	Ultra Labs	
Primaderm	Absorbent Cotton	
Synthaderm	Corporation	

HYDROCOLLOID DRESSINGS

Comfeel Pressure Relief Dressing	Kendall	Dressing change required about every 4 to 7 days or PRN for leakage; relatively impermeable to gas and vapor exchange; use with caution in deep, full-thickness wounds because it may foster anaerobic infection
Comfeel Ulcer Care Dressing	Kendall	
Cutinova Hydro	Beiersdorf Medical	
Duoderm and Duoderm CGF	ConvaTec	
Hydropad	Baxter	
Intact	Bard Home Health	
Johnson & Johnson Ulcer Dressing	Johnson & Johnson	
Restore	Hollister	
Tegasorb	3M	
Ultec	Sherwood Medical	

HYDROGEN DRESSINGS

Intrasite gel	Smith-Nephew	Available in gel or sheet gel form; normalize wound humidity; sterile as packaged
Vigilon	Bard Home Health	
Geliperm	E. Furgera & Co.	

Continued

Table 4-1   Dermal wound care products—cont'd

HYDROGEN DRESSINGS—CONT'D		
Nugel	Johnson & Johnson	
Elastogel	Southwest Technologies	Hydrophilic powder dressing that becomes a gel when contact is made with the wound surface
HYDROPHILLIC POWDER DRESSINGS		
Chronicure	ABS LifeScience	
Multidex	Lange Medical Products	
TOPICAL DEBRIDING AGENTS		
Debrisan	Johnson & Johnson	Absorbs wound drainage and bacteria
DuoDerm Paste	ConvaTec	Physiologic debrider
Elase	Parke-Davis	Indicated for slough and eschar
Santyl	Knoll	Indicated for slough and eschar
Silvadine Cream	Marion Labs	Physiologic debrider with antimicrobial properties; bacterial and fungicidal action maintained for about 12 hours; change twice each day
Travase	Flint Labs	Indicated for eschar; moisten only with sterile water or saline; not appropriate for pregnant women

TOPICAL MOISTURIZERS

Carrington Gel	Carrington Labs	Available in gel, granulate, or sheet form
Dermagran	Dermasciences	
DuoDerm Paste	ConvaTec	
Geliperm Wet	E. Furgera & Co.	
Second Skin	Spence	

TRANSPARENT FILL (ADHESIVE)

Acuderm	Acme United	Semipermeable; dressing change required about every 4 to 7 days or PRN; may be used to protect skin against friction
Bio-Occlusive	Johnson & Johnson	
Ensure	Desert	
Opraflex	Professional Medical Products	
Op-Site	Smith-Nephew	
Polyskin	Kendall	
Tegaderm	3-M	
Uniflex	Acme United	

Continued

Table 4-1 Dermal wound care products—cont'd

TRANSPARENT FILL (NONADHESIVE)

Jobskin	Jobst	Clings to superficial open wounds without the need of adhesive; topicals may be applied to the dressing; removal—when the dressing falls off or by flushing with normal saline solution
Omiderm	Dermatologic Research Laboratories (D. R. Labs)	

MISCELLANEOUS (TRADITIONAL)

Karaya	Generic	Absorbent, adhesive, and hydrophilic properties; promotes wound bed
Insulin	Generic	Enhances protein synthesis by skin; observe for hypoglycemia; apply at meal times
Stomahesive	ConvaTec	Useful in debriding thick, hard necrotic tissue
Sugar	Generic	Hypertonic sugar solutions absorb moisture and debris, which may enhance wound healing; use with caution because sugar may provide a medium for bacterial growth

MISCELLANEOUS (CONTEMPORARY)

Biobrane	Woodruff Labs	Silicone membrane coated with collagen and hydrophilic peptide; drying and sticking to wound bed may damage healthy tissue; often used for burns
Procurren	Curatec	Platelet-derived formula containing growth factors to increase healing of severe and chronic wounds

CHAPTER 5

Gastroenterologic and Ostomy Care

Bowel Training

PURPOSE

- To promote control of bowel evacuation on a regular basis
- To prevent decubiti and skin breakdown
- To improve the patient's self-esteem and body image
- To promote self-care in the home

RELATED PROCEDURES

- Administration of Medications: General Guidelines (see Chapter 9)
- Bladder Training
- Enema Administration (see Chapter 9)
- Fecal Impaction: Manual Removal
- Skin Care (see Chapter 4)

GENERAL INFORMATION

Nursing measures to restore or promote normal bowel function include (1) dietary modification, (2) increasing fluid intake, and (3) increasing the patient's activity level.

EQUIPMENT

1. Suppositories, tap-water enema, stool softeners as prescribed by the physician
2. Water-soluble lubricant
3. Bedpan, bedside commode, and toilet
4. Soap and warm water, basin, tissues, washcloth, and towels
 5. Disposable nonsterile gloves and an impermeable plastic trash bag (see *Infection Control*)

PROCEDURE

1. Explain the procedure to the patient/caregiver.
2. Assemble the equipment at a convenient work area.
3. Obtain the history of the patient's previous bowel habits, and establish regular evacuation times to correspond to the preillness pattern.
4. Assess the patient's bowel function to include the following:
   a. Type and frequency of stool
   b. Date of the last bowel movement
   c. Auscultate for presence of bowel sounds
   d. Palpate abdomen for tenderness, firmness, and presence of mass
   e. Evaluate the medication profile for medicine-induced constipation
5. Perform perineal care as needed.
6. Consult with the physician regarding the use of stool softeners, enemas, stimulants, and bulk producers.
7. Evaluate for and remove fecal impaction.
8. Consult with the physician for activity orders. Encourage maximum mobility and physical activity within limits of the patient's ability.
9. Consult with the physician regarding recommendations for the patient's fluid intake. Encourage an adequate fluid intake. (Approximately 2000 to 3000 ml each day unless the patient is ordered on fluid restriction.)
10. Consult with the physician regarding diet orders. Instruct the patient to eat a well-balanced diet, with increases in fiber and bulk to promote regular bowel movement. (Approximately 4 to 6 g of fiber is needed each day to facilitate normal bowel function.)
11. Provide patient comfort measures.
12. Clean and replace the equipment. Discard disposable items according to *Standard Precautions.*

NURSING CONSIDERATIONS

Evaluate the program for 4 to 6 weeks; if it is not successful, consult with the physician for readjustment of prescribed activity, diet, and medications.

Institute a skin-care regimen for problems with incontinence.

DOCUMENTATION GUIDELINES

Document the following on the visit report:
- The procedure and patient toleration
- Condition of the patient's skin
- Patient's ability to establish control of the bowels
- Color, amount, and consistency of stool
- Any patient/caregiver instructions and response to teaching
- Physician notification, if applicable
- *Standard Precautions*
- Other pertinent findings

Document medications on the medication record.
Update the plan of care.

Colostomy Irrigation

PURPOSE

- To empty the colon of feces, gas, mucus
- To establish a regular pattern of evacuation
- To prevent constipation
- To promote self-care in the home

RELATED PROCEDURES

- Ostomy Care
- Pouch Change

EQUIPMENT

1. Irrigating bag with tubing
2. Irrigating sleeve with belt
3. Water-soluble lubricant
4. Plastic garbage bag or Chux
5. Ostomy appliance (pouch)
6. Bedpan or large bowl if the patient is bedbound
7. Soap and warm water, basin, washcloths, and towels
8. Disposable nonsterile gloves, disposable protective apron, and an impermeable plastic trash bag (see *Infection Control*)

STOP

PROCEDURE

1. Explain the procedure to the patient/caregiver.
2. Assemble the equipment at a convenient work area.
3. Assist the patient to sit on the toilet or in a chair facing the toilet.
4. Fill the irrigation bag with 500 to 1000 ml of water.
5. Flush the tubing with water to empty it of air.
6. Hang up the irrigation bag on the bathroom door hook, or raise the bag 18 inches above the stoma before irrigation.
7. Take off the pouch and the soiled colostomy bag.
8. Remove any stool or drainage from the stoma with toilet paper. Gently clean with soap and warm water as needed.
9. Inspect the skin and stoma for changes in appearance; notify the physician as appropriate.
10. Place the ring and irrigation sleeve over the stoma, and adjust the belt for a snug fit (a mild soapy solution may be squirted into the sleeve for easier cleaning).
11. Put the bottom of the sleeve into the toilet.
12. Attach the cone tip to the irrigation tubing and lubricate.
13. Gently insert the cone into the stoma for a snug fit (Fig. 5-1). If there is resistance, perform a lubricated digital examination to remove feces. **Never** use force because this could perforate the bowel.
14. Open the clamp and let the water flow in for 15 minutes.

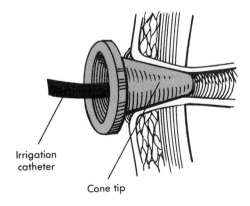

Irrigation catheter

Cone tip

Fig. 5-1   Insertion of colostomy cone into the stoma. (From Phipps WJ, Long BC, Woods NF, Cassmeyer VL: *Medical-surgical nursing: concepts and clinical practice,* ed 4, St Louis, 1991, Mosby.)

Press on the cone just firmly enough to keep water from running back out. If cramps occur, turn off the water with the clamp, and wait until the cramps subside before proceeding. If the water backs up into the tubing, shut off the water with the clamp. Wait a few minutes, then open the clamp and continue the irrigation (lower the bag to decrease the flow of water, or raise the bag to increase the flow).

15. Close the bottom of the sleeve with the clamp when most of the water has come back out (about 10 to 20 minutes).
16. Instruct the patient to walk around if able for about 30 minutes to complete the emptying of the bowel. Instruct patients who are not ambulatory to lean forward or massage their abdomen to complete emptying of the bowel.
17. Take off sleeve. Wash around the stoma or have the patient shower to remove fecal drainage. Rinse and dry area thoroughly. Put on a new pouch.
18. Clean the irrigation sleeve, cone tip, and irrigation bag with soap and water. Allow them to air dry, and store them in the patient's bathroom.
19. Provide patient comfort measures.
20. Clean and replace the equipment. Discard disposable items according to *Standard Precautions.*

NURSING CONSIDERATIONS

Encourage the patient/caregiver to perform the procedure with minimal assistance from you on the next visit.

Consider referral to social services for assistance with ostomy supplies or relaxation therapy techniques.

If the patient is confined to the bed, turn the patient to uncover the colostomy and to elevate the head. Protect the bed with a plastic garbage bag or Chux, and drain the irrigation solution into a bedpan or a large clean bowl. Perform peristomal care, and apply the pouch.

Report signs of skin irritation or a dark/purplish or pale colored stoma to the physician as appropriate (the stoma should be red or bright pink).

Consult with the physician if the stoma structure prohibits cone insertion; consider irrigating the stoma with a soft silicone catheter gently inserted into the bowel no more than 5 cm (2 to 3 inches); never force the catheter into the bowel because this could perforate it.

DOCUMENTATION GUIDELINES

Document the following on the visit report:
- The procedure and patient toleration
- Results, including the amount and color of stool
- Condition of the stoma and the surrounding skin
- Any psychosocial concerns regarding the stoma
- Any patient/caregiver instructions and response to teaching, including the ability to perform the colostomy irrigation
- Physician notification, if applicable
- *Standard Precautions*
- Other pertinent findings

Update the plan of care.

Fecal Impaction: Manual Removal

PURPOSE

- To remove hardened feces and promote bowel function
- To relieve abdominal discomfort

RELATED PROCEDURES

- Bowel Training
- Enema Administration (see Chapter 9)

GENERAL INFORMATION

Fecal impaction is common in the elderly when diet and limited activity may alter normal patters of defecation. Signs and symptoms of fecal impaction include absence of stools, complaints of abdominal or rectal pain, fecal oozing, and a persistent urge to defecate with no results.

EQUIPMENT

1. Bedpan
2. Water-soluble lubricant
3. Plastic trash bag or Chux pad
4. Soap and warm water, basin, tissues, washcloths, and towels

5. Disposable nonsterile gloves and an impermeable plastic trash bag (see *Infection Control*)

PROCEDURE

1. Assess for signs or symptoms of fecal impaction. Ask when the patient's last bowel movement occurred.
2. Explain the procedure to the patient/caregiver.
3. Assemble the equipment at a convenient work area.
4. Place a plastic trash bag or Chux under the patient's buttocks.
5. Assist patient to a left lateral Sims' position; flex the patient's knees. Drape the patient so that the anus is exposed.
6. Perform perineal care as needed.
7. Lubricate the index finger of your dominant hand.
8. Gently insert index finger past the anus into the rectum.
9. Palpate for the fecal mass.
10. Push the index finger into the feces, remove the feces, and place in bedpan. If possible, instruct patient to bear down while extracting feces to facilitate removal.
11. Clean the perineal and anal area; replace the patient's clothes.
12. Provide patient comfort measures.
13. Clean and replace the equipment. Discard disposable items according to *Standard Precautions*.

NURSING CONSIDERATIONS

Consult with the physician when fecal impaction is suspected. Report concerns about diet, immobility, or patient neglect.

It is advisable to obtain an enema order when requesting a fecal disimpaction order. Perform disimpaction first.

Removal of fecal impaction may be contraindicated in patients with severe cardiac disease, in those who have undergone colorectal or gynecologic surgery, or in those with bleeding tendencies. If bleeding occurs during the procedure or if the patient complains of severe pain, stop and notify the physician.

DOCUMENTATION GUIDELINES

Document the following on the visit report:
* The procedure and patient toleration
* Results obtained
* When the patient had his or her last bowel movement

- Any patient/caregiver instructions and response to teaching
- Physician notification, if applicable
- *Standard Precautions*
- Other pertinent findings
Update the plan of care.

Gastrostomy Tube Care: General Guidelines

PURPOSE
- To provide guidelines for gastrostomy management in the home
- To promote self-care in the home

RELATED PROCEDURES
- Administration of Medications: General Guidelines (see Chapter 9)
- Dressing Changes: Hydrocolloid Dressings and Transparent Adhesive Films (see Chapter 4)
- Gastrostomy Tube Feedings
- Gastrostomy Tube Replacement

EQUIPMENT
1. Soft-bulb syringe
2. Water in a small container
3. 4- × 4-inch gauze sponge and dressing supplies, if necessary
4. Hypoallergenic tape, if necessary
5. pH strips
6. Cotton-tip applicators, soap and warm water, basin, washcloth, and towels
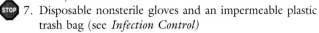 7. Disposable nonsterile gloves and an impermeable plastic trash bag (see *Infection Control*)

PROCEDURE
1. Explain the procedure to the patient/caregiver.
2. Assemble the equipment at a convenient work area.

3. Position the patient to expose the gastrostomy tube.
4. Inspect the skin at the gastrostomy site for redness, tenderness, swelling, irritation, or for presence of drainage or gastric leakage; notify the physician as appropriate.
5. Gently cleanse the peristomal area with soap and water daily. Use a spiral pattern beginning at the stoma site and work outward. Use a cotton-tip applicator to clean hard-to-reach areas around the stoma site. Rise and pat dry.
6. Apply a dry dressing with hypoallergenic tape if leakage is a problem. Instruct the patient/caregiver to change the dressing if it becomes wet. (A transparent adhesive film may be used around the gastrostomy site to protect the skin from gastric leakage; change the film daily if there is a possibility of leakage underneath it.) **Avoid using a dressing in most cases because this promotes skin maceration.**
7. Assist the patient to a sitting position with his or her head elevated at least 45 degrees during feeding and for 1 hour after feeding to prevent aspiration. Pillows may be used to support the patient.
8. Auscultate the abdomen for the presence of bowel sounds; assess for abdominal distention or discomfort. Delay the feeding or instillation of medication, and notify the physician if no bowel sounds are present or if the patient complains of abdominal discomfort.
9. Assess tension of the gastrostomy tube and make adjustments in the following manner:
   a. Check the balloon volume every 7 to 10 days to prevent accidental tube removal because of balloon leakage. (It is normal for small amounts to leak from balloon over time.) Replace fluid to the original amount or to a maximum of 20 ml to prevent accidental tube removal.
   b. Decrease the balloon size in increments of 2 ml to avoid excessive tension, which could result in erosion of gastric mucosa. (The tube should be able to rotate 360 degrees and move slightly in and out of the stoma; if there is no movement, the balloon is too tight against the stomach wall.)
   c. Discourage the patient from pulling on the tube. (Consider using hand mittens or soft restraints if the patient is confused.)
   d. Avoid taping the gastrostomy tube to the patient's ab-

domen; if the tube must be taped to prevent tugging, use hypoallergenic tape

10. Verify tube placement *before* feeding:
    a. Listen with a stethoscope over the left upper quadrant while injecting 10 to 15 cc of air into the tube. A bubbling or "whooshing" sound should be present.
    b. Assess the amount of gastric residual before feeding. Reinstall the gastric aspirate. Hold the tube feeding and notify the physician of continued gastric residual greater than 100 ml or twice the hourly feeding rate, absence of bowel sounds, or complaints of abdominal discomfort.

11. Do not give medication with feedings. Crush medicines into a fine powder, and mix with 5 ml of water. Administer the medicine with a syringe. Multiple medications should be given one at a time.

12. Flush the tube with 50 ml of warm water before and after feeding, after medication administration, or when checking residuals.

13. Close the feeding port caps. If the caps are not present, plug or clamp the end of the gastrostomy tube.

14. If the gastrostomy tube is accidentally dislodged, replace it as soon as possible to prevent tract closure.

15. Evaluate for tube feeding complications, such as tube blockage, aspiration, nausea, vomiting, diarrhea, fluids and electrolyte imbalances, as well as gastrostomy site infection or complications with placement. Notify the home health agency clinical supervisor and physician as necessary.

16. Provide patient comfort measures, including nose and mouth care.

17. Clean and replace the equipment. Discard disposable items according to *Standard Precautions.*

NURSING CONSIDERATIONS

Do **not** feed patient if tube position is in doubt.

Consider gently irrigating the tube with cola or cranberry juice to clear it. Reinforce with the family that regular flushing with water is the best way to prevent tube clogging.

Consult with the physician regarding changing the gastrostomy tube, because some tubes require periodic replacement to prevent tissue adhesions.

Consider replacing the gastrostomy tube when chronic leakage around the stoma site occurs.

It is imperative that the patient/caregiver understand the importance of sitting the patient up during feedings and also 1 hour after feedings to prevent aspiration, as well as during operation of equipment and management of the gastrostomy tube.

Instruct the patient/caregiver to measure the gastric pH daily (expected range for gastric fluid is 1 to 4).

DOCUMENTATION GUIDELINES

Document the following on the visit report:
- The procedure and patient toleration
- The patient's general physical status, including abdominal assessment
- Condition of the gastrostomy site and patency of the tube
- Any patient/caregiver instructions and response to teaching
- Physician notification, if applicable
- *Standard Precautions*
- Other pertinent findings

Document the amount, type, and frequency of tube feedings and medications administered on the medication record.

Update the plan of care.

Gastrostomy Tube Feedings

PURPOSE

- To provide long-term nutritional support
- To regulate the flow of liquid nourishment by bolus, by continuous and intermittent feeding, or by the feeding-pump method
- To promote self-care in the home

RELATED PROCEDURES

- Gastrostomy Care
- Administration of Medications: General Guidelines (see Chapter 9)

EQUIPMENT

1. Tube feeding (warmed to room temperature) as prescribed by the physician
2. Soft-bulb syringe or feeding bag
3. Feeding pump
4. Water in a small container
5. 4- × 4-inch gauze dressing and dressing supplies if necessary
6. pH strips
7. Cotton-tip applicators, soap and warm water, basin, washcloth, and towels
8. Disposable nonsterile gloves and an impermeable plastic trash bag (see *Infection Control*)

❖ Bolus Feeding

PROCEDURE

1. Explain the procedure to the patient/caregiver.
2. Assemble the equipment at a convenient work area.
3. Assist the patient to sit up with his or her head elevated at least 45 degrees. Pillows may be used to support the patient.
4. Expose the gastrostomy tube. Place the basin under the tube, and uncap the tube or remove the plug.
5. Aspirate for stomach contents to verify placement. Reinstill the gastric aspirate. If gastric residual is greater than 100 ml, delay the feeding for 30 minutes to 1 hour, and check again. Auscultate the abdomen for the presence of bowel sounds. Notify the physician of high gastric residuals, absence of bowel sounds, or patient complaints of abdominal discomfort *before* administering tube feedings.
6. Pour warm water into a cup. Draw 50 ml of warm water into the soft-bulb syringe.
7. Gently irrigate the tube with the water. If the patient coughs or appears to be choking, do not administer feeding and notify the physician. (Flush the gastrostomy tube with 50 ml of water every 8 hours to prevent clogging.)
8. Draw up the gastrostomy feeding into the syringe and administer 200 to 300 ml over 10 to 15 minutes. Follow the feeding with 50 ml of warm water.
9. Clamp the tube before it empties, and remove the syringe.

10. Close the feeding port caps. If the caps are not present, clamp or plug the end of the gastrostomy tube.
11. Clean the peristomal area with soap and water. Use a spiral pattern beginning at the stoma site and work outward. Use cotton-tip applicators to clean hard-to-reach creases around the stoma site. Rinse and pat dry. (Avoid placing a dressing on the site if possible. Change the dressing as soon as it becomes moist to prevent skin irritation or infection.)
12. Provide patient comfort measures.
13. Clean and replace the equipment. Discard disposable items according to *Standard Precautions.*

❖ Continuous or Intermittent Feeding

PROCEDURE

1. Follow steps *1* through *7* of the procedure for *Bolus Feeding.*
2. Administer feeding by gravity in the following manner:
   a. Hang a container of feeding solution on an IV pole about 18 inches above the patient's shoulders
   b. Adjust the delivery rate with the flow regulator
3. Refill the feeding bag before the container is empty for continuous infusion.
4. Add 50 ml of warm water to the bag when the last of the formula has reached the feeding tube to clear the tube.
5. Close the feeding port caps or clamp the feeding tube to prevent a return flow of feeding when changing the bag or when the feeding is near completion.
6. Clean the feeding bag with liquid soap and water. Rinse well, and air dry. The feeding bag may be cleaned and reused 3 or 4 times.
7. Follow steps *11* through *13* of the procedure for *Bolus Feeding.*

❖ Feeding Pump

PROCEDURE

1. Follow steps *1* through *7* of the procedure for *Bolus Feeding.*
2. Suspend the container from the feeding pump, and thread the tubing through the pump.

3. Make sure the pump is turned off, and put the feeding into the container.

4. Turn the pump on at the prescribed flow rate, and allow the feeding to flow through the tubing. Turn off the feeding pump.

5. Connect the free end of the feeding bag tubing to the gastrostomy tube; unclamp the tube and turn on the pump.

6. Intermittently, observe the flow to make sure that the tubing is not blocked or kinked, in which case the pump alarm should sound.

7. Refill the feeding bag before the container is empty.

8. Add 50 ml of warm water to the bag to clear the tube when the last of the formula has reached the feeding tube.

9. Close the feeding port caps or clamp the tube to prevent a return flow of formula when you are changing the bag or when the feeding is near completion.

10. Clean the feeding bag with liquid soap and water. Rinse well, and air dry. The feeding bag may be cleaned and reused 3 or 4 times.

11. Follow steps *11* through *13* of the procedure for *Bolus Feeding*.

NURSING CONSIDERATIONS

Do not give feeding if tube position is in doubt.

Check the expiration date of the gastrostomy feedings.

Discard the feeding solution 24 hours after the container has been opened.

Discard the old, continuous feedings after 8 hours and administer a fresh feeding. Do not mix old and new feedings.

Administer feedings at room temperature.

Store the tube feedings in the refrigerator.

The patient may need antidiarrheal medication (Kaopectate) for diarrhea or liquid stools; consult with the physician as needed.

It is imperative that the patient/caregiver understand the importance of sitting the patient up during feedings and 1 hour after feedings to prevent aspiration, as well as for management of the gastrostomy tube. Instruct the caregiver to check the gastrostomy tube position every 4 hours when continuous feeding, before every intermittent feeding, and before administering medication. Reinforce the idea that regular water flushing has been shown to be the best way to prevent tube clogging.

Instruct the patient/caregiver to keep a log of the amount, time, frequency, and patient toleration to feedings. The patient/caregiver should know to delay feedings and notify the home health agency clinical supervisor and physician if the gastrostomy tube should come out or if the patient has choking or discomfort with the feeding.

Instruct the patient/caregiver to measure gastric pH daily (the expected range for gastric fluid is from 1 to 4).

DOCUMENTATION GUIDELINES

Document the following on the visit report:

- The procedure and patient toleration
- The patient's general physical status, including abdominal assessment
- Condition of the gastrostomy site and patency of the tube
- Amount and character of any gastric return
- Tube patency
- Gastrostomy site care
- Any patient/caregiver instructions and response to teaching, including the ability to administer gastrostomy tube feedings
- Physician notification, if applicable
- *Standard Precautions*
- Other pertinent findings

Document the type, amount, and frequency of tube feedings and medications administered on the medication record.

Update the plan of care.

Gastrostomy Tube Replacement

PURPOSE
- To access the gastrointestinal tract
- To prevent skin adhesions and strictures
- To prevent infection

GENERAL INFORMATION
It is recommended that the first gastrostomy tube insertion be performed by the physician. Thereafter, the home health nurse may replace certain types of gastrostomy tubes as needed.

EQUIPMENT
1. Prescribed gastrostomy tube and water-soluble lubricant
2. Luer-tip syringe
3. Sterile water or saline solution
4. Hypoallergenic tape
5. Cotton-tip applicators, soap and warm water, basin, washcloth, and towels

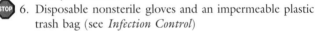 6. Disposable nonsterile gloves and an impermeable plastic trash bag (see *Infection Control*)

PROCEDURE
1. Consult with the physician and evaluate the need for gastrostomy tube replacement in the following manner:
   a. Determine how long the old tube has been in place because placement of more than 2 months for certain types of gastrostomy tubes may cause complications with adhesions of tissue to the tube.
   b. Review the manufacturer's recommendations for gastrostomy tube replacement.
   c. Replace accidentally dislodged tubes as soon as possible to prevent tract closure or strictures.
   d. Inspect the tube for inward or outward migration. When the tube is initially inserted, measure and record the length of the tube in centimeters from the insertion site to the proximal end, or mark the tube at skin entry point with indelible ink; some tubes have graduation markings for reference. If at some point the tube is

longer or if the mark is farther out, reconfirm the tube placement at that time.

2. Explain the procedure to the patient/caregiver.

3. Assemble the equipment at a convenient work area. Obtain the correct French size of the replacement tube appropriate to the stoma size before removing the old tube. Fill the balloon of the new tube with 10 to 20 ml of water to check for patency and leakage; then deflate.

4. Assist the patient to lie down in a comfortable position, and expose the tube.

5. Remove the old gastrostomy tube in the following manner:
   a. Deflate the balloon
   b. Rotate the tube 360 degrees between your thumb and index finger to loosen any crustations
   c. Gently pull the gastrostomy tube out of the stoma
   d. Do not force the removal of the gastrostomy tube; if resistance is felt, you are unable to pull it out, or the patient complains of pain, contact the physician because the patient may need medical intervention to remove the old tube

6. Replace the gastrostomy tube in the following manner:
   a. *Tube with a balloon*—Insert the Luer-tip syringe into the balloon port of the existing tube, and remove the fluid from the balloon. Gently twist and rotate the old tube to assess if it will come out; with an upward twisting motion, gently remove the existing tube. Cleanse the stoma site with soap and water; use a spiral pattern to cleanse the area, beginning at the stoma site and working outward. Use cotton-tip applicators to clean the hard-to-reach areas around the stoma site; rinse, and pat dry thoroughly. Apply a small amount of water-soluble lubricant to the tip of the new tube and stoma; do **not** use petroleum-based lubricant. Gently insert the tip of the tube into the stoma and guide it through the tract into the stomach with a slight twisting motion. Fill the balloon with 10 to 20 ml of water (use the amount necessary to keep the tube securely in the stomach; the maximum amount is 20 ml). **Never** use air to fill the balloon. Gently tug the tube to make sure that there is a snug fit that allows for some in-and-out play (some in-and-out play of the tube is needed to minimize pressure-related complications, such as necrosis).

b. *Percutaneous endoscopic gastrostomy* (PEG) *tube*—This type of tube is usually removed by the physician endoscopically; the physician may replace this type of tube with a balloon type.

c. *Mushroom or button type*—This type of tube is usually removed by the physician; it may be replaced with the balloon type if desired.

d. *Flexi-Flo gastrostomy tube*—Follow the guidelines in step *6a* to remove and replace the tube. Gently snug the balloon up against the gastric mucosa and slide the skin disc down against the skin to provide secure placement. Slide the disc back up to the nearest cm marking to allow for a slight in-and-out play.

7. Aspirate gastric contents with a syringe to assess placement. Reinstill gastric aspirate, and rinse with 50 ml of water.

8. Close the feeding ports. If caps are not present, clamp or plug the end of the tube.

9. If possible, avoid using tape to secure the tube to the patient's abdomen. If the tube must be taped to prevent tugging, use hypoallergenic tape.

10. Provide patient comfort measures.

11. Clean and replace the equipment. Discard disposable items according to *Standard Precautions*.

NURSING CONSIDERATIONS

Do not force the gastrostomy tube to come out.

If resistance is met after deflating the balloon, notify the home health agency supervisor and physician because the patient will require medical evaluation.

If possible, avoid applying a dressing to the stoma. If a dressing is used, it should not be placed under a skin disc, and it must be changed promptly if it is moist to prevent skin irritation or infection.

DOCUMENTATION GUIDELINES

Document the following on the visit report:

• The procedure and patient toleration
• Type of gastrostomy tube inserted and ml capacity of balloon
• French size of tube inserted and ml capacity of balloon
• Amount of normal saline solution used to fill the balloon
• Marking of tube or cm marking of skin disc

- Condition of the gastrostomy site and patency of the tube
- Physician notification, if applicable
- *Standard Precautions*
- Other pertinent findings

Update the plan of care.

Nasogastric Tube Feeding

PURPOSE

- To provide short-term nutrition support through a tube into the alimentary tract
- To administer medicine
- To promote self-care in the home

RELATED PROCEDURES

- Administration of Medications: General Guidelines (see Chapter 9)
- Nasogastric Tube Insertion

EQUIPMENT

1. Nasogastric tube feeding (warmed to room temperature) as prescribed by the physician
2. Soft-bulb syringe or tube feeding bag
3. Water in a small container
4. Stethoscope
5. Rubber bands
6. Safety pin
7. IV pole
8. 4- × 4-inch gauze dressing
9. pH strips
10. Mouthwash, tissues, and towel
11. Disposable nonsterile gloves and an impermeable plastic trash bag (see *Infection Control*)

PROCEDURE

1. Explain the procedure to the patient/caregiver.
2. Assemble the equipment at a convenient work area.

3. Offer mouthwash, and administer oral care.
4. Assist the patient to a sitting position with the head elevated at least 45 degrees to prevent aspiration. Drape a towel over the patient's chest.
5. Auscultate for bowel sounds; hold the feeding, and notify the physician if no bowel sounds are present or if the patient complains of nausea, abdominal distention, or pain.
6. Assess the nasogastric tube placement, using one of the following methods:
   a. Attach the barrel of a syringe to the end of the nasogastric tubing; open the clamp and aspirate gastric contents; reinstill gastric aspirate
   b. Submerge the distal end of the tube in the water, and observe for air bubbles (air bubbles indicate that the tube is not in the stomach); hold the feeding until the nasogastric tube can be reinserted into the stomach
   c. Place the stethoscope on the patient's abdomen, and inject 20 cc of air into the nasogastric tube; a *whooshing* sound indicates that the air bolus has entered the stomach and that placement is correct
7. Check the amount of gastric residual before each intermittent feeding or approximately every 2 hours during continuous feeding. If the gastric residual is greater than 100 ml, delay the feeding for 30 minutes to 1 hour, and then check it again. Reinstill the gastric aspirate. Notify the physician of a high residual.
8. Administer the feeding in the following manner:
   a. Bolus method—draw up the prescribed feeding into the syringe, and administer the amount to be given; administer the feeding slowly because this helps prevent nausea, vomiting, and diarrhea
   b. Continuous and intermittent method—administer the tube feeding in a nasogastric bag attached to the nasogastric tube; hang the feeding bag on an IV pole approximately 18 inches above the patient's shoulders; regulate the flow of the tube feeding by adjusting the flow regulator on the tube feeding bag
9. Allow 20 to 30 minutes for a 200 to 300 ml feeding.
10. Do not give medications with feedings. Crush medicines into a fine powder, and mix them with 5 ml of water. Administer the medications with a syringe. Multiple medications should be given one at a time.

11. Follow the feeding or medications with 50 ml of water. (Flush the nasogastric tube with 50 ml of water every 8 hours to prevent clogging.)
12. Clamp the tube before it empties, and remove the syringe or feeding bag; this procedure prevents air from entering the stomach.
13. Clamp or plug the end of the nasogastric tube.
14. Loop a rubber band around the nasogastric tube, and secure it to the patient's shirt or gown with a safety pin to prevent tugging.
15. Position the patient in an upright position with the head elevated at least 45 degrees for 1 hour after feeding to prevent aspiration.
16. Notify the home health agency clinical supervisor, and consult with the physician if the patient experiences diarrhea, constipation, or tube blockage. Observe for pressure necrosis at the nares and signs of gastrointestinal bleeding.
17. Provide patient comfort measures.
18. Clean and replace the equipment. Discard disposable items according to *Standard Precautions.*
    a. Wash nasogastric feeding bag or syringe with soap and water daily; rinse well and air dry

NURSING CONSIDERATIONS

Check the expiration date on formulas.

Discard the formula 24 hours after the container has been opened.

Discard old continuous feedings after 8 hours, and administer a fresh feeding.

Do not mix old and new feedings.

Administer the feedings at room temperature.

Store tube feedings in the refrigerator.

It is imperative that the patient/caregiver understand the importance of sitting the patient up during feedings and for 1 hour after feedings or medication administration to prevent aspiration, as well as for management of the nasogastric tube.

Instruct the patient/caregiver to keep a log of the amount, time, and frequency of tube feedings and patient toleration of feedings.

The patient/caregiver should know to delay the feedings and notify the home health agency clinical supervisor and physician if the nasogastric tube should come out if the patient has choking or discomfort with the feeding.

Instruct the patient/caregiver to measure the gastric pH daily (the expected range of gastric fluid is 1 to 4).

DOCUMENTATION GUIDELINES

Document the following on the visit report:
- The procedure and patient toleration
- Abdominal assessment
- Intake and output
- Any patient/caregiver instructions and response to teaching, including the ability to administer nasogastric tube feedings
- Physician notification, if applicable
- *Standard Precautions*
- Other pertinent findings

Document the type, amount, and frequency of the tube feeding as well as any medications administered on the medication record.

Update the plan of care.

Nasogastric Tube Insertion

PURPOSE
- To provide guidelines for nasogastric tube insertion
- To access the gastrointestinal tract to provide nutritional support and to administer medication when normal swallowing is impaired
- To decompress the stomach

RELATED PROCEDURE
- Nasogastric Tube Feeding

GENERAL INFORMATION

Nasogastric tubes commonly used in the home include the Levin tube and the double-lumen Salem sump tube (Fig. 5-2). These tubes are used to remove fluid and gas from the stomach

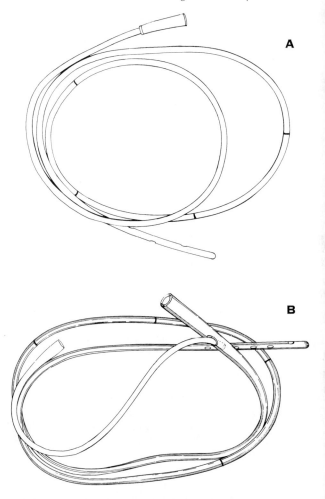

Fig. 5-2 Nasogastric tubes. **A,** Levin tube. **B,** Salem sump tube. (From Phipps WJ, Long BC, Woods NF, Cassmeyer VL: *Medical-surgical nursing: concepts and clinical practice,* ed 4, St Louis, 1991, Mosby.)

(decompression) and to administer tube feedings on a short-term basis.

Use intermittent or low pressure with the Levin tube because the single lumen may adhere to the stomach wall and cause trauma. The larger lumen of the Salem sump tube drains the stomach, whereas the smaller lumen provides a continuous flow of air at atmospheric pressure, preventing adherence to the stomach wall. For this reason the air vent of the Salem sump tube should not be clamped off or connected to suction.

EQUIPMENT

1. Nasogastric tube
2. Soft-bulb syringe
3. Water in a small container
4. Stethoscope
5. Water-soluble lubricant
6. Rubber bands
7. Safety pin
8. 4- × 4-inch gauze dressing
9. Hypoallergenic tape
10. Paper towels
11. Disposable nonsterile gloves and an impermeable plastic trash bag (see *Infection Control*)

PROCEDURE

1. Explain the procedure to the patient/caregiver.
2. Assemble the equipment at a convenient work area.
3. Assist the patient to a sitting position with the head elevated at least 45 degrees. Place a towel under the chin for protection.
4. Offer mouthwash, and assist with oral care as needed.
5. Assess the patency of the nares. Instruct the patient to close each nostril alternately and then breathe. Identify the nostril for nasogastric insertion.
6. Cut 2- to 3-inch lengths of tape, and set aside.
7. Put a small amount of lubricant on the paper towel.
8. Measure the correct length of tubing for placement by measuring the tube from the patient's tip of nose, to the ear lobe, and then to the xiphoid process (approximately 18 inches) (Fig. 5-3).

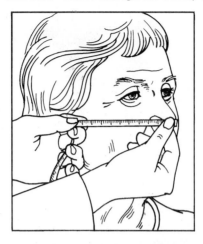

Fig. 5-3 Measuring the length of the nasogastric tube. (From Beare PG, Myers JL: *Adult health nursing,* ed 2, St Louis, 1994, Mosby.)

9. Instruct the patient to tilt his or her head back, and insert the tube in the following manner:
   a. Apply ice to the gastric tube to stiffen it for insertion, if needed
   b. Dip the end of the tubing in lubricant
   c. Insert the tubing slowly through the nostril with a 180-degree rotation motion
   d. Raise the tube slightly; if it meets resistance, aim it back and toward the ear; do **not** force the tube
   e. Instruct the patient to swallow if possible because this will facilitate insertion; if swallowing is not possible, the patient may be given ice chips to suck on during the procedure; advance the tube each time the patient swallows
10. Tape the tubing to the nose (Fig. 5-4). Instruct the patient/caregiver to make sure that the tape adheres to the patient's nose to prevent dislodgment of the tube.
11. Assess placement in the following manner:
    a. Assess for signs and symptoms of respiratory distress; ask the patient to talk
    b. Place the tube in a glass of water, and observe for air

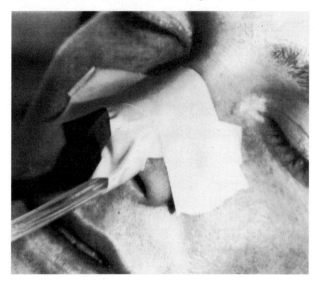

Fig. 5-4 Nasogastric tube taped to the patient's nose. (From Hirsch J, Hannock L, editors: *Mosby's manual of clinical nursing procedures,* St Louis, 1981, Mosby.)

       bubbles; if no air bubbles are apparent, the tube is placed correctly

  c. Inject 20 cc of air with a soft-bulb syringe through the tubing while listening with the stethoscope; if the tubing is placed correctly, you will hear a *whooshing* sound of air bolus injected into the stomach

  d. Aspirate the gastric contents with a soft-bulb syringe while it is connected to the tube; if it is placed correctly, you should obtain gastric contents; advance the tube 1 or 2 inches if you are unable to aspirate the gastric contents; reinstill the gastric aspirate

12. Clamp or plug the end of the tube.
13. Loop a rubber band around the nasogastric tube, and secure it to the patient's shirt or gown with a safety pin.
14. Provide patient comfort measures.
15. Clean and replace the equipment. Discard disposable items according to *Standard Precautions.*

DOCUMENTATION GUIDELINES

Document the following on the visit report:
- The procedure and patient toleration
- Size of the inserted tube
- Placement verification of the tube
- Any patient/caregiver instruction and compliance with the procedure, including the ability to manage nasogastric tube feedings at home
- Physician notification, if applicable
- *Standard Precautions*
- Other pertinent findings

Update the plan of care.

Ostomy Care

PURPOSE

- To maintain cleanliness and good skin care
- To permit examination of the skin around the stoma
- To provide education for patient self-care
- To assist in controlling odors
- To prevent leakage
- To promote self-care in the home

RELATED PROCEDURES

- Colostomy Irrigation
- Pouch Change

EQUIPMENT

1. Ostomy appliance pouch
2. Protective cover
3. Plastic bag or Chux
4. Soap and warm water, basin, washcloth, and towels
5. Disposable nonsterile gloves and an impermeable plastic trash bag (see *Infection Control*)

PROCEDURE

1. Explain the procedure to the patient/caregiver.
2. Assemble the equipment at a convenient work area.

3. Place the patient in a comfortable position with the abdominal area exposed.
4. Place a plastic bag or Chux under the patient if he or she is bedbound.
5. Remove the appliance and discard it.
6. Cleanse the peristomal area with soap and water. Use a spiral pattern at the stoma site, and work outward. Rinse, and pat dry.
7. Examine the stoma for integrity versus any signs of necrosis or infection. Report any abnormal findings to the physician.
8. Position the appliance to fit well around the stoma. (The appliance will depend on the type of stoma.)
9. Provide patient comfort measures.
10. Clean and replace the equipment. Discard disposable items according to *Standard Precautions.*

NURSING CONSIDERATIONS

Consider referral to the enterostomal therapist to establish a stoma and peristomal care regimen.

Reassure the patient, and be supportive.

Encourage the patient to talk about his or her feelings of the altered body image, sexuality, or self-esteem.

Help the patient to adjust to life with a stoma, and encourage her or him to return to normal patters of socialization.

DOCUMENTATION GUIDELINES

Document the following on the visit report:
- The procedure and patient toleration
- Color, shape, and size of stoma
- Type of stoma
- Condition of the surrounding skin
- Function, character, and amount of drainage
- Any patient/caregiver instructions and response to teaching, including the patient's reaction and ability to perform ostomy care
- Physician notification, if applicable
- *Standard Precautions*
- Other pertinent findings

Update the plan of care.

Ostomy Pouch Change

PURPOSE
- To contain odor and effluence
- To protect the skin
- To promote self-care in the home

RELATED PROCEDURES
- Colostomy Irrigation
- Ostomy Care

EQUIPMENT
1. Flange skin barrier
2. Convex insert, if needed
3. Ostomy appliance (pouch)
4. Stomadhesive paste
5. Soap and warm water, basin, washcloth, and towels
6. Disposable nonsterile gloves and an impermeable plastic trash bag (see *Infection Control*)

PROCEDURE
1. Explain the procedure to the patient/caregiver.
2. Assemble the equipment at a convenient work area.
3. Place the patient in a comfortable sitting or semi-reclining position, and uncover the stoma. Assess the integrity of the stoma.
4. Cut a 1-inch dice opening in the skin barrier (e.g., Hollister, Premium Wafer). Cut a skin barrier to fit one-eighth of an inch around the stoma.
5. Place the convex insert inside the flange skin barrier, and press down under the flange until the insert is *seated* under the flange.
6. Attach the ostomy pouch to the flange. Make sure that the flange and pouch are secure.
7. Remove the backing paper from the back of the skin barrier.
8. Squeeze a thin ribbon of stomadhesive paste around the cut edge of the skin barrier or onto the skin around the stoma.

9. Remove the old flange skin barrier from around the stoma.

10. Wash the skin and stoma with soap and water. Rinse well, and pat dry.

11. Center the ostomy pouch over the stoma. Press down firmly on all sides. Instruct the patient to be still for about 5 minutes to improve adherence of the flange. Consider use of an ostomy belt to further secure the flange and pouch.

12. Clamp the bottom of the pouch.

13. Provide patient comfort measures.

14. Clean and replace the equipment. Discard disposable items according to *Standard Precautions.*

 NURSING CONSIDERATIONS

To empty the pouch, instruct the patient/caregiver to tilt the bottom of the pouch upward and remove the pouch clamp. Hold up a portion of the lower end of the pouch and allow the contents to drain into the toilet or bedpan. Wipe off the bottom of the pouch and reclamp. Release flatus through the gas-release valve if the pouch has one. Otherwise, tilt the pouch bottom upward and unclamp to release flatus.

Reassure the patient and encourage increasing involvement in self-care of the ostomy.

 DOCUMENTATION GUIDELINES

- The procedure and patient toleration
- Condition of the stoma site and surrounding skin
- Any patient/caregiver instructions and response to teaching, including the ability to change the pouch and manage the ostomy at home
- Physician notification, if applicable
- *Standard Precautions*
- Other pertinent findings

Update the plan of care.

Rectal Tube Insertion

PURPOSE
- To relieve abdominal distention
- To assist the patient to pass flatus

EQUIPMENT
1. No. 22 or 24 rectal tube
2. Water-soluble lubricant
3. Bedpan or container with approximately 30 ml of water
4. Soap and warm water, basin, tissues, washcloth, and towels
5. Disposable nonsterile gloves and an impermeable plastic trash bag (see *Infection Control*)

PROCEDURE
1. Explain the procedure to the patient/caregiver.
2. Assemble the equipment at the bedside or a convenient work area.
3. Assist the patient to lie on the left side and expose the anal area. Drape the patient for privacy.
4. Place the outflow tip of the rectal tube into the bedpan or container so that it is covered with water.
5. Lubricate the tip of the rectal tube.
6. Gently insert the rectal tube into the rectum (approximately 3 to 5 inches; do not force the tube).
7. Leave the rectal tube in place for approximately 20 minutes.
8. Observe/listen for expulsion of flatus.
9. Gently remove the rectal tube.
10. Provide patient comfort measures.
11. Clean and replace the equipment. Discard disposable items according to *Standard Precautions*.

DOCUMENTATION GUIDELINES
Document the following on the visit report:
- The procedure and patient toleration
- Results obtained
- Physician notification, if applicable
- *Standard Precautions*
- Other pertinent findings
Update the plan of care.

CHAPTER 6

Head, Eyes, Ears, Nose, Throat (HEENT) Care

Care of the Patient with an Artificial Eye

PURPOSE

- To provide eye prothesis cleaning
- To cleanse the eye and irrigate the socket
- To prevent infection
- To promote self-care in the home

RELATED PROCEDURE

- Eye Instillation and Irrigation (see Chapter 9)

EQUIPMENT

1. Eye prosthesis cup
2. Soap and warm water, basin, washcloth, towel, and/or a prescribed irrigation solution for cleaning the eye socket
3. Disposable nonsterile gloves (optional) and an impermeable plastic trash bag (see *Infection Control*)

PROCEDURE

1. Explain the procedure to the patient/caregiver.
2. Assemble the equipment at a convenient work area.
3. Assist the patient to a sitting or side-lying position.
4. Remove the eye prosthesis by pulling down the lower lid and by applying slight pressure along the lower lid with the thumb (Fig. 6-1, *A*). Then raise the upper lid slightly with the index finger to break the suction (Fig 6-1, *B*). The eye prosthesis should pop out. (Some patients may have a small suction device to remove the eye prosthesis. Clean the suction device, and apply it to the eye prosthesis. Gently rock the prosthesis back and forth to break the suction.)

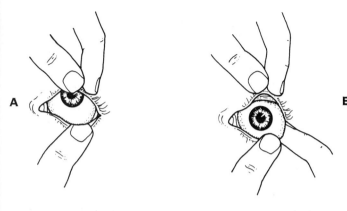

Fig. 6-1 Removal of artificial eye. **A,** Applying slight pressure to the lower lid. **B,** Raising the upper lid to break suction.

5. Place the eye prosthesis into a cup. Gently clean it with mild soap and water, unless another cleaning solution is ordered by the physician.
6. Inspect the eye prosthesis for signs of chips or cracks. Assess the condition of the eye socket, and evaluate it for drainage or signs of infection.
7. Assess the condition and appearance of the other eye.
8. Irrigate and clean the eye socket as ordered by the physician.
9. Replace the eye prosthesis by pulling down the lower lid and slipping the lower edge of the prosthesis gently into the socket. Draw the upper lid over the upper edge of the eye prosthesis.
10. Evaluate the patient's comfort level once the eye prosthesis is reinserted.
11. Provide patient comfort measures.
12. Clean and replace the equipment. Discard disposable items according to *Standard Precautions.*

NURSING CONSIDERATIONS

Encourage the patient to perform the procedure of removing and cleansing the prosthesis and irrigating the eye socket daily.

The eye is not a sterile area, but good handwashing and hygiene are to be emphasized.

DOCUMENTATION GUIDELINES

Document the following on the visit report:
- The procedure and patient toleration
- Condition of the eye prosthesis and eye socket
- Any patient/caregiver instructions and response to teaching, including the ability to care for the artificial eye
- Physician notification, if applicable
- *Standard Precautions*
- Other pertinent findings

Update the plan of care.

Care of the Patient with Cataract or Retinal Surgery

PURPOSE

- To provide eye care for postsurgical patients
- To treat, cleanse, and remove exudate from the eyes of patients who have recently undergone cataract or retinal surgery
- To relieve discomfort

RELATED PROCEDURES

- Eye Instillation and Irrigation (see Chapter 9)
- Administration of Medications: General Guidelines (see Chapter 9)

GENERAL INFORMATION

Eyelids should be kept dry and clean. Moisture on the lid predisposes the eye to inflammation and infection. Avoid shining light into the patient's eyes.

EQUIPMENT

1. Prescribed eye medication
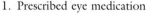 2. Disposable nonsterile gloves (optional) and impermeable plastic trash bag (see *Infection Control*)

PROCEDURE

1. Explain the procedure to the patient/caregiver.
2. Strictly adhere to prescribed activity restrictions and physical limitations when providing care, such as turning, combing hair, brushing teeth, and shaving.
3. Instruct the patient not to bend over or lift anything until activity restrictions are discontinued by the physician.
4. Instruct the patient to remain on his or her back unless otherwise ordered by the physician.
5. Protect the operated eye(s) at all times. If the physician orders, the patient may wear either an eye shield or glasses during the day. At night the patient should wear an eye shield over the operated eye(s).
6. Notify the physician immediately if the patient coughs frequently; is nauseated; or complains of a sudden, sharp pain in the operated eye.
7. Instill eye drops or ointment as ordered.
8. Provide patient comfort measures.
9. Clean and replace the equipment. Discard disposable items according to *Standard Precautions.*

NURSING CONSIDERATIONS

Prescribed eye medication for adults can be kept at the patient's bedside unless the medication requires refrigeration or children are in the home.

If the patient is receiving both eye drops and ointment, apply the eye drops first.

Always announce yourself when entering and leaving the room of a patient with impaired vision.

Explain all procedures before beginning.

Patients who have both eyes covered **must** have the bed siderails up or have the bedside protected in some way.

Evaluate the patient for constipation or straining, and take corrective action.

DOCUMENTATION GUIDELINES

Document the following on the visit report:
- The procedure and patient toleration
- Condition of the eye
- Any incidence of pain or problems with instillation of medication

- Any patient/caregiver instructions and compliance with the procedure
- Physician notification, if applicable
- *Standard Precautions*
- Other pertinent findings

Document medications on the medication record.

Update the plan of care.

Care of the Patient with Contact Lenses

PURPOSE

- To maintain the integrity of the prescribed artificial lens
- To prevent infection

EQUIPMENT

1. Hard or soft contact lenses as prescribed by the optometrist
2. Storage container for contact lenses
3. Saline solutions and prescribed drops
4. Thermal disinfecting kit (optional)
5. Contact lens disinfectant and/or enzyme solution, surfactant cleaner, disposable nonsterile gloves (optional), and an impermeable plastic trash bag (see *Infection Control*)

PROCEDURE

1. Review the physician's orders or the manufacturer's recommendations for storing, rinsing, cleaning, wetting, and lubricating lenses.
2. Explain the procedure to the patient/caregiver.
3. Assemble the equipment at a convenient work area where the patient is comfortable.
4. Place the patient in a sitting or supine position.
5. If the patient is able, instruct him or her to look upward.
6. *Inserting a clean, hard lens*—Wet it with the appropriate solution immediately before insertion. Place the hard lens with the concave side up on the tip of your right index finger. Then separate the patient's eyelids with your left

thumb and index finger. Place the hard lens directly over the cornea of the patient's eye.

    a. Evaluate the patient's comfort level and vision after the lens is inserted.

7. *Removing a hard lens*—Separate the patient's eyelids to expose the lens. Apply a slight pressure toward the bony orbit above and below the patient's eye. (Use both thumbs. Do not touch the eye.) Move the lower and upper lids toward the lens, applying slight pressure to the lower lid to tilt the lens (Fig. 6-2). Continue to bring the lids together until the lens slips from the patient's eye. Grasp the lens as it slips from the eye.

    a. Clean and disinfect the lenses according to the physician's orders or the manufacturer's recommendations

    b. Center the lenses in a storage container, with the convex side down. Make sure that the lenses are placed in proper storage containers: "R" for right lens and "L" for left lens

8. *Inserting a clean, soft lens*—Wet it with the appropriate solution immediately before insertion. Hold the lens with

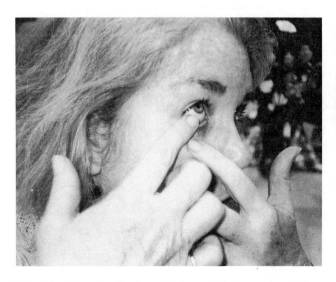

Fig. 6-2 Removing hard contact lenses. (Photo courtesy Robyn Rice.)

your right thumb and index finger. Then separate the patient's eyelids with your left thumb and index finger. Place the soft lens directly over the cornea of the patient's eye.

a. Evaluate the patient's comfort level and vision after the lens is inserted.

b. If the lens is not centered over the cornea, instruct the patient to close the eye, roll it toward the lens, and then blink a few times.

9. *Removing a soft lens*—Retract the patient's lower lid. Put a few drops of sterile saline solution into the patient's eye. With the tip of your index finger on the lower part of the lens, slide the lens off the cornea and onto the lower part of the eye (Fig. 6-3). Slightly squeeze the lens with your thumb and index finger to create suction. Gently pinch the lens and lift out.

a. Discard the disposable lens. Clean and disinfect the lenses according to the physician's orders or the manufacturer's recommendations. Be careful not to scratch the lenses with your fingernail.

b. Place the lenses in a storage container, and fill the container with storage solution ordered by the physician or recommended by the manufacturer.

10. Provide patient comfort measures.

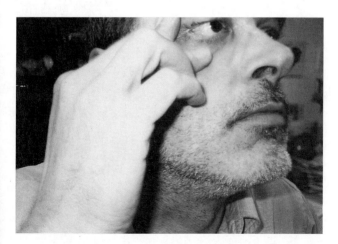

Fig. 6-3   Removing soft contact lenses. (Photo courtesy Robyn Rice.)

11. Clean and replace the equipment. Discard disposable items according to *Standard Precautions.*

NURSING CONSIDERATIONS

Instruct the patient on how to insert and remove contact lenses without assistance.

To prevent eye infections, emphasize the importance of **hand-washing** and the regular cleaning of lenses, as well as checking the expiration date of cleaning solutions.

Instruct the patient not to wear hard lenses longer than 12 hours without interruption.

The time for wearing soft lenses vary. (Follow the manufacturer's recommendations.)

DOCUMENTATION GUIDELINES

Document the following on the visit report:
- The procedure and patient toleration
- Any patient/caregiver instructions and response to teaching, including the ability to manage contact lenses
- Physician notification, if applicable
- *Standard Precautions*
- Other pertinent findings

Update the plan of care.

Care of the Patient with Depressed Corneal Reflex

PURPOSE

- To protect the eye and the surrounding tissue and structures in the presence of decreased lacrimation and/or decreased corneal sensation and muscle movement

RELATED PROCEDURES

- Administration of Medications: General Guidelines (see Chapter 9)
- Eye Instillation and Irrigation (see Chapter 9)

GENERAL INFORMATION

The corneal reflex can be tested by stroking the patient's eyelashes with a cotton ball. The stimulus to the cornea should result in a blink.

EQUIPMENT

1. Irrigation solution as prescribed by the physician
2. Prescribed eye drops with eyedropper
3. Ophthalmologic or paper tape
4. Warm water, basin, washcloth, and towels
5. Disposable nonsterile gloves and an impermeable plastic trash bag (see *Infection Control*)

PROCEDURE

1. Explain the procedure to the patient/caregiver.
2. Assemble the equipment at a convenient work area.
3. Assess the patient's eyes each visit for redness and mucopurulent or purulent discharge.
4. Gently clean crust or drainage along the eyelid with a damp washcloth.
5. Irrigate the eye with a prescribed irrigation solution every 2 to 4 hours or as ordered by the physician.
6. Instill prescribed eye drops.
7. If the patient's eyes are to be taped shut, use a strip of ophthalmologic or paper tape. Turn the tape back at the top and bottom edges to protect the patient's eyebrows and to facilitate removal (Fig. 6-4).
8. Provide patient comfort measures.
9. Clean and replace the equipment. Discard disposable items according to *Standard Precautions.*

NURSING CONSIDERATIONS

The corneas must be kept moist to maintain the integrity of the eye.

Encourage caregivers to tape the eyelids of unconscious patients with no corneal reflexes and/or conscious patients who are unable to close their eyelids—especially at night.

Instruct the patient/caregiver to avoid eye patches or shields because they can become dislodged and abrade the cornea.

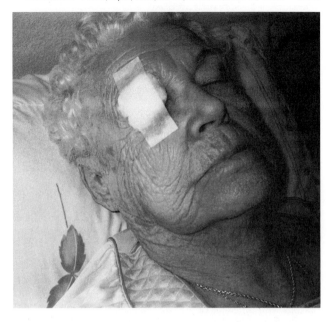

Fig. 6-4 Taped eye of a patient with a depressed corneal reflex. (Photo courtesy Robyn Rice.)

DOCUMENTATION GUIDELINES

Document the following on the visit report:
- The procedure and patient toleration
- Condition of the eyes and corneas
- Any patient/caregiver instructions and response to teaching
- Physician notification, if applicable
- *Standard Precautions*
- Other pertinent findings

Document medications on the medication record.

Update the plan of care.

Care of the Patient with Hearing Aid

PURPOSE
- To maintain the integrity and correct the working order of the patient's hearing aid
- To optimize the hearing-impaired patient's ability to communicate
- To promote self-care in the home

GENERAL INFORMATION
There are three types of hearing aids commonly seen in the home setting. The in-the-canal (ITC) aid is the newest, smallest, and least visible aid on the market. It fits entirely in the ear canal (Fig. 6-5). The ITC has cosmetic appeal and does not interfere with most activities of daily living. However, it requires manual dexterity to operate, to insert and remove, and to change batteries. Also, cerumen tends to plug up this model more than the others. The ITC aid is OT recommended for persons with moisture or skin problems in the ear canal. An in-the-ear (ITE), or intraaural, aid fits into the external auditory ear and allows more fine-tuning (Fig. 6-6). It is more powerful and is more useful for a wider range of hearing loss than the ITC aid. The ITE is the most common type of aid worn today. A behind-the-ear (BTE), or postaural, aid hooks around and behind the ear and is connected by a short, clear, hollow plastic

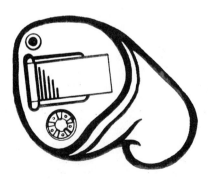

Fig. 6-5 In-the-canal (ITC) hearing aid. (From Sigler BA, Schuring LT: *Ear, nose, and throat disorders,* St Louis, 1993, Mosby.)

tube to an ear mold inserted into the external auditory canal (Fig. 6-7). It is useful for patients with manual dexterity difficulties and rapidly progressive hearing loss.

EQUIPMENT

1. Hearing aid
2. Batteries
3. Brush or wax loop
4. Storage container
5. Soft towel and washcloth
6. Disposable nonsterile gloves (optional) and an impermeable plastic trash bag (see *Infection Control*)

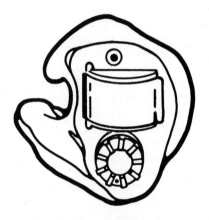

Fig. 6-6 In-the-ear (ITE) hearing aid. (From Sigler BA, Schuring LT: *Ear, nose, and throat disorders,* St Louis, 1993, Mosby.)

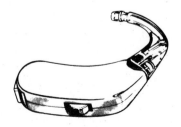

Fig. 6-7 Behind-the-ear (BTE) hearing aid. (From Sigler BA, Schuring LT: *Ear, nose, and throat disorders,* St Louis, 1993, Mosby.)

PROCEDURE

1. Explain the procedure to the patient/caregiver.
2. Assemble the equipment at a convenient work area.
3. Assess the patient's knowledge of operating the hearing aid. Explain the mechanism of the instrument and the adjustment of the controls for best results.
4. Store the hearing aid in an appropriate container when not in use and in a safe place, such as the patient's bedside table drawer. Instruct the patient to always keep spare batteries available.
5. Check the batteries if the hearing aid is not functioning:
   a. Turn the volume up to high
   b. Cup your hand over the ear mold
   c. If no sound is heard, replace the batteries, matching the plus (+) and minus (−) signs. Batteries usually need replacing after 1 week of daily wear
6. Examine the cord of the BTE aid for breaks, and replace it as necessary.
7. Disconnect the ear mold from the hearing aid to clean it.
8. Wash the ear mold with soap and water. (Do not wash any other part of the hearing aid.) Use a wax loop or brush (supplied with the aid) to clean the holes in the aid. Do not jam the wax deeper into the holes; this action could cause damage to the aid. Dry the aid thoroughly.
9. Snap the dry mold back into the hearing aid.
10. Assist the patient to insert the hearing aid in the following manner:
    a. Turn the hearing aid off and the volume down
    b. Hold the aid so that the bore (i.e., the long portion with the hold[s]) is at the bottom; guiding it along the patient's cheek, bring the aid to the ear
    c. Insert the bore into the canal first; use the other hand to pull up and back on the outer ear; gently twist and push the aid into the ear until it is in place and fits snugly
    d. Gently bring the cannula of the BTE aid up and over the ear and toward the back to prevent kinking
11. Turn on the hearing aid. Adjust the volume gradually to a comfortable level for talking to the patient in a regular voice at a distance of 3 to 4 feet. Volume controls are commonly adjusted by rotating the control. Rotate the volume

control toward the nose to increase the volume and away from the nose to decrease the volume.

12. Evaluate the patient's comfort level and the patient's ability to hear once the hearing aid is functioning.
13. Provide patient comfort measures.
14. Clean and replace the equipment. Discard disposable items according to *Standard Precautions.*

NURSING CONSIDERATIONS

Evaluate the need for written safety precautions: Is the patient unable to hear fire alarms or the telephone?

Instruct the patient to avoid the use of hair sprays while wearing a hearing aid because this can cause malfunction.

Do not leave the aid in the storage container near a stove, heater, or sunny window.

Store batteries in a cool, dry place.

Instruct the patient to avoid extremes of hot or cold temperatures or exposure to rain or bath water while wearing the hearing aid.

DOCUMENTATION GUIDELINES

Document the following on the visit report:
- The procedure and patient toleration
- Patient's ability to hear with the hearing aid on
- Any patient/caregiver instructions and response to teaching, including ability to manage the hearing aid
- Physician notification, if applicable
- *Standard Precautions*
- Other pertinent findings

Update the plan of care.

Care of the Patient with Visual Impairment

PURPOSE
- To maximize visual function
- To encourage the optimal level of independence
- To promote self-care in the home

GENERAL INFORMATION
Provide dim lighting for patients after cataract removal. Provide average lighting for patients with glaucoma. Provide bright lighting for patients with peripheral cataracts.

EQUIPMENT
1. Eye glasses
2. Appropriate lighting
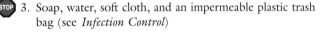 3. Soap, water, soft cloth, and an impermeable plastic trash bag (see *Infection Control*)

PROCEDURE
1. Explain the procedure to the patient/caregiver.
2. Assemble the equipment at a convenient work area.
3. Keep the patient's area equipped with proper lighting to provide increased illumination of the entire area.
4. Keep the glasses clean, using soap, warm water, and a soft cloth. Do not use hot water because it may damage the glasses.
5. To avoid breakage or damage, store the glasses in a case when they are not being used. Have the patient's name imprinted on both the frames and the case to prevent loss.
6. Check for irritation on the patient's nose and behind the ears. (Report to the optometrist for adjustment, if necessary.)
7. Encourage activities and interaction with friends and family within the patient's limitations. Offer encouragement and praise to support home independence.
8. Use other sensory stimulation, such as the following, for patients with complete loss of vision, sound, or touch:
   a. Always allow the blind patient to take your arm and follow.

   b. Acquaint the patient with his or her surroundings as to the location of the telephone, furniture, doors, and household rooms.

   c. Instruct the patient on how to use the telephone and call the physician or home health agency clinical supervisor, as well as how to access emergency assistance if needed.

   d. Always indicate your presence by speaking to the patient when entering or leaving the room.

   e. Keep the doors closed or wide open, flush with the wall, to prevent accidents. Do not rearrange furniture or the patient's belongings without letting the patient know of the changes.

   f. When serving food to the patient, explain the contents of the tray, and place the contents in a clockwise position.

9. Evaluate the patient's progress and adjustment to visual impairment at each visit.

10. Provide patient comfort measures.

11. Clean and replace the equipment. Discard disposable items according to *Standard Precautions.*

NURSING CONSIDERATIONS

Evaluate the patient for social service needs, regarding adjustment to vision loss, and refer the patient to community services for the visually impaired.

DOCUMENTATION GUIDELINES

Document the following on the visit report:

- The procedure and patient toleration
- Degree of diminished visual perception
- Lighting requirements
- Condition of the eyes
- Level of independence
- Use of visual aids
- Home safety precautions
- Any patient/caregiver instructions regarding the procedure and response to teaching.
- Physician notification, if applicable
- *Standard Precautions*
- Other pertinent findings

Update the plan of care.

CHAPTER 7

Intravenous Therapy Procedures

Administration of Intravenous Therapy: General Guidelines

PURPOSE

- To provide guidelines for home management of intravenous (IV) therapy

RELATED PROCEDURES

- Administration of Medications: General Guidelines (see Chapter 9)
- Discontinuation and Removal of Peripheral Intravenous Fluids
- Infusions (see Chapter 8)
- Peripheral Intravenous Management

PROCEDURE

1. Check for any known allergies.
2. Obtain an appropriate home health agency consent form and have the patient sign it **before** initiating IV therapy.
3. The patient/caregiver must have access to a telephone.
4. The patient/caregiver must be **willing** and **able** to administer home IV therapy (see the Patient Education Guidelines box, *Home IV Therapy,* on pp. 281-282). The nurse, as well as the patient/caregiver, **must** use aseptic technique.
5. A reliable and capable caregiver **must** be available during the infusion to maintain and discontinue fluids if the patient is unable to do these.

6. An IV infusion may be initiated by the physician or nurse. The nurse should have advanced training (i.e., IV certification) for job requirements beyond the basic procedures.

7. IV therapy may be initiated with verbal orders. These orders must be validated with written orders signed by the patient's physician. Written orders must be in the chart within 14 days of service or according to state regulations.

8. The physician's order for intravenous therapy must include the type of solution, any medication additives with the dose specified, and the total 24-hour volume to be infused and/or the hourly flow rate. IV fluids typically used in home care include normal saline solution, lactated Ringer's with or without dextrose, and dextrose and sterile water combinations.

9. The home health admissions department will contact the home infusion company for supplies, medications, fluids, and equipment.

10. Consider the purpose for which the infusion is being administered, and select the most appropriate type of needle or catheter and tubing. A 20- to 22-gauge catheter is commonly used for hydration fluids.

11. Preferred sites for peripheral IV therapy are the veins of the hand and forearm (Fig. 7-1).

12. Examine the catheter insertion site for signs or symptoms of phlebitis or infiltration each visit and before initiating, during, and after discontinuing IV therapy. If redness, swelling, or leakage around the catheter site occurs, discontinue the IV and restart at another site.

13. Change the gauze dressings at the IV catheter site at least 3 times a week. Change transparent or occlusive dressings at the IV catheter site 1 to 2 times a week.

14. Change both the primary and secondary tubing every 48 hours or upon suspected contamination.

15. Change the injection cap(s) weekly or twice a week if frequently accessed.

16. Change peripheral IV catheters every 48 to 72 hours or sooner if the IV is leaking from the catheter exit site or if infiltration or phlebitis occurs.

17. Check all IV solutions for the expiration date, presence of cracks, discoloration, or particulate matter before they are hung.

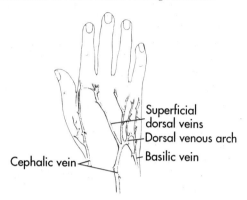

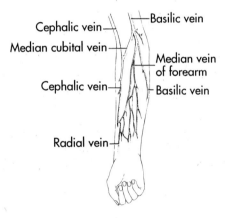

Fig. 7-1   Preferred sites for peripheral IV therapy. (From Perry AG, Potter PA: *Clinical nursing skills and techniques,* ed 4, St Louis, 1997, Mosby.)

18. Check all IV labels for the correct patient name, medication, dosage, and expiration date.
19. Discard all IV solutions, including those with medication additives, 24 hours after the seal has been broken.
20. Label all IV solutions with the medication additive (if any).
21. The first dose of antibiotic therapy **must** be initiated in a controlled setting where emergency medical services are available.

Box 7-1

PATIENT/CAREGIVER IV SKILLS CHECKLIST

Administration and management of IV fluids

Irrigation and/or heparinization of the catheter

Discontinuation of IV therapy

Dressing change

Complications of IV therapy: recognition and trouble-shooting

Medications: purpose, action, dosage, schedule, side effects

Operation and maintenance of IV pump

Standard Precautions

Documentation: solution, rate, status of IV site, tubing change, use of pump

When to call the home health agency clinical supervisor or the physician

22. The home health agency **must** provide 24-hour, on-call nurses for patients who are receiving home IV therapy. Consider a plan of action for possible complications.
23. Notify the home health agency clinical supervisor and the physician with the following documentation:
    a. Abnormal laboratory values (see Appendix II, *Laboratory Values*)
    b. Fever, transfusion reaction, complications from IV or unstable cardiopulmonary status
    c. Noncompliant or unsafe patient/caregiver behaviors or unavailable patient/caregiver
    d. Patient/caregiver inability to start an IV after 3 sticks
    e. Occluded central venous access device

NURSING CONSIDERATIONS

Patient/caregiver education is crucial to the safe administration of home IV therapy infusion (Box 7-1).

Written guidelines and return demonstrations are needed for all aspects of care (see the Patient Education Guidelines box, *Home IV Therapy*, on pp. 281-282).

Storage requirements, infusion preparation administration, discontinuation, equipment management, and disposal of supplies must be completely understood by the patient/ caregiver for safe home IV therapy.

The patient/caregiver also needs information on possible adverse side effects of IV therapy, troubleshooting potential problems, and when to call the home health agency clinical supervisor or physician.

DOCUMENTATION GUIDELINES

Document the following on the visit report:
- The procedure and patient toleration
- Size and length of IV catheter
- IV site selection and the appearance of the catheter exit site
- Use of an IV pump or equipment to regulate the IV flow
- Type of dressing applied
- Any patient/caregiver instructions and response to teaching, including the ability to safely manage home IV therapy
- Physician notification, if applicable
- *Standard Precautions*
- Other pertinent findings

Document the following on the medication or IV record: solution infused, expiration date, the amount and hourly rate for each 24-hour volume, IV medications, and initials of the person who hung the infusion.

Update the plan of care.

Central Venous Catheter Management

PURPOSE
- To administer intravenous fluids
- To sample blood for laboratory analysis
- To maintain the patency of the catheter
- To prevent infection

RELATED PROCEDURES
- Administration of Intravenous Therapy: General Guidelines
- Groshong Catheter Management
- Implantable Vascular Access Device Management
- Multiple-Lumen Nontunneled Catheter Management

- Peripheral Inserted Central Catheter: Insertion Guidelines
- Peripheral Intravenous Management
- Specimen Labeling and Transport (see Chapter 12)

GENERAL INFORMATION

Central venous catheters (CVCs) are required for patients with a variety of medical conditions, including cancer and bowel disease. These catheters are used for long-term venous access and spare the patient repeated venipunctures. Central venous catheters are commonly used in the home to administer all types of IV therapy, including antimicrobial agents, hyperalimentation, chemotherapy, narcotics, and blood components. Central venous catheters are also used for blood sampling.

Common CVCs used in home care are subclavian catheters (e.g., Hohn or Deseret triple lumen catheters); tunneled catheters (e.g., Hickman and Broviac or Groshong catheters); implantable vascular access devices (IVADs) (e.g., PORT-A-Cath); and peripheral venous access systems (e.g., PAS port or a peripheral inserted central catheter line). Use 1-inch needles whenever injections are made through the Luer-Lok injection cap because this reduces the possibility of damaging the catheter. Consult the manufacturer's recommendations if you are using a needleless system to access the CVC and to initiate IV therapy.

❖ Blood Sampling

EQUIPMENT

1. Blood specimen tubes
2. Occlusion hemostat or Kelly-Bulldog clamp if needed (most CVSs have preattached clamps)
3. 10 cc and 20 cc syringes with 1-inch, 20-gauge needles for blood sampling
4. Laboratory requisition, labels
5. Antiseptic and alcohol wipes
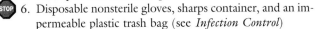 6. Disposable nonsterile gloves, sharps container, and an impermeable plastic trash bag (see *Infection Control*)

PROCEDURE

1. Explain the procedure to the patient/caregiver.
2. Assemble the equipment at a convenient work area.
3. Assist the patient to a comfortable position to access the catheter.

4. Review the orders for laboratory specimens, and obtain the correct blood tubes.
5. Clean the injection cap(s) with an antiseptic wipe, then use an alcohol wipe; air dry.
6. Attach the syringe, then release the clamp. (Most Hickman and Broviac catheters come with preattached clamps and reinforced clamping sleeves. The Groshong catheter does not have a clamp.)
7. Gently aspirate 7 ml of blood from the catheter. Reclamp the catheter. Place the needle syringe with blood in a sharps container.
8. Connect a 20 cc syringe to the injection cap. Unclamp the catheter, and gently withdraw the appropriate amount of blood needed for blood sampling.
9. Follow the procedure for *Irrigation* to clear the line and to prevent occlusion.
10. Clamp the catheter over the reinforced clamping sleeve.
11. Label and prepare the blood tube(s) for transport.
12. Provide patient comfort measures.
13. Clean and replace the equipment. Discard disposable items according to *Standard Precautions*.

❖ Cap Change

EQUIPMENT

1. Injection cap(s)
2. Occlusion hemostat or Kelly-Bulldog clamp (many CVCs are preattached clamps)
3. Sterile normal saline solution, heparin flush solution (100 U/ml)
4. 10 cc syringes with 1-inch, 23-gauge needles
5. Antiseptic and alcohol wipes
6. Disposable nonsterile gloves, sharps container, and an impermeable plastic trash bag (see *Infection Control*)

PROCEDURE

1. Follow steps *1* through *3* of the procedure for *Blood Sampling*. Using aseptic technique, prime a new injection cap with 0.9% normal saline solution.
2. Make sure that the catheter is clamped with either a preattached clamp or a toothless, smooth-edge clamp. (The Groshong catheter does not have a clamp.)

3. Don gloves. Grasp the end of the catheter between the index finger and the thumb. Clean the connection with an antiseptic wipe and then an alcohol wipe; air dry.
4. Using aseptic technique, remove the old injection cap, and discard it. Pick up the new cap, touching only the outside rubber port. Then remove the protective covering from the end of the new injection cap, and discard it.
5. Attach the new injection cap onto the catheter. Be careful not to touch the tip of the catheter or the injection cap.
6. Attach the syringe of the heparin flush, release the clamp, and flush slowly.
7. Clamp the catheter, maintaining positive pressure on the syringe plunger, and then remove the syringe.
8. Loop the catheter with the cap pointing upward on the dressing. Secure with tape to prevent tugging or accidental dislodgment.
9. Follow steps *12* and *13* of the procedure for *Blood Sampling*.

❖ Dressing Change

EQUIPMENT

1. Disposable CVC dressing tray (includes alcohol swab sticks [3], antiseptic swab sticks [3], benzoin swab stick [1], antibiotic ointment [if ordered], tape, and face mask)
2. Two transparent adhesive dressings
3. Disposable nonsterile and sterile gloves, sharps container, and an impermeable plastic trash bag (see *Infection Control*)

PROCEDURE

1. Follow steps *1* through *3* of the procedure for *Blood Sampling*.
2. Place the dressing tray on a clean, dry surface. Unwrap the tray, including the sterile gloves, without touching the inner sterile contents.
3. Don nonsterile gloves and the face mask. Remove the old dressing, being careful not to dislodge the catheter. Discard the dressing.
4. Examine the catheter exit site for signs of infection (redness or drainage). Report to the physician as appropriate.
5. Discard the nonsterile gloves. Don the sterile gloves. Use

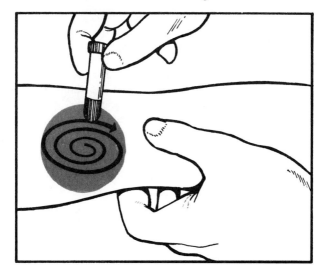

Fig. 7-2 Cleaning the venipuncture site. (From LaRocca JC, Otto SE: *Pocket guide to intravenous therapy,* ed 3, St Louis, 1997, Mosby.)

aseptic technique to clean the catheter exit site in the following manner:

a. Remove an antiseptic swab stick from its package and use it to clean the area, starting at the catheter exit site and moving outward in a spiral motion to cover an area 4 to 6 cm in diameter (Fig. 7-2); discard the swab, and select a new one (never go back to the catheter exit site with a swab stick or a wipe that has touched skin away from the site)

b. Repeat step *5a* two additional times with antiseptic swab sticks; air dry

c. Clean the area thoroughly with alcohol swab sticks as described in step *5a;* air dry

6. Apply the benzoin swab to the perimeters of the dressing as a skin preparation.

7. Apply transparent adhesive dressing. If desired, picture frame the perimeters of dressing with tape (Fig. 7-3).

8. Loop the catheter, with the cap pointing upward, on the dressing. Secure with tape to prevent tugging or accidental dislodgment.

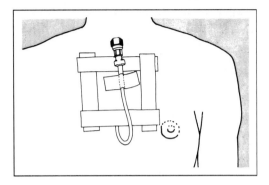

Fig. 7-3 Securing the transparent adhesive dressing. (Courtesy Bard Access Systems, Salt Lake City, Utah.)

9. Date and time the dressing change on the tape.
10. Perform injection *Cap Change* and catheter *Irrigation* as needed (see the following procedures for CVC injection: *Cap Change* and *Irrigation*).
11. Instruct the patient to contact the home health agency if the dressing becomes loosened or soiled.
12. Follow steps *12* through *13* of the procedure for *Blood Sampling*.

❖ Irrigation and Heparinization

EQUIPMENT

1. 100 U/ml heparin solution as prescribed by the physician
2. Sterile normal saline solution as prescribed by the physician
3. 10 cc syringes with 1-inch, 23-gauge needle
4. Antiseptic and alcohol wipes

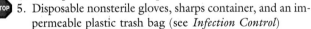

5. Disposable nonsterile gloves, sharps container, and an impermeable plastic trash bag (see *Infection Control*)

PROCEDURE

1. Follow steps *1* through *3* of the procedure for *Blood Sampling*.
2. Clean the injection cap(s) with an antiseptic wipe, followed by an alcohol wipe; air dry.
3. Connect the syringe of normal saline and unclamp the cath-

eter. (Most Hickman and Broviac catheters come with pre-attached clamps and reinforced clamping sleeves. The Groshong catheter does not have a clamp.)

4. Irrigate the lumen with the ordered amount of normal saline solution; clamp the catheter between syringes, then flush with the ordered amount of heparin solution. Inject the heparin into the catheter no faster than ½ ml per second.

5. Clamp the catheter, and, while maintaining positive pressure on the syringe plunger, remove the syringe.

6. Loop the catheter, with the cap pointing upward, on the dressing. Secure with tape to prevent tugging or accidental dislodgment.

7. Follow steps *12* and *13* of the procedure for *Blood Sampling*.

 NURSING CONSIDERATIONS

If the catheter cannot be irrigated, do not force the solution into the catheter. Instruct the patient to change his or her body position, to cough, to deep breathe, or to raise his or her arm above the head. If you are still unable to irrigate and flush the catheter, notify the home health agency clinical supervisor and physician for further orders.

Refer to specific catheter procedures for further irrigation guidelines. Groshong catheters do not require heparinization.

 DOCUMENTATION GUIDELINES

Document the following on the visit report:
- The procedure and patient toleration
- The condition of the catheter exit site, including any signs of redness, swelling, or drainage
- Irrigation and patency of the catheter lumen(s)
- Blood sampling and designated laboratory for delivery
- Any patient/caregiver instructions and response to teaching, including the ability to safely manage the central venous catheter at home
- Physician notification, if applicable
- *Standard Precautions*
- Other pertinent findings

Document IV medications/solutions infused on the medication or IV record.

Update the plan of care.

Changing Intravenous Solutions

PURPOSE
- To administer IV fluids
- To prevent infection

RELATED PROCEDURE
- Administration of Intravenous Therapy: General Guidelines

EQUIPMENT
1. Bag of IV solution as prescribed by the physician
2. Time tape
 3. Disposable nonsterile gloves and an impermeable plastic trash bag (see *Infection Control*)

PROCEDURE
1. Explain the procedure to the patient/caregiver.
2. Assemble the equipment in a convenient work area.
3. Position patient to access the IV.
4. Prepare a new bag of IV solution for changing by removing the protective cover from the bag's IV tubing port.
5. Move the roller clamp to stop the flow rate from the old IV bag.
6. Remove the old IV bag from the IV pole.
7. Holding the IV bag upside down, quickly remove the spike from the old IV bag and, without touching it, spike the new IV bag.
8. Hang the new bag of IV solution on the IV pole.
9. Gently squeeze the drip chamber until it is one-third to one-half full. If the drip chamber is too full, pinch off the IV tubing just below the drip chamber. Turn the container upside down and squeeze the drip chamber so that the solution goes back into the IV bag. Then hang up the bag and tubing.
10. Examine the tubing. Small bubbles can usually be removed by closing the roller clamp, stretching the tubing downward, and flicking the tubing with the finger (the bubbles should rise to the drip chamber). For a large amount of air,

insert a needle and syringe into a port below the air bubbles and allow the air to enter the syringe.
11. Adjust the flow rate as ordered by the physician.
12. Time tape the new IV bag.
13. Provide patient comfort measures.
14. Clean and replace the equipment. Discard disposable items according to *Standard Precautions.*

NURSING CONSIDERATIONS

Change IV fluids daily.

DOCUMENTATION GUIDELINES

Follow the documentation guidelines for the procedure for *Administration of Intravenous Therapy: General Guidelines.*
Update the plan of care.

Changing Intravenous Tubing

PURPOSE
- To change IV tubing for a peripheral IV
- To prevent infection

RELATED PROCEDURE
- Administration of Intravenous Therapy: General Guidelines

EQUIPMENT
1. Infusion tubing
2. Sterile 2- × 2-inch gauze dressing
3. Disposable nonsterile gloves and an impermeable plastic trash bag (see *Infection Control*)

PROCEDURE
1. Explain the procedure to the patient/caregiver.
2. Assemble the equipment in a convenient work area.
3. Position the patient to access the IV.
4. Using aseptic technique, place a sterile 2- × 2-inch gauze dressing near the patient.
5. If the needle or catheter hub is not visible, remove the old

dressing (do not remove tape that is holding the IV needle or catheter in place).

6. For an IV infusion, do the following:
   a. Move the roller clamp to "off" on the new IV tubing
   b. Slow the rate of infusion "to keep open" on the old tubing
   c. With the old tubing in place, compress and completely fill the drip chamber
   d. Remove the old tubing from the IV solution; hang or tape the old tubing on the IV pole
   e. Spike the new tubing into the IV solution
   f. Squeeze the drip chamber on the new tubing until one-third to one-half full
   g. Open the roller clamp; remove the protective cap from the needle adapter (if necessary) and flush the tubing

7. Place the needle adaptor of the new tubing, with the protective cap off, on the sterile 2- × 2-inch gauze pad already placed near the patient.

8. Hold the IV catheter in place and gently disconnect the old IV tubing. Quickly insert the needle adaptor of the new tubing into the hub of the IV catheter and secure with a Luer-Lok.

9. Open the roller clamp of the new tubing. Allow the solution to run rapidly for about 30 seconds. Adjust the IV flow rate as required.

10. Provide patient comfort measures.

11. Clean and replace equipment. Discard disposable items according to *Standard Precautions.*

NURSING CONSIDERATIONS

Change primary IV tubing every other day. Whenever possible, change the primary IV tubing when changing IV solution bags.

If an infusion pump is used, remove the old tubing from the pump and replace with new tubing.

Follow manufacturer's guidelines when using a **needleless** IV system.

DOCUMENTATION GUIDELINES

Follow the documentation guidelines for the procedure for *Administration of Intravenous Therapy: General Guidelines.*

Update the plan of care.

Declotting an Implantable Vascular Access Device

PURPOSE
- To declot and clear the PORT-A-Cath with thrombolytic agents

RELATED PROCEDURES
- Administration of Intravenous Therapy: General Guidelines
- Administration of Medications: General Guidelines (see Chapter 9)
- Implantable Vascular Access Device Management

GENERAL INFORMATION
Adhere to the manufacturer's recommendations for administration of thrombolytic agents. According to the *Intravenous Nursing Society in the Intravenous Nursing Standards of Practice,* the volume of thrombolytic agent instilled should approximate the volume of the catheter, thus ensuring that the agent is retained in the catheter and is not instilled into the bloodstream.

EQUIPMENT
1. Thrombolytic agent (e.g., Urokinase) as prescribed by the physician
2. Sterile normal saline solution as prescribed by the physician
3. 10 cc syringes with 1-inch, 20-gauge needles, straight noncoring needle with integrated extension tubing and clamp for the implantable vascular access device (IVAD)
4. Antiseptic and alcohol wipes
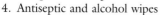 5. Disposable nonsterile gloves, sharps container, and an impermeable plastic trash bag (see *Infection Control*)

PROCEDURE
1. Explain the procedure to the patient/caregiver.
2. Assemble the equipment at a convenient work area.
3. Assist the patient to a comfortable position to access the catheter.

4. Clean the injection cap(s) or the area of skin over the septum of the vascular access device with an antiseptic wipe, followed by an alcohol wipe; air dry.
5. Follow specific catheter protocols to access the catheter.
6. Draw up the ordered amount of Urokinase into a 10 cc syringe (use a smaller syringe to draw up small amounts, then transfer to 10 cc syringe).
7. Connect the syringe to the integrated extension tubing on a noncoring needle. Unclamp the tubing.
8. Slowly inject the Urokinase into the occluded lumen and port of the vascular access device. Wait 10 minutes.
9. Attempt aspiration of the residual clot.
10. Repeat the procedure with a 20-minute dwell time if patency is not achieved.
11. Notify the physician for further orders if you are unable to aspirate from the catheter.
12. Provide patient comfort measures.
13. Clean and replace the equipment. Discard disposable items according to *Standard Precautions.*

DOCUMENTATION GUIDELINES

Document the following on the visit report:
- The procedure and patient toleration
- Patency of the vascular access device
- Condition of the catheter exit site
- Physician notification, if applicable
- *Standard Precautions*
- Other pertinent findings

Document the thrombolytic agent on the medication record. Update the plan of care.

Discontinuation and Removal of Peripheral Intravenous Fluids

PURPOSE

To discontinue an IV infusion
To prevent infection

RELATED PROCEDURE

• Administration of Intravenous Therapy: General Guidelines

EQUIPMENT

1. Sterile 2- × 2-inch gauze dressing or adhesive bandage
2. Hypoallergenic tape
3. Antiseptic and alcohol wipes
🛑 4. Disposable nonsterile gloves and an impermeable plastic trash bag (see *Infection Control*)

PROCEDURE

1. Explain the procedure to the patient/caregiver.
2. Assemble the equipment at a convenient work area.
3. Assist the patient to a comfortable position to access the IV.
4. Clamp the IV tubing with the flow regulator.
5. Remove the patient's dressing, and loosen the tape that is securing the catheter.
6. Place a 2- × 2-inch sterile gauze dressing over the catheter exit site.
7. Exert pressure on the site, and withdraw the catheter at the same time. Continue to apply pressure to the site for 2 to 3 minutes to prevent bleeding.
8. Cleanse the area with an antiseptic wipe, followed by an alcohol wipe; air dry.
9. Place a gauze dressing or an adhesive bandage over the catheter exit site, and secure it with tape.
10. Provide patient comfort measures.
11. Clean and replace the equipment. Discard disposable items according to *Standard Precautions.*

DOCUMENTATION GUIDELINES

Document the following on the visit report:
- The procedure and patient toleration
- Other pertinent findings

Record discontinuation of IV medications on the medication record. Record discontinuation of IV fluids on the IV record or visit report.

Update the plan of care.

Groshong Catheter Management

PURPOSE

- To administer IV fluids
- To sample blood for laboratory analysis
- To maintain patency of the catheter
- To prevent infection

RELATED PROCEDURES

- Administration of Intravenous Therapy: General Guidelines
- Central Venous Catheter Management
- Specimen Labeling and Transport (see Chapter 12)

GENERAL INFORMATION

The Groshong catheter is a long-term central venous access device. It can be used to administer total parenteral nutrition (TPN), chemotherapy, IV fluids, blood and blood products, and antibiotic therapy; it also may be used for blood sampling.

The Groshong is a small-diameter, silicone-rubber catheter that has a patented, three-position valve that eliminates the need for heparinization and clamping (Fig. 7-4). The tip of the catheter is placed in the superior vena cava via one of the large central veins (e.g., right subclavian) and tunneled subcutaneously to the exit site (upper abdominal area).

The Groshong catheter has a small Dacron cuff that fibroses to the surrounding tissue. This secures the catheter in place and acts as a physical barrier for bacterial migration. The

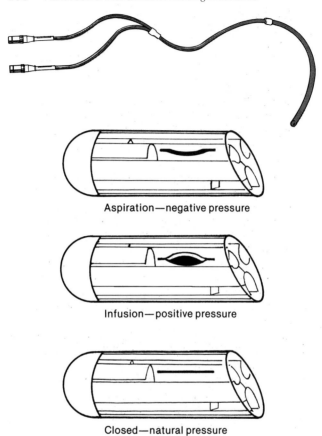

Aspiration—negative pressure

Infusion—positive pressure

Closed—natural pressure

Fig. 7-4 Three-position Groshong valve and Groshong central venous catheter. (Courtesy Bard Access Systems, Salt Lake City, Utah.)

three-position valve near the closed tip opens outward during infusion and inward during blood withdrawal. The valve automatically closes when it is not in use. As a result of hydrostatic pressure, venous blood pressure is not sufficient to spontaneously open the valve inward; this prevents blood from backing up into the lumen and occluding the catheter with a clot.

EQUIPMENT

1. Sterile normal saline solution as prescribed by the physician
2. 10 cc, 20 cc, or 30 cc syringes with 1-inch, 20-gauge needles
3. Blood specimen tubes
4. Laboratory requisition, labels
5. Antiseptic and alcohol wipes
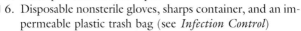 6. Disposable nonsterile gloves, sharps container, and an impermeable plastic trash bag (see *Infection Control*)

❖ Blood Sampling

PROCEDURE

1. Explain the procedure to the patient/caregiver.
2. Assemble the equipment at a convenient work area.
3. Assist the patient to a comfortable position to access the catheter.
4. Ask the patient/caregiver whether any problems exist with the catheter. Evaluate the dressing and injection cap change.
5. Review the order for the laboratory specimens, and obtain correct blood tubes.
6. Remove the injection cap from the end of the catheter and clean it with an antiseptic wipe, followed by alcohol wipes; air dry.
7. Connect the 10 cc syringe, then aspirate 5 to 10 ml of blood (slowly withdraw the blood). Discard the syringe into a sharps container.
8. Attach a 20 cc syringe directly to the catheter tubing, and withdraw the amount of blood needed for laboratory analysis.
9. Flush the Groshong catheter with 20 ml of normal saline solution, using 1 ml at a time for the first 10 ml. Then, briskly push the remaining 10 ml to remove residual blood.
10. Maintain positive pressure on the syringe plunger as the syringe is removed.
11. Using aseptic technique, attach a new sterile injection cap. (See the procedure for *Central Venous Catheter Management*.)
12. Label and prepare the blood tube(s) for transport.
13. Provide patient comfort measures.

14. Clean and replace the equipment. Discard disposable items according to *Standard Precautions*.

❖ Irrigation

PROCEDURE

1. Follow steps *1* through *4* of the procedure for *Blood Sampling*.
2. Clean the injection cap with an antiseptic wipe, followed by an alcohol wipe; air dry.
3. Draw up the required amount of normal saline solution in the syringe.
4. Connect the syringe to the injection cap; then irrigate the catheter in the following manner:
   a. Briskly irrigate the Groshong catheter with 10 ml of normal saline solution
      (1) Before and after antibiotic therapy
      (2) Weekly, when the catheter is not in use
   b. Briskly irrigate the Groshong catheter with 20 ml of normal saline solution
      (1) After blood sample withdrawal
      (2) After blood transfusions
      (3) After administration of blood products
      (4) If blood is observed in the catheter
   c. Irrigate the Groshong catheter with 30 ml of normal saline solution
      (1) After TPN infusion
5. Maintain positive pressure on the syringe plunger as the needle is removed from the injection cap.
6. Follow steps *11* through *14* of the procedure for *Blood Sampling*.

NURSING CONSIDERATIONS

Routine clamping of the Groshong catheter is not needed. Heparin is not required to keep the catheter open.

DOCUMENTATION GUIDELINES

Document the following on the visit report:
- The procedure and patient toleration
- Blood sampling and designated laboratory for delivery
- Amount of normal saline solution used for irrigation
- Condition of catheter exit site

- Dressing and cap change (if done)
- Any patient/caregiver instructions and response to teaching, including the ability to safely manage the Groshong catheter at home
- Physician notification, if applicable
- *Standard Precautions*
- Other pertinent findings

Document IV medications/solutions infused on the medication or IV record.

Update the plan of care.

Implantable Vascular Access Device Management

PURPOSE
- To administer IV fluids
- To sample blood for laboratory analysis
- To maintain the patency of the implantable vascular access device
- To prevent infection

RELATED PROCEDURES
- Administration of Intravenous Therapy: General Guidelines
- Central Venous Catheter Management
- Specimen Labeling and Transport (see Chapter 12)

GENERAL INFORMATION

The implantable vascular access device (IVAD) is implanted under the skin with the attached catheter surgically tunneled into the cephalic or external jugular vein. The catheter tip sits in the superior vena cava near the right atrium, much like other central venous catheters. Flush the port of the IVAD with 10 ml of normal saline solution after intravenous infusion or blood sampling. Then heparinize the IVAD with 5 ml of heparin solution. Heparinize the IVAD every 30 days when it is not in use.

EQUIPMENT

1. 100 U/ml heparin solution as prescribed by the physician
2. Sterile normal saline solution as prescribed by the physician
3. (1) Right-angle, noncoring needle with integrated extension tubing with clamp
4. 5 cc syringes, 10 cc syringes, and (1) 20 cc syringe for blood sampling
5. Blood specimen tubes
6. Laboratory requisition, labels
7. Antiseptic and alcohol wipes
8. Disposable sterile gloves, sharps container, and an impermeable plastic trash bag (see *Infection Control*)

STOP

❖ Blood Sampling

PROCEDURE

1. Explain the procedure to the patient/caregiver.
2. Review the orders for laboratory specimens, and obtain the correct blood tubes.
3. Assemble the equipment at a convenient work area, using aseptic technique.
4. Assist the patient to a comfortable position to access the IVAD.
5. Don sterile gloves and cleanse the skin over the IVAD septum (injection site) with antiseptic wipes. Start at the site of the needle entrance, and work in a circular motion 4 to 6 cm outward. Discard the wipe.
6. Repeat step 5 two additional times with antiseptic wipes.
7. Clean the area with an alcohol wipe; air dry.
8. Attach the syringe with 10 ml of normal saline solution to the extension tubing; prime the extension tubing and noncoring needle. (Only special noncoring needles can be used when entering the port.)
9. Palpate the location of the IVAD septum to access the portal septum.
10. Firmly push the needle through the skin and portal septum at a 90-degree angle, until it hits the bottom of the portal chamber (Fig. 7-5). You may hear a click as the needle touches the bottom of the portal chamber.
11. Flush the system with 10 ml of normal saline solution to confirm that fluid flows through the system.

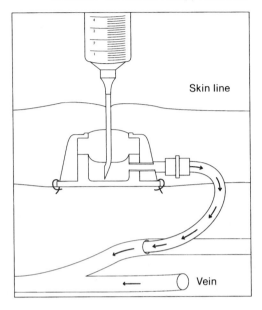

Skin line

Vein

Fig. 7-5 Position of the needle through the skin. (Courtesy Pharmacia Deltec, St Paul, Minnesota.)

12. Aspirate 5 ml of blood, then discard.
13. Clamp the extension tubing, then remove the syringe and discard it in a sharps container.
14. Attach a 20 cc syringe. Unclamp the extension tubing, and withdraw the appropriate amount of blood for a sample.
15. Repeat steps *13* and *14* until the appropriate amount of blood sample is obtained.
16. When the blood sampling is completed, clamp the tubing and remove the syringe. Discard the syringe in a sharps container.
17. Attach the syringe containing 10 ml of normal saline solution. Unclamp the extension tubing, and irrigate the IVAD.
18. Clamp the extension tubing, and remove the syringe. Discard the syringe.
19. Attach the syringe containing the 5 ml of heparin solution. Unclamp the extension tubing, and flush the system.
20. Maintain positive pressure on the syringe plunger as the syringe is removed to prevent backflow of blood into the

portal septum and to ensure a heparin lock (Fig. 7-6). Hold the port in place while removing the needle. Discard the needle, tubing, and syringe.

21. Cleanse the injection site with an antiseptic wipe, followed by an alcohol wipe; air dry.
22. Label and prepare the blood tube(s) for transport.
23. Provide patient comfort measures.
24. Clean and replace the equipment. Discard disposable items according to *Standard Precautions*.

❖ Bolus Injection

PROCEDURE

1. Access the IVAD as described in the procedure for *Blood Sampling*.
2. Flush the system with 10 ml of normal saline solution to ensure patency. Secure the noncoring needle with tape.
3. Clamp the extension tubing, and remove the syringe. Discard the syringe.
4. Attach the syringe with the drug to be injected into the extension tubing.
5. Inject the medication.
6. When the injection is complete, clamp the extension tubing. Remove the syringe, and discard it.

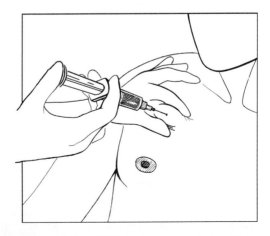

Fig. 7-6 Maintaining positive pressure as needle is withdrawn. (Courtesy Pharmacia Deltec, St Paul, Minnesota.)

7. Irrigate the IVAD with 10 ml of normal saline solution, followed by 5 ml of heparin flush. (Be careful to clamp the tubing when exchanging syringes.)
8. Maintain positive pressure on the syringe plunger as you withdraw the noncoring needle to prevent backflow of blood into the portal septum and to ensure a heparin lock.
9. Follow steps 23 and 24 of the procedure for *Blood Sampling.*

❖ Continuous Infusion

PROCEDURE

1. Access the IVAD as described in the procedure for *Blood Sampling.* Use a right-angle, noncoring needle with an extension tubing.
2. Clamp the extension tubing.
3. Attach the syringe with 10 ml of normal saline solution to the extension tubing. Unclamp the extension tubing, and flush the portal septum.
4. Clamp the extension tubing, and remove the syringe.
5. Connect the IV set or infusion to the extension tubing.
6. Unclamp the extension tubing and begin the infusion.
7. Secure the needle placement with sterile Steri-Strips or with ½-inch tape. Roll a 2- × 2-inch piece of sterile gauze under the needle to stabilize it, if needed. Apply transparent adhesive dressing, and tape all connections.
8. Loop the extension tubing on the dressing, and secure it with tape.
9. Follow steps 23 and 24 of the procedure for *Blood Sampling.*

NURSING CONSIDERATIONS

Use a sterile needle and tubing for each bolus access.

Change the sterile needle and tubing for continuous infusion every 7 days or per agency protocol.

Follow the manufacturer's recommendations for blood sampling for PAS PORT and PICC lines.

A dressing is not required when the port is not accessed.

DOCUMENTATION GUIDELINES

Document the following on the visit report:
- The procedure and patient toleration
- Blood sampling and designated laboratory for delivery
- Patency of the IVAD
- Condition of the skin over the IVAD

- Any patient/caregiver instructions and response to teaching, including the ability to safely manage the IVAD at home
- Physician notification, if applicable
- *Standard Precautions*
- Other pertinent findings

Document IV medications/solutions infused on the medication or IV record.

Update the plan of care.

Multiple-Lumen Nontunneled Catheter Management

PURPOSE
- To administer IV fluids
- To sample blood for laboratory analysis

RELATED PROCEDURES
- Administration of Intravenous Therapy: General Guidelines
- Central Venous Catheter Management
- Specimen Labeling and Transport (see Chapter 12)

GENERAL INFORMATION
The multiple- or triple-lumen catheter typically has three ports. The white and blue lumens are of equal diameter. The red-rust colored lumen is slightly larger and should be used for infusion of blood and for obtaining blood specimens. This central venous catheter is for short-term use only.

Irrigate all accessed ports of the multiple-lumen catheter with normal saline solution, followed by heparin flush before or after use and daily to maintain patency of the lumens. Follow the manufacturer's recommendations for a needleless system.

❖ Blood Sampling
EQUIPMENT
1. Sterile normal saline solution as prescribed by the physician

2. 100 U/ml heparin solution as prescribed by the physician
3. Syringes with 1-inch, 20-gauge needles
4. Blood tubes
5. Laboratory requisitions and labels
6. Antiseptic and alcohol wipes
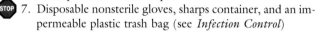
7. Disposable nonsterile gloves, sharps container, and an impermeable plastic trash bag (see *Infection Control*)

PROCEDURE

1. Explain the procedure to the patient/caregiver.
2. Assemble the equipment at a convenient work area.
3. Assist the patient to a comfortable position to access the IV.
4. Review the physician's order for laboratory specimens, and obtain the correct blood tubes.
5. Stop infusions through all ports being used for IV infusion.
6. Clean the injection cap of the red-rust–colored lumen with antiseptic wipes, followed by alcohol wipes; air dry.
7. Draw the blood specimen in the following manner:
   a. Attach a 10 cc syringe, unclamp the catheter, and withdraw at least 6 ml of blood, then discard the syringe and needle into a sharps container
   b. Attach a syringe—the size required for obtaining specimens—then withdraw enough blood for the specimens needed (use this method for drawing antibiotic levels); clamp the lumen
8. Transfer blood into the test tube appropriate for the laboratory collection. Discard the used syringe (and needle, if used) in a sharps container.
9. Unclamp the catheter lumen.
10. Irrigate the lumen with 10 ml of normal saline solution, then flush with the ordered amount of heparin solution, remembering to clamp the lumen in between flushing.
11. Maintain positive pressure on the syringe plunger as you withdraw the needle to prevent a backflow of blood into the catheter tip and to ensure a heparin lock. Then clamp the lumen.
12. Resume infusion(s) to the other lumens if they are stopped.
13. Label and prepare the test tube(s) for transport.
14. Provide patient comfort measures.
15. Clean and replace the equipment. Discard disposable items according to *Standard Precautions*.

❖ Intermittent Infusion

EQUIPMENT

1. 100 U/ml heparin solution as prescribed by the physician
2. Sterile normal saline solution as prescribed by the physician
3. (3) 5 cc syringes with 1-inch, 23-gauge needles
4. Antiseptic and alcohol wipes

🛑 5. Disposable nonsterile gloves, sharps container, and an impermeable plastic trash bag (see *Infection Control*)

PROCEDURE

1. Follow steps *1* through *3* of the procedure for *Blood Sampling*.
2. Clean the injection cap with an antiseptic wipe, followed by alcohol wipes; air dry.
3. Unclamp the selected lumen for infusion.
4. Flush the lumen with 5 ml of normal saline solution.
5. Begin the infusion, using a small-bore needle to puncture the injection cap.
6. Secure the needle to the injection cap with tape.
7. Tape the connection, making tabs on the ends of the tape by folding them back ½ inch. (The tabs on the end of the tape will enable you to remove it easily.)
8. Irrigate the catheter lumen with 5 ml of normal saline solution, then flush with 2.5 ml of heparin solution when the infusion is complete.
9. Maintain a positive pressure on the syringe plunger as you remove the needle to prevent a backflow of blood into the catheter tip cap and to ensure a heparin lock.
10. Clamp the lumen with the slide guard.
11. Follow steps *14* and *15* of the procedure for *Blood Sampling*.

NURSING CONSIDERATIONS

Irrigate all accessed ports of the multiple-lumen catheter with normal saline solution, followed by the heparin flush before and after use and daily to maintain patency of lumens.

It may not be possible to aspirate blood if it is drawn too quickly or if the syringe used is smaller than 20 cc.

It may be necessary to clamp the lumen with the slide guard and to remove the Luer-Lok injection cap to obtain blood.

Do not draw clotting studies (prothrombin time [PT], partial thromboplastin time [PTT]) from the catheter. Draw clotting studies peripherally before the catheter is heparinized because circulating heparin affects the PTT results up to 4 hours after the catheter has been heparinized.

DOCUMENTATION GUIDELINES

Document the following on the visit report:
- The procedure and patient toleration
- Catheter exit site and the condition of the catheter, including the patency of all lumens
- Blood sampling and designated laboratory of delivery
- Any patient/caregiver instructions and response to teaching, including the ability to safely manage the multiple-lumen catheter at home
- Physician notification, if applicable
- *Standard Precautions*
- Other pertinent findings

Document IV medications/solutions infused on the medication or IV record.

Update the plan of care.

Peripheral Inserted Central Catheter: Insertion Guidelines

PURPOSE

- To provide guidelines and a standardization of procedure for the peripheral insertion of a central venous catheter, referred to as a peripheral inserted central catheter (PICC) line

GENERAL INFORMATION

Insertion of PICC lines should be done by a PICC-certified nurse. Before the PICC line is placed, the patient's chart should be reviewed for (1) the physician's order, (2) site restrictions, (3) coagulation status, and (4) medical allergies. A post-insertion chest x-ray is recommended to verify the catheter tip position, if it is being placed in the superior vena cava. A patient permit is required before placement.

PICC lines can be used for administration of blood products, chemotherapy, antibiotics, fluids, and controlled narcotic infusions. Superior vena cava placement is required for the infusion of TPN or any irritating or sclerosis agents. PICC lines should never be used for high-pressure injection (i.e., diagnostic procedure or bolus emergency drugs). Do not use a syringe smaller than 5 cc with PICC lines. The alarm feature of the infusion pumps should not exceed 40 psi for 3 French catheters or larger.

EQUIPMENT

1. PICC tray (single-lumen 3 French or double-lumen 4 French each)
2. Sterile 5 cc or 10 cc syringes with needles (2)
3. Sterile Luer-Lok injection cap or reflux valve
4. Sterile 3-inch Luer-Lok extension set
5. Vial of 100 U/ml heparin solution as prescribed by the physician
6. Vial of 10 ml bacteriostatic 0.9% sodium chloride as prescribed by the physician
7. Transparent occlusive dressing
8. Tourniquets (2)
9. Sterile 2- × 2-inch gauze dressings (2)
10. Sterile 4- × 4-inch gauze dressings (4)
11. Antiseptic and alcohol wipes
12. Two pairs of disposable sterile gloves, mask with an eye shield, gown, sharps container, and an impermeable plastic trash bag (*see Infection Control*)

PROCEDURE

1. Explain the procedure to the patient/caregiver. Obtain a written consent for the procedure.
2. Assemble the equipment at a convenient work area.
3. Assist the patient to a comfortable position to insert the IV.
4. Apply a tourniquet and evaluate the antecubital veins for venipuncture. Remove the tourniquet.
5. Using a tape measure, measure the patient for the desired final catheter tip location. Position the patient's arm at a 45-degree angle from the body.
   a. **Subclavian vein:** Measure and record the distance from the insertion site to the sternal notch; if the catheter is

to be inserted with no amount of the catheter left out from the site, cut the catheter 1 inch shorter than the distance from the insertion site to the sternal notch; if 1 inch of the catheter is to be left out from the exit site, cut the full length from the insertion site to the sternal notch

b. **Superior vena cava (SVC):** If 1 inch of the catheter is to be left out at an exit site, measure from 1 inch below the insertion site to the second intercostal space; if the intercostal spaces are not palpable, one-third of the distance from the sternal notch to the xiphoid process may be used as an estimate; a catheter entering from the left arm will be slightly longer because it crosses over the chest and into the SVC, which is along the right border of the sternum; (a post-insertion x-ray examination is required to verify superior vena cava placement; therefore, SVC placement should be done while the patient is in the hospital)

c. **Midaxillary:** Measure from the insertion site to the desired tip location, allowing for the amount of the catheter that is to be left out from the exit site as appropriate

6. Measure the bilateral arm circumference midway between the elbow and the shoulder, and record for future reference.

7. Clean the work area, scrub the hands, and put on a mask and eye protection. Open a sterile PICC tray, and add sterile items to the PICC tray.

8. Prepare the patient for the following procedure:
   a. Head of the bed is as flat as possible
   b. Linen protector is under the arm to be cannulated
   c. Provide adequate work space and lighting
   d. Tourniquet is in place but is **not** tied

9. Don sterile gloves and gown.

10. Place a large sterile drape under the patient's arm.

11. Prepare the insertion site for 3 minutes with alcohol wipes, and follow in 3 minutes with povidone iodine (Betadine) wipes. Vigorously cleanse the antecubital area from the center outward in a circular motion.

12. If necessary, shorten the catheter in the following manner:
    a. Do not touch the catheter with gloved hands; always use forceps to handle the catheter

    b. Pull the guidewire out of the catheter ¼ to ½ inch short of the desired length; bend the guidewire at the hub to prevent movement

    c. Cut the catheter at a 45-degree angle. Do **not** trim the guidewire or stylet.

13. Draw up 5 ml of normal saline solution and 5 ml of heparin flush. Prime the extension tubing.

14. Place a fenestrated drape over the prepared puncture site, and add sterile 4- × 4-inch gauze around the site as needed to absorb the blood flow.

15. Tighten the tourniquet, placing sterile 4- × 4-inch gauze on the tails to prevent contamination when releasing the tourniquet. Don a second set of sterile gloves.

16. Perform venipuncture in the following manner:

    a. Venipuncture is verified by a flashback of blood into the hub or the syringe (if used)

    b. Advance the introducer sheath into the vein approximately ¼ inch

    c. Remove the needle; to control the blood flow, apply pressure above the introducer with the fifth finger or with 2- × 2-inch gauze, and occlude the end of the introducer

    d. Release the tourniquet with the 4- × 4-inch gauze

17. The catheter is advanced in the following manner:

    a. Thread the catheter through the introducer with forceps in short, controlled steps

    b. After 5 to 7 inches of the catheter is placed, remove the introducer according to manufacturer's guidelines, and allow 3 inches of the catheter to remain outside the vein to facilitate removal of the introducer

    c. Advance the remainder of the catheter

18. If the catheter is placed centrally, instruct the patient to touch his or her chin to the shoulder of the arm being cannulated to promote insertion while threading in the catheter.

19. The catheter guidewire is removed in the following manner:

    a. Stabilize the catheter with one hand, and gently pull out the guidewire; do not pull vigorously or suddenly

    b. After the guidewire is removed, immediately place the thumb over the hub to prevent an ingress of air

c. Place the extension set with the syringe attached on the hub, and secure the connection

d. Flush 3 ml of saline solution into the catheter; withdraw blood into the extension set to confirm that the catheter tip is within the vascular system; flush the remaining saline solution into the catheter

e. Heparinize the catheter with 3 to 5 ml of 100 U/ml heparin solution

20. Apply a sterile occlusive dressing in the following manner:

a. Cleanse the site with antiseptic wipes

b. Pull the catheter out 1 inch and L-shaped to prevent kinking and occlusion at the bend of the arm; secure with Steri-Strips

c. Place 2- × 2-inch gauze pads folded under the length of the hub and extension tubing

d. Cover with two 10- × 14-cm transparent dressings so that the site is covered from 1½ inches above the exit site

21. Provide patient comfort measures. Dry warmth may be applied to the area of insertion immediately after the line is secured and the dressing is applied. Continue warmth for 24 to 48 hours as tolerated by the patient.

22. Clean and replace the equipment. Discard disposable items according to *Standard Precautions.*

NURSING CONSIDERATIONS

Teach the caregiver/patient to watch for signs/symptoms of mechanical phlebitis, including edema, red streaks from the insertion site and cording, and intense and continuous pain in the arm of insertion. Dry warmth should resolve this common problem.

DOCUMENTATION GUIDELINES

Document the following on the visit report:
- The patient verification and/or chart review of allergy
- The procedure and patient toleration
- Catheter type, gauge, lot number, total length, and length inserted
- Insertion site
- Catheter tip position
- Application of occlusive dressing

- Complications or problems encountered
- Physician notification, if applicable
- *Standard Precautions*
- Other pertinent findings

Update the plan of care.

Peripheral Inserted Central Catheter: Removal of the Catheter

PURPOSE

- To provide guidelines for PICC removal

RELATED PROCEDURE

- Peripheral Insertion of a Central Catheter

GENERAL INFORMATION

It is recommended that an IV-certified registered nurse remove the PICC catheter (preferably an IV nurse who has attended a PICC certification course).

EQUIPMENT

1. Sterile normal saline as prescribed by the physician
2. 10 cc syringe with needle
3. Antiseptic ointment if prescribed by the physician
4. A towel or protective barrier 5. Sterile 2- × 2-inch gauze dressing
5. Hypoallergenic tape
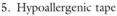 6. Sterile disposable gloves, sharps container, and an impermeable plastic trash bag (see *Infection Control*)

PROCEDURE

1. Explain the procedure to the patient/caregiver.
2. Assemble the equipment in a convenient work area.
3. Assist the patient to a comfortable position to remove the IV.
4. Place the towel or protective barrier under the patient's arm.

5. Remove the old dressing, and discard.
6. Examine the catheter exit site for signs of redness or infection; report to the physician as needed.
7. If the catheter is patent, flush with 3 cc of normal saline solution before removal.
8. Grasp the catheter near the exit site, and pull the catheter out with a slow, steady motion. Continue to remove the catheter by regrasping the catheter near the exit site until it is completely removed.
9. If the patient complains of severe pain or if abnormal resistance to removal is felt, stop the procedure. Secure the catheter with tape; apply a sterile 2- × 2-inch dressing over the insertion site and notify the physician for further orders.
10. Apply pressure with a 2- × 2-inch gauze dressing until any bleeding stops.
11. When the bleeding has stopped, apply antiseptic ointment (if ordered) to the site and cover with a new sterile 2- × 2-inch gauze dressing; secure with tape. (Vaseline gauze may also be used to cover the insertion site to minimize the possibility of air entering the central venous system through the open insertion site.)
12. Measure the length of catheter removed and compare to note with length inserted.
13. Clean and replace equipment. Discard disposable items according to *Standard Precautions.*

NURSING CONSIDERATIONS

Instruct the patient/caregiver to leave the dressing in place for 24 hours.

Instruct the patient/caregiver to report any fever or unusual pain or discomfort to the physician.

DOCUMENTATION GUIDELINES

Document the following on the visit report:
- The procedure and patient toleration
- The condition of the catheter exit site
- Size of the catheter and gauge and length of the catheter removed; if the length of catheter removed is not the same as that inserted, notify the physician and follow any further orders
- The condition of the catheter

- Assess the type of the catheter for any tearing or other damage; notify the physician of any noted damage
- Any patient/caregiver instructions and response to teaching
- Physician notification, if applicable
- *Standard Precautions*
- Other pertinent findings

Update the plan of care.

Peripheral Intravenous Management

PURPOSE

- To administer IV fluids
- To hydrate the patient
- To sample blood for laboratory analysis
- To heparin lock an IV for intermittent infusion of fluids and/or medications

RELATED PROCEDURES

- Administration of Intravenous Therapy: General Guidelines
- Specimen Labeling and Transport (see Chapter 12)

GENERAL INFORMATION

When choosing a site to start an IV, select the largest convenient vein most distal to an extremity. Choose a site below the patient's elbow to increase comfort. Avoid cannulation over joints or previous IV sites because this predisposes to infiltration. The wing-tip or scalp needle is useful for accessing small or fragile veins for blood sampling. Heparin lock the IV for intermittent infusion of IV fluids and/or medications.

EQUIPMENT

1. IV fluids as prescribed by the physician
2. IV administration set
3. Tourniquet
4. Arm board (optional)
5. Number 18- to 22-gauge needle, catheter or wing-tip needle with integrated extension tubing

6. Transparent adhesive dressing or sterile 2- × 2-inch gauze dressing
7. Hypoallergenic tape
8. IV pole
9. Blood specimen tubes; 5 cc to 10 cc syringes with 1-inch, 20-gauge needles; laboratory requisition labels for blood sampling
10. Antiseptic and alcohol wipes
11. Disposable nonsterile gloves, sharps container, and an impermeable plastic trash bag (see *Infection Control*)

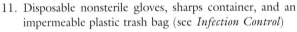

❖ Insertion of a Peripheral IV and Initiation of Hydration Fluids

PROCEDURE

1. Explain the procedure to the patient/caregiver.
2. Assemble the equipment at a convenient work area.
3. Assist the patient to a comfortable position to initiate or access the IV.
4. Use aseptic technique to set up IV fluids in the following manner:
   a. Clamp the tubing with the flow regulator
   b. Spike the container with tubing; hang the container on the IV pole
   c. Squeeze the drip chamber until it is one-half full
   d. Open the flow regulator, and prime the tubing; reclamp the tubing to prevent fluid flow
   e. Time tape the IV bag if the pump is not used
5. Apply a tourniquet, and select the vein.
6. Cleanse the selected site with antiseptic wipes. Start at the point of needle insertion, and clean outward in a circular motion, approximately 3 to 4 cm. Repeat with alcohol wipes; air dry.
7. Stretch the skin tight. Insert the needle with the bevel up at a 30-degree angle and parallel to the skin. Decrease the angle, and move the needle forward until the needle enters the vein.
8. Observe for blood flow to indicate correct needle placement.
9. Pull the needle back slightly; advance the catheter, and release the tourniquet.
10. Attach the IV tubing to the catheter hub. Open the flow regulator.

11. Slowly start the IV infusion. Assess the site for infiltration. If infiltration occurs, discontinue the IV, and restart the IV at an alternative site. Adjust the prescribed flow rate once the correct placement of the catheter has been established.

12. Tape the catheter to prevent accidental dislodgement. Avoid taping directly over the catheter because this may impede blood flow.

13. Apply transparent adhesive or 2- × 2-inch gauze dressing. Picture frame the dressing with tape to secure the site so that early signs of phlebitis or infiltration can be detected.

14. Secure the IV tubing to the patient's arm with tape to prevent tugging.

15. Instruct the patient/caregiver in the management of home IV therapy (see the Patient Education Guidelines box, *Home IV Therapy,* on pp. 281-282).

16. Provide patient comfort measures.

17. Clean and replace the equipment. Discard disposable items according to *Standard Precautions.*

NURSING CONSIDERATIONS

If the venipuncture is unsuccessful, reattempt it with a new catheter. If unsuccessful after 3 attempts, notify the physician for further orders.

Label the catheter insertion site with the catheter guage, date and time of insertion, and initials of the nurse.

❖ Inserting a Winged-Tip Needle for Blood Sampling

PROCEDURE

1. Follow steps *1* through *5* of the procedure for *Insertion of a Peripheral IV and Initiation of Hydration Fluids.* Keep the cap on the needle. Attach the 10 cc syringe to the hub of the integrated extension tubing on the wing-tip needle.

2. Remove the cap from the winged-tip needle. Point the needle in the direction of the blood flow, and hold it at a 45-degree angle above the skin, with the bevel facing up.

3. Pinch the wings tightly together. Pierce the patient's skin at a point slightly to one side of the vein, approximately ½ inch below the spot where you plan to puncture the vein wall.

4. Decrease the needle angle, until the needle is almost level with the skin surface, and direct it toward the selected vein.

5. Puncture the vein. Observe for blood backflow.

6. Lift the bevel of the needle off the vein floor, and advance it, until the needle is inserted into the vein.
7. Remove the tourniquet.
8. Withdraw the blood sample into the syringe.
9. Discontinue the IV once the blood sample has been obtained.
10. Apply a 2- × 2-inch gauze dressing or adhesive bandage to the venipuncture site.
11. Attach a 20-gauge needle onto the syringe with blood sample. Then push the needle through the rubber stopper to fill the blood specimen tube(s). Label blood tubes and transport.
12. Follow steps *16* and *17* of the procedure for *Insertion of a Peripheral IV and Initiation of Hydration Fluids.*

NURSING CONSIDERATIONS

If the winged-tip needle has an integrated extension set with a two-way needle hub, attach the Vacutainer to the two-way needle hub. Slide the blood specimen tube(s) into the Vacutainer and onto the two-way needle once the vein is accessed to obtain blood samples.

❖ Managing a Heparin Lock: Initiating a Heparin Lock

EQUIPMENT

1. Sterile normal saline solution as prescribed by the physician
2. 100 U/ml heparin solution as prescribed by the physician
3. Sterile Luer-Lok injection cap
4. Number 18- to 22-gauge catheter and venipuncture supplies
5. Sterile 3 cc syringes with 1-inch, 23- to 25-gauge needles
6. Kelly clamp
7. Antiseptic and alcohol wipes
8. Disposable nonsterile gloves, sharps container, and an impermeable plastic trash bag (see *Infection Control*)

PROCEDURE

1. Follow steps *1* through *3* of the procedure for *Insertion of a Peripheral IV and Initiation of Hydration Fluids.*
2. Draw up 1 ml of heparin solution and 2 ml of normal saline solution into separate syringes.

3. Cleanse the rubber stopper on the Luer-Lok injection cap with antiseptic wipes, followed by alcohol wipes; air dry.
4. Prime the Luer-Lok injection cap with normal saline solution.
5. Perform venipuncture. See the procedure for *Initiation of a Peripheral IV and Initiation of Hydration Fluids.*
6. Attach the saline-filled Luer-Lok injection cap into the cannula, then flush with 2 ml of normal saline solution.
7. Observe the catheter exit site for signs of infiltration or leakage. If the catheter is patent, flush the Luer-Lok injection cap with 1 ml of heparin solution.
8. Maintain the positive pressure on the syringe plunger as you withdraw the needle to prevent the backflow of blood into the catheter tip and to ensure a heparin lock.
9. Tape to secure the catheter and to prevent accidental dislodgement.
10. Apply a sterile 2- × 2-inch gauze or transparent adhesive dressing. Picture frame with tape as needed to secure the dressing. Date and time the dressing.
11. Follow steps *16* and *17* of the procedure for *Insertion of a Peripheral IV and Initiation of Hydration Fluids.*

❖ Managing a Heparin Lock: Transferring a Continuous Infusion to a Heparin Lock

EQUIPMENT

1. 100 U/ml heparin solution as prescribed by the physician
2. Sterile normal saline solution as prescribed by the physician
3. Sterile Luer-Lok injection cap
4. Kelly clamp
5. Sterile 3 cc syringes with 1-inch, 23- to 25-gauge needles
6. Antiseptic and alcohol wipes
7. Disposable nonsterile gloves, sharps container, and an impermeable plastic trash bag (see *Infection Control*)

PROCEDURE

1. Follow steps *1* through *3* of the procedure for *Insertion of a Peripheral IV and Initiation of Hydration Fluids.*
2. Clamp off the intravenous tubing with a flow regulator.
3. Disconnect the tubing, using a Kelly clamp to stabilize the catheter hub.

4. Remove the protective covering from the Luer-Lok injection cap and aseptically insert it into the hub of the catheter.
5. Slowly flush with 2 ml of normal saline solution, and assess for infiltration to ascertain the catheter position. Flush with 1 ml of heparin solution if no swelling or leakage is noted.
6. Maintain positive pressure on the syringe plunger as you withdraw the needle to prevent backflow into the catheter tip and to ensure a heparin lock.
7. Follow steps *16* and *17* of the procedure for *Insertion a Peripheral IV and Initiation of Hydration Fluids*.

❖ Managing a Heparin Lock: Stopping/ Discontinuing a Continuous Infusion

EQUIPMENT

1. Same as the procedure for *Transferring a Continuous Infusion to a Heparin Lock*

PROCEDURE

1. Follow steps *1* through *3* of the procedure for *Insertion of a Peripheral IV and Initiation of Hydration Fluids*.
2. Draw up 2 ml of normal saline solution and 1 ml of heparin solution in separate syringes.
3. Clamp off the IV tubing with the flow regulator.
4. Remove the needle and tubing from the heparin lock by one of the following methods:
   a. Remove the needle from the Luer-Lok injection cap; carefully remove the needle from the end of the tubing and place it in the sharps container; discard the tubing and IV bag
   b. Cut the IV tubing 3 inches above the needle; place the needle and the connecting tubing in a sharps container; discard the remainder of the tubing and IV bag
5. Irrigate the Luer-Lok injection cap and the IV catheter with 2 ml normal saline solution, then flush with 1 ml of heparin solution.
6. Maintain positive pressure on the syringe plunger as you withdraw the needle to prevent backflow of blood into the catheter tip and to ensure a heparin lock.
7. Evaluate for dressing change.
8. Follow steps *16* and *17* of the procedure for *Insertion a Peripheral IV and Initiation of Hydration Fluids*.

DOCUMENTATION GUIDELINES

Document the following on the visit report.
- The procedure and patient toleration
- Type and number of the catheter that has been inserted
- Condition of the catheter exit site
- Blood specimen drawn and designated laboratory for delivery
- Any patient/caregiver instructions and response to teaching, including the ability to safely manage home IV therapy
- Physician notification, if applicable
- *Standard Precautions*
- Other pertinent findings

Document IV medications/solutions infused on the medication of IV record.

Update the plan of care.

Patient Education Guidelines
Home IV Therapy

1. Wash your hands before and after IV care.
2. Check your IV site. If it is red or painful, do not administer IV fluids, and call the home health agency clinical supervisor. Your home health agency's number is _____.
3. Flush your IV catheter with _____ ml of normal saline solution before administering IV fluids or medications, such as antibiotics.
4. When preparing your IV fluids, close the roller clamp on the IV tubing. Then attach the IV tubing to the IV bag without touching the sterile surfaces. *Keep the tubing and connections as germ-free as possible.*
5. Squeeze the drip chamber on the IV tubing until it is about one-half full. Always remember to flush air from the IV tubing.
6. If you have an IV pump, follow your nurse's instructions to hook up your IV tubing and to operate the pump.
7. Connect the IV fluids to the catheter. Open the roller clamp. You should see fluid flow through the drip chamber.
8. Turn on the IV pump or adjust the roller clamp on the IV tubing to adjust the drops per minute as your physician has ordered. Your drops per minute are _____.
9. Watch the rate of flow of your IV fluids every hour, and do not let the bag of IV fluids run dry because this can cause the catheter to clog up.
10. Administer your IV fluids and medications at the correct dose and time.
11. Stop the IV infusion when it has been completed. Irrigate and flush your catheter as your nurse has shown you to keep your IV line open. Flush with _____ of normal saline solution and _____ of heparin solution. Check with your nurse because some catheters do not require a heparin flush.
12. If you have a central line, keep your catheter clamped at all times when it is not in use.

Continued

Patient Education Guidelines

Home IV Therapy—cont'd

13. Change your IV dressing if it becomes loose or soiled.

14. Clean the entry site of your IV with an antiseptic wipe. Start at the center and move outward about 1 to 2 inches in a circular motion. Do this two more times with fresh antiseptic wipes. Never return to the entry site of your IV with the same wipe because this could spread germs into your IV.

15. Cover your IV with a gauze dressing, and secure it with tape. Tape your IV catheter to prevent tugging or to prevent it from accidentally coming out.

16. If your IV catheter accidentally gets torn, clamp it to prevent leakage or air embolism, and notify the home health agency clinical supervisor.

17. If the IV catheter accidentally comes out, cover the site with a gauze dressing to prevent bleeding. Hold pressure to the area for 5 minutes, and then notify the home health agency clinical supervisor.

18. If you should feel short of breath or dizzy, notify the Emergency Medical Services (EMS) for emergency assistance. Your local EMS number is _____.

19. Carefully place used needles in a sharps container. Always avoid touching the needle. Keep your sharps container out of the reach of children. When your sharps container is full, call your home IV supplier for a new sharps container or other IV supplies.

20. Record the date and time that you hang a bag of IV fluids.

21. Call the home health agency clinical supervisor if the following circumstances occur:
    - Dressing supplies are needed
    - You have questions or problems regarding your IV
    - You are hospitalized

CHAPTER 8

Infusions

Antibiotic Therapy: Intermittent Infusion

PURPOSE
- To provide guidelines for intermittent administration of intravenous (IV) antibiotics
- To treat infection

RELATED PROCEDURES
- Administration of Intravenous Therapy: General Guidelines (see Chapter 7)
- Administration of Medications: General Guidelines (see Chapter 9)
- Central Venous Catheter Management (see Chapter 7)
- Peripheral Intravenous Management (see Chapter 7)
- Specimen Labeling and Transport (see Chapter 12)

GENERAL INFORMATION
Antibiotics act by inhibiting bacterial-wall synthesis or by altering the intracellular function of bacteria, such as deoxyribonucleic acid (DNA) binding and reproduction. Categories of antibiotics that are used most widely include the cephalosporins, the aminoglycosides, and penicillins.

Antibiotic therapy is usually administered through intermittent drug infusion. The medication is diluted in a small bag of dextrose 5% water (D5W) or normal saline (NS) solution and is administered for approximately 30 minutes. Administration time varies according to the volume of solution to be infused.

Since adverse side effects are possible with the use of any antibiotics (Table 8-1), the first dose should be administered in a controlled setting, where emergency medical services are available. Antibiotics may be administered via peripheral or central venous access devices. Administer specific medications accord-

Table 8-1 Adverse side effects of antibiotics

Aminoglycosides	Nephrotoxicity, ototoxicity, neuromuscular blockade, and respiratory depression
Cephalosporins	Anaphylaxis, diarrhea, neutropenia, and altered liver function
Penicillins	Anaphylaxis, diarrhea, nephrotoxicity, central nervous system changes, and cutaneous reactions

ing to the manufacturer's instructions. It is recommended that IV-certified nurses administer antibiotic therapy in the home.

Consult with the physician or the home infusion service's pharmacist regarding serum level monitoring of antibiotics. Electrolyte, liver panel, blood urea nitrogen (BUN), and serum creatinine levels may be required for therapy lasting at least 5 days. In addition, serum peak and trough levels are usually monitored for aminoglycoside or vancomycin therapy (Table 8-2).

Before administering an antibiotic, ascertain the patency of the IV with a normal saline flush. The typical sequence of antibiotic administration is saline flush, antibiotic, saline flush, heparinization, which is known as the *SASH* method. Change the tubing every day. Use a new needle on the tubing with each antibiotic administration. Review the manufacturer's recommendations if a *needleless* system is being used.

EQUIPMENT

1. Antibiotic medication as prescribed by the physician
2. Sterile normal saline solution as prescribed by the physician
3. 100 U/ml heparin solutions as prescribed by the physician
4. Syringes (follow specific catheter procedures for irrigation, heparinization, and blood sampling)
5. Two 1-inch 21- to 23-gauge needles
6. IV pole
7. IV administration set
8. Blood tubes, labels, and laboratory requisition for blood sampling if required

Table 8-2 Antibiotic drug classification and suggested laboratory tests

Drug classification	Suggested test and frequency
Aminoglycosides: gentamicin, amikacin tobramycin Vancomycin/clindamycin	Audiogram weekly if therapy lasts longer than 2 weeks Sequential multiple analysis-6 (SMA-6), peak and trough twice each week
Beta-lactam cephalosporins: includes cefazolin (Ancef), ceftriaxone, ceftazidime	Complete blood count (CBC), SMA-6 once each week
Penicillins: ampicillin, penicillin G, penicillin V	CBC, SMA-6, serum glutamic oxaloacetic transaminase (SGOT) twice each week
Antifungals: amphotericin B	SMA-6, magnesium (Mg), CBC twice each week for therapy of more than 3 times each week; blood urea nitrogen (BUN), creatine each week
Sulfonamides: trimethoprim/ sulfamethoxazole (Bactrim)	CBC, SMA-6 once each week

Modified from Rice R: *Home health nursing practice: concepts and application,* ed 2, St Louis, 1996, Mosby.

9. Antiseptic and alcohol wipes

 10. Disposable nonsterile gloves, sharps container, and an impermeable plastic trash bag (see *Infection Control*)

PROCEDURE

1. Explain the procedure to the patient/caregiver.
2. Assemble the equipment at a convenient work area.
3. Assist the patient to a comfortable position to access the IV. Perform the necessary laboratory work.
4. Close the roller clamp on the IV tubing. Remove the protective cap from the antibiotic bag, and spike the bag with the IV tubing.
5. Hang the antibiotic bag on the IV pole. Squeeze the drip

chamber until it is half full. Open the roller clamp to expel air from the tubing.

6. Using aseptic technique, attach the needle to the hub of the tubing; leave the cap on.
7. Cleanse the injection port of the indwelling IV with an antiseptic wipe, followed by an alcohol wipe; air dry.
8. Flush the catheter with normal saline solution to ascertain patency.
9. Uncap and insert the needle into the injection port of the indwelling IV.
10. Secure the needle to the injection port with 1-inch tape. Tape the IV tubing to the patient's arm to prevent tugging.
11. Open the roller clamp, and begin the infusion at the prescribed rate.
12. Discontinue the IV after infusion. Place the needle in the sharps container; replace with a sterile-capped needle for the next infusion.
13. Clean the catheter injection port of the indwelling IV with an antiseptic wipe, followed by an alcohol wipe; air dry.
14. Flush the catheter with normal saline solution and heparinize according to specific catheter protocols.
15. Provide patient comfort measures.
16. Clean and replace the equipment. Discard disposable items according to *Standard Precautions.*

NURSING CONSIDERATIONS

Antibiotics may be administered simultaneously with compatible IVs; consult with the home infusion pharmacist for a compatibility check.

If the antibiotic is piggybacked into a continuous infusion, hang the medication container above the primary IV, and infuse at the prescribed rate. The secondary set may remain attached to the IV or may be removed until the next dose of antibiotic therapy. If the antibiotic line is removed, cap the end of the line with a new needle.

Instruct the patient/caregiver to store antibiotic medication bags in the refrigerator. Take the antibiotic out of the refrigerator 20 to 30 minutes before administration.

DOCUMENTATION GUIDELINES

Document the following on the visit report:
• The procedure and patient toleration
• Condition of catheter exit site

- Patency of the catheter
- Blood sampling and designated laboratory for delivery
- Any patient/caregiver instructions and response to teaching, including the ability to manage home antibiotic therapy safely
- Physician notification if applicable
- *Standard Precautions*
- Other pertinent findings

Document medications on the medication record.

Update the plan of care.

Chemotherapy

PURPOSE

- To provide guidelines for IV chemotherapy administration
- To treat cancer

RELATED PROCEDURES

- Administration of Intravenous Therapy: General Guidelines (see Chapter 7)
- Administration of Medications: General Guidelines (see Chapter 9)
- Central Venous Catheter Management (see Chapter 7)
- Specimen Labeling and Transport (see Chapter 12)

GENERAL INFORMATION

Chemotherapy is used to treat cancer. Chemotherapeutic drugs act primarily by inhibiting the growth of frequently dividing cells. Normal cells affected by chemotherapeutic drugs include red and white blood cells, hair follicles, the mucosal lining of the gastrointestinal tract, skin, and germinal cells (sperm and ova). Chemotherapy is administered according to a schedule to allow recovery of the body's normal cells. In addition, chemotherapy is commonly given in combination with other drugs to enhance tumor cell destruction.

It is recommended that only chemotherapy-certified nurses administer chemotherapeutic medications. The pharmacy will prepare and deliver all chemotherapeutic medications to the patient's home. In addition, the patient/caregiver must be provided with spill kits. Volumetric pumps must be used for all infusions. Administer bolus injections through the side arm of a running intravenous infusion. Review the manufacturer's recommendations if a *needleless* system is being used.

EQUIPMENT

1. Chemotherapeutic medication(s) and infusion fluids as prescribed by the physician
2. Antiemetic if prescribed by the physician
3. Sterile normal saline solution and 100 U/ml heparin solution or catheter flush solution per specific catheter protocols as prescribed by the physician
4. IV infusion set
5. IV infusion pump
6. Syringes for catheter flush
7. 5 cc syringes with 23-gauge needles and extravasation antidote as required; hot or cold compresses as recommended by the physician for extravasation
8. Blood tubes, labels, and laboratory requisition for blood sampling if required
9. Antiseptic and alcohol wipes to initiate chemotherapy or to access the IV catheter
10. Chemotherapy gloves or double nonsterile gloves, goggles, a resealable plastic bag, spill kit, sharps container, impermeable plastic trash bag, and a puncture- and leak-proof container (see *Infection Control*)

PROCEDURE

1. Explain the procedure to the patient/caregiver.
2. Verify allergies that the patient may have.
3. Explain the side effects of possible hair loss, nausea and vomiting, anorexia, stomatitis, constipation, diarrhea, and skin and hemopoietic changes.
4. Obtain a signed consent form before administering chemotherapy.
5. Obtain the necessary laboratory work.
6. Plan and intervene for the following possible chemotherapy side effects:
   a. Review home health agency cardiopulmonary resuscitation (CPR) guidelines

b. Consult with the physician, and consider pain medication for aches and pains

c. Instruct the patient to wear a wig, scarf, or turban for hair loss; (reassure the patient that hair loss is temporary and that the hair will regrow when the drug is stopped)

d. Instruct the patient to eat small and frequent meals that are high in protein for appetite loss

e. Instruct the patient to increase fiber in the diet to alleviate constipation; consult with the physician, and consider the use of a stool softener

f. Consult with the physician, and instruct the patient to increase fluid intake up to 2 to 3 quarts daily for cystitis

g. Consider psychiatric home health nurse referral for problems with depression or changes in mood or affect

h. Implement bleeding precautions for thrombocytopenia

i. Instruct the patient to maintain good personal hygiene

j. Instruct the patient to use a soft toothbrush or swab toothettes frequently to minimize the risk of oral mucosa breakdown

k. Premedicate with antiemetics before nausea begins or administer around the clock (for example, **before** administration of chemotherapeutic medication or meals)

l. Monitor the complete blood count, including platelets, liver function tests, baseline cardiac studies, urine creatinine clearance, and serum electrolytes, as ordered by the physician; notify the physician of abnormal clinical findings and laboratory values before the administration of the chemotherapeutic drug

7. Assist the patient to a comfortable position to access the IV.

8. Initiate the peripheral IV, or access the central venous catheter. (Vesicant drugs must be delivered via a central venous catheter.)

9. Don gloves; wear goggles.

10. Administer chemotherapeutic medication(s).

11. Evaluate the patient for signs of extravasation during the infusion. Be aware that tissue necrosis may not occur until 1 to 5 weeks after the drug extravasation. If extravasation is suspected or occurs, consult with the physician and consider the following:

a. Immediately **stop** the infusion of the chemotherapeutic drug as soon as extravasation of a cytotoxic or irritant agent is suspected or occurs

   b. Leave the needle in place

   c. Aspirate any residual drug from the IV tubing or the catheter and infiltration site

   d. Instill the prescribed antidote specific for the cytotoxic drug

   e. Remove the needle if it is clotted off, and inject the prescribed antidote subcutaneously clockwise into the infiltrated site, using a 25-gauge needle; change the needle with each new injection

   f. Apply sterile occlusive dressing

   g. Elevate the extremity

   h. Apply hot or cold compresses as ordered by the physician

12. Discontinue the IV after the medication(s) is (are) administered.

13. Flush the catheter according to specific protocols.

14. Provide patient comfort measures.

15. Clean and replace the equipment. Immediately clean up any chemotherapy spills. Be careful not to touch the spill. Place disposable items in a resealable bag, and discard. Place used needles and syringes in a puncture-proof, leak-proof container. **All chemotherapy materials, including bags and tubing, must be discarded in a leak-proof container.**

NURSING CONSIDERATIONS

Prepare chemotherapeutic agents for administration at a bathroom or kitchen counter on a plastic-backed field (e.g., on a plastic trash bag). The area should be washed thoroughly before and after preparation with soap and water or with 70% alcohol, and then allowed to dry.

Instruct the patient and family to wear gloves when handling linen contaminated with chemotherapeutic agents or excreta. Wash the contaminated linen **separately** from all other linens.

Follow local, state, and Environmental Protection Agency (EPA) recommendations for disposal of hazardous waste and chemotherapeutic medications and supplies.

DOCUMENTATION GUIDELINES

Document the following on the visit report:
- The procedure and patient toleration
- Side effects and therapeutic actions

- Blood sampling and designated laboratory for delivery
- Extravasation management
- IV catheter site before and after infusion or injection of chemotherapeutic medication(s)
- Catheter size and type
- Drug sequence and administration technique
- Any chemotherapy medications
- Any patient/caregiver instructions and response to teaching, including the ability to safely manage home chemotherapy
- Physician's notification, if applicable
- *Standard Precautions*
- Other pertinent findings

Document IV medications on the medication record. Document IV fluids on the IV record.

Consider an incident report for problems with extravasation.

Update the plan of care.

Lasix Intravenous Push

PURPOSE

- To promote diuresis
- To relieve edema

RELATED PROCEDURES

- Administration of Intravenous Therapy: General Guidelines (see Chapter 7)
- Administration of Medications: General Guidelines (see Chapter 9)
- Edema (see Chapter 2)
- Injections (see Chapter 9)
- Intake and Output (see Chapter 2)
- Peripheral Intravenous Management: Inserting a Winged-Tip Needle for Blood Sampling (see Chapter 7)
- Specimen Labeling and Transport (see Chapter 12)

GENERAL INFORMATION

Lasix (furosemide) intravenous push (IVP) is given to patients for whom oral Lasix is no longer effective. Careful monitoring of the patient's intake and output, serum potassium level, and weight are important in order to evaluate the efficacy of the Lasix.

EQUIPMENT

1. Lasix as prescribed by the physician
2. Sterile normal saline solution as prescribed by the physician
3. Number 21 or 23 winged-tip needle and a tourniquet
4. 3 cc syringes with 1-inch needles
5. Antiseptic wipes
6. 2- × 2-inch gauze dressing
7. Hypoallergenic tape
8. Blood tubes, labels, and laboratory requisition for blood sampling if required
9. Disposable nonsterile gloves, sharps container, and impermeable plastic trash bags (see *Infection Control*)

PROCEDURE

1. Explain the procedure to the patient/caregiver.
2. Assemble the equipment at a convenient work area.
3. Assist the patient to a comfortable sitting or supine position.
4. Assess the patient's cardiopulmonary status. Obtain the patient's vital signs (record blood pressure before and after the procedure).
5. Evaluate the fluid and electrolyte status.
   a. Weigh the patient
   b. Assess the patient's compliance with the low-salt diet or with fluid restrictions if ordered by the physician
6. Verify the medication with the patient's medication record, and check the patient's identity.
7. Prepare the medication from an ampule or a vial as described in the procedure for *Injections*. Replace the protective needle cap on the syringe.
8. Select the site for venipuncture. Use a large vein in the hand or forearm.
9. Apply a tourniquet above the venipuncture site.

10. Clean the venipuncture site with an antiseptic wipe. Begin at the venipuncture site, and proceed in an outward circular motion for approximately 4 to 5 cm.
11. Perform venipuncture using a winged-tip needle, with the bevel up at a 45-degree angle.
12. Flush the needle with 2 ml normal saline solution to check for infiltration. (Discontinue the IV, and repeat the procedure for problems with swelling or leaking around the IV site.)
13. Pinch the winged-tip needle tubing to stop the flow of blood.
14. Disconnect the saline syringe, and attach the syringe of Lasix to the tubing hub.
15. Slowly inject Lasix during a 5-minute period.
16. Once the medication has been administered, withdraw the needle and apply pressure over the site with an antiseptic wipe. Apply a dressing as needed.
17. Reassess the blood pressure and the level of consciousness.
18. Provide patient comfort measures.
19. Clean and replace the equipment. Discard disposable items according to *Standard Precautions.*

NURSING CONSIDERATIONS

Consider the use of a central venous access device or heparin lock for patients who require frequent Lasix IVP.

DOCUMENTATION GUIDELINES

Document the following on the visit report:
- The procedure and patient toleration
- Cardiopulmonary status, including blood pressure before and after the procedure
- Patient weight
- Blood sampling and designated laboratory for delivery as appropriate
- Intake and output
- Any patient/caregiver instructions and response to teaching, including the adherence to medications and diet
- Physician notification, if applicable
- *Standard Precautions*
- Other pertinent findings

Document IV medications on the medication record.
Update the plan of care.

Total Parenteral Nutrition and Intralipid Administration

PURPOSE
- To provide guidelines for total parenteral nutrition (TPN)/ intralipids administration
- To provide nutritional support for patients who are unable to eat or swallow appropriately

RELATED PROCEDURES
- Administration of Intravenous Therapy: General Guidelines (see Chapter 7)
- Administration of Medications: General Guidelines (see Chapter 9)
- Central Venous Catheter Management (see Chapter 7)
- Specimen Labeling and Transport (see Chapter 12)

GENERAL INFORMATION

Use a central venous line for TPN infusion. TPN infusions must be delivered by some type of volumetric pump. Review manufacturer's instructions for IV equipment administration guidelines. (The infusion is usually cycled during the nighttime to allow the patient greater freedom during the day.) Change TPN tubing and the bag at the same time. The physician usually orders tapering at the beginning and the end of the infusion to prevent metabolic complications. A full chemistry panel, including magnesium, is usually monitored when a home TPN infusion is provided. When they are ordered, intralipids are commonly mixed in the TPN solution. Use a 1.2 micron filter for solutions containing lipids. Review the manufacturer's recommendations if a *needleless* system is being used.

Remove TPN solutions from the refrigerator 2 hours before infusing them. Multivitamins and other medication additives with short stability may be added before infusion.

EQUIPMENT
1. TPN and intralipid solution as prescribed by the physician
2. Multivitamins if prescribed by the physician

3. Sterile normal saline solution and 100 U/ml heparin solution for irrigation and flush as prescribed by the physician

4. Intravenous tubing with a 1.2 micron filter

5. Occlusion clamp if needed (most central venous catheters have an in-line clamp)

6. Infusion pump

7. Patient refrigerator for storage of bags of TPN

8. 12 cc syringe with at least 1-inch needle

9. Blood tubes, labels, and laboratory requisition for blood sampling if required

10. Antiseptic and alcohol wipes

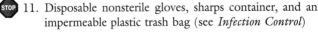 11. Disposable nonsterile gloves, sharps container, and an impermeable plastic trash bag (see *Infection Control*)

PROCEDURE

1. Explain the procedure to the patient/caregiver.

2. Assemble the equipment at a convenient work area.

3. Assist the patient to a comfortable position to access the IV. Perform necessary laboratory work.

4. Examine the TPN bag for leaks and an expiration date.

5. Cleanse the medication port with antiseptic wipes, followed by alcohol wipes; air dry.

6. Use aseptic technique to draw up multivitamins and additives with a 12 cc syringe, and inject through the medication port. (Be careful not to pierce the TPN bag with the needle.)

7. Turn the TPN bag upside down to mix the multivitamins and medication additives with the TPN solution.

8. Label the TPN bag, indicating the addition of multivitamins and medication additives.

9. Pull the protective cap off the TPN bag, and spike the tubing into the IV bag. Hang the TPN bag on the IV pole.

10. Follow the manufacturer's recommendations to hook up the tubing and cassette to the IV pump. Fill the intravenous drip chamber half full, and prime the cassette and IV tubing. Set the desired infusion rate.

11. Irrigate with normal saline solution, and access the central line as described in the procedure for *Central Venous Catheter Management* in Chapter 8. Tape all connections. Begin the infusion.

12. When the infusion is complete, discontinue the fluids.

Then irrigate and flush the central line as described in the procedure for *Central Venous Catheter Management* in Chapter 8.

13. Provide patient comfort measures.
14. Clean and replace the equipment. Discard disposable items according to *Standard Precautions.*

NURSING CONSIDERATIONS

Weigh the patient each visit.

Instruct the patient/caregiver to store TPN bags in the refrigerator and take the bags out to warm them to room temperature 1 hour before administration.

See Appendix II, *Laboratory Values,* at end of the text.

DOCUMENTATION GUIDELINES

Document the following on the visit report:
- The procedure and patient toleration
- Blood sampling and designated laboratory for delivery as appropriate
- Weight
- Vital signs
- Condition of catheter exit site
- Any patient/caregiver instructions and response to teaching, including the ability to safely manage home TPN therapy
- Physician notification, if applicable
- *Standard Precautions*
- Other pertinent findings

Document TPN, intralipids, and any IV medication additives on the medication/IV record.

Update the plan of care.

CHAPTER 9

Medications

Administration of Medications: General Guidelines

PURPOSE

- To provide safe and accurate medication administration
- To instruct the patient/caregiver in the therapeutic regimen
- To promote self-care in the home

RELATED PROCEDURES

- Antibiotic Therapy (see Chapter 8)
- Bladder Instillation and Irrigation
- Chemotherapy (see Chapter 8)
- Coumadin Administration: Bleeding Precautions
- Ear Instillation and Irrigation
- Eye Instillation and Irrigation
- Injections
- Lasix IVP (see Chapter 8)
- Metered Dose Inhaler Use (see Chapter 3)
- Instillation of Nose Drops
- Patient/Caregiver Self-Medication Errors at Home
- Prefilling Insulin Syringes
- Suppositories
- Topical Medications
- Total Parenteral Nutrition (TPN) (see Chapter 8)
- Tuberculin (TB) Skin Test

PROCEDURE

1. Obtain a physician's order for the patient's medication. It should include the following information:
   a. Name of the patient
   b. Name of the medicine

     c. Medication dose, route, and frequency of administration

2. Check the patient's known allergies.
3. Inscribe the physician's order on the medication record with start and stop date and time. Update records as needed.
4. Review *The Five Rights* to verify the physician's order for the medication:
   a. Right medication
   b. Right patient
   c. Right time
   d. Right method of administration
   e. Right amount
5. Administer medication according to the home health agency policies and state nurse practice acts. Recheck all calculations. Do not administer medicines or treatments that are not ordered by the physician.
6. Ask to see all medicines that the patient is taking. Check the labels on all medicine containers; compare these with the prescribed medication regimen. Inform the physician of any over-the-counter medicines that are not written on the patient's medication record and that may have been prescribed by other physicians.
7. Instruct the patient/caregiver on the current medication regimen:
   a. Assess the patient's/caregiver's understanding of the medicines, including the following: purpose, actions, side effects, dosage, and time to take medicine
   b. Instruct the patient/caregiver to verbalize information or to give a return demonstration of the administration technique
   c. Perform medication teaching each visit, until the patient/caregiver is knowledgeable about and can safely administer all medications; reinforce information if learning difficulties or problems with comprehension are noted
   d. Instruct the patient/caregiver in any new medication ordered by the physician or in changes in dosage of medications
   e. Provide instructional handouts, teaching guides, and patient education materials as needed

8. Assist the patient/caregiver to adhere with the medication regimen in the following manner:
   a. Set up the patient's pills in advance
   b. Prefill the insulin syringes
   c. Organize medicines for simple administration; place the medicines in envelopes; use a chart or medication dispenser from the pharmacy; use **large print** instructions
   d. Instruct the caregiver to administer medicines if the patient is unable to do so
9. Evaluate the therapeutic effects of the medicine; assess it for adverse side effects and for patient compliance with the medication regimen.
10. Provide patient comfort measures.

NURSING CONSIDERATIONS

Administer Food and Drug Administration (FDA) approved drugs within the recommended dosages and amounts found in the *Physician's Desk Reference (PDR)* or other acceptable drug references.

Consult with the home health agency medical director for guidelines regarding drugs not approved by the FDA.

To prevent patient confusion regarding the medication regimen as well as potential adverse side effects of a multiple medication regimen, consult with the physician to try to limit the patient to 6 medicines at a time.

Encourage the patient to use the same pharmacist for all medications.

Be aware that the physician may give the patient/caregiver changes or updates in medications over the phone or during office visits—therefore it is important to assess what medications that patient is taking **each** visit.

DOCUMENTATION GUIDELINES

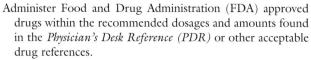

Document the following on the visit report:
- The procedure and patient toleration
- Patient response to the medication regimen
- Learning difficulties or problems with patient comprehension if reinforcement of medication teaching is necessary
- Any patient/caregiver instructions and response to teaching, including the ability to safely administer medications
- Physician notification, if applicable

- *Standard Precautions*
- Other pertinent findings

Document the medication's name, dosage, route, frequency of administration, and administration site as appropriate on the medication record.

Keep the medication record current.

Obtain written physician's orders for changes in the dosages of medications or for new medications.

Sign your full name and professional credentials on the medication record.

Complete an incident report as appropriate for medication errors.

Update the plan of care.

Bladder Instillation and Irrigation

PURPOSE
- To instill medication into the bladder
- To prevent obstruction or to dislodge clots

RELATED PROCEDURES
- Administration of Medications: General Guidelines
- Closed Urinary Drainage Management (see Chapter 13)
- Indwelling Foley Catheter Insertion and Care (see Chapter 13)
- Intermittent Straight Catheterization: Sterile Technique (see Chapter 13)

EQUIPMENT
1. Indwelling Foley catheter or sterile catheter (size ordered by the physician)
2. Irrigation solution or medication as prescribed by the physician
3. Urinary collection bag with drainage tubing as needed
4. 60 cc sterile irrigation syringe
5. Sterile connector cap or 4- × 4-inch gauze dressing and rubber band
6. Disposable sterile catheter plug

7. Basin or bowl
8. Antiseptic wipes
9. Soap and warm water, washcloth, and towels
 10. Disposable sterile gloves and an impermeable plastic trash bag (see *Infection Control*)

PROCEDURE

1. Explain the procedure to the patient/caregiver.
2. Assemble the equipment at a convenient work area.
3. Assist the patient to a supine position, with the knees flexed and separated. Place a towel or waterproof pad underneath the buttocks.
4. Wash the perineal area with soap and water; dry it. Drape the patient for privacy.
5. Insert the catheter if it is not already in place.
6. If the catheter is in place, scrub the outside of the connection with an antiseptic wipe.
7. Disconnect the drainage tubing from the catheter by twisting them in opposite directions and carefully pulling them apart without pulling on the catheter.
8. Apply a sterile catheter plug to the end of the catheter.
9. Apply a sterile cap to the end of the drainage tubing, or cover it with a sterile 4- × 4-inch gauze dressing and secure it with a rubber band to prevent contamination.
10. Fill the irrigation syringe with 30 to 60 ml of irrigation solution.
11. Position a basin to collect the return solution.
12. Unplug the catheter.
13. Insert the irrigation syringe into the end of the catheter. Be careful not to let the catheter end touch anything but the syringe.
14. **Gently** inject the irrigation solution into the bladder, approximately 30 ml at a time.
15. Remove the syringe from the catheter, and allow the irrigation solution to return to the basin by gravity.
16. Repeat steps *14* and *15* until all of the prescribed irrigation solution is used.
17. Clamp or plug the catheter if the solution is to dwell in the bladder for a specific amount of time.
18. Remove the connector cap from the drainage tubing. Cleanse the end of the tubing and catheter with antiseptic wipes.
19. Reconnect the drainage tubing to the catheter.

20. Provide patient comfort measures.
21. Clean and replace the equipment. Discard disposable items according to *Standard Precautions.*

NURSING CONSIDERATIONS

Instruct the patient/caregiver to notify the home health agency clinical supervisor if urine does not flow within 2 hours after the procedure.

If clots are not a problem, keep the system closed and use a needle and syringe with a clamp on the drainage tubing for instillation of medication.

Do **not** attempt to force the irrigation solution into the bladder if resistance is felt; notify the physician as appropriate.

Obtain physician's orders to remove and replace a totally obstructed catheter.

DOCUMENTATION GUIDELINES

Document the following on the visit report:
• The procedure and patient toleration
• Perineal hygiene
• Color, odor, amount, and characteristics of the patient's urine
• Amount and type of irrigation solution used and amount of return solution
• Physician notification, if applicable
• *Standard Precautions*
• Other pertinent findings

Document medications on the medication record.

Update the plan of care.

Coumadin Administration: Bleeding Precautions

PURPOSE

- To prevent complications of thrombosis or pulmonary emboli
- To instruct the patient/caregiver in bleeding precautions
- To promote self-care in the home

RELATED PROCEDURE

- Administration of Medications: General Guidelines

GENERAL INFORMATION

Coumadin (warfarin) is used for long-term anticoagulant therapy. Weekly monitoring of prothrombin time (PT) is recommended. Obtain the baseline liver and renal function studies before administration. See Appendix II, *Laboratory Values*, at end of the text.

EQUIPMENT

1. Coumadin as prescribed by the physician.

PROCEDURE

1. Explain the procedure to the patient/caregiver.
2. Verify the medication with the patient's clinical record, and check the patient's identity. Confirm that the patient is taking the prescribed amount of Coumadin correctly. (See the patient instruction recommendations in the procedure for *Administration of Medications: General Guidelines.*)
3. Do not give intramuscular (IM) injections unless absolutely necessary.
4. Apply pressure to all venipuncture sites for 10 minutes or until the bleeding has stopped.
5. Instruct the patient/caregiver in Coumadin administration to include the following **bleeding precautions:**
   a. No rectal temperatures, enemas, or suppositories
   b. Do not use a straight razor or nail clippers
   c. Use a soft toothbrush
   d. Wear slippers when ambulatory; protect the feet
   e. Do not pick at scabs or wounds

    f. Avoid activities that may cause cuts or bruising

    g. Avoid aspirin-containing drugs; take Coumadin at the same time each day

6. Instruct the patient to wear a MedicAlert bracelet to indicate that an anticoagulant is being taken.

7. Limit the diet according to the following instructions:

    a. Provide a list of foods containing vitamin K that should be avoided during the therapy

    b. Instruct the patient/caregiver **not** to take/administer over-the-counter multiple vitamins that contain vitamin K unless ordered by the physician

    c. Restrict alcohol intake

8. Instruct the patient/caregiver to report any bleeding; black, tarry stools; or blood in the urine.

9. If bleeding occurs, instruct the patient/caregiver to hold a pressure dressing to the site and to notify the home health agency and physician.

10. Provide patient comfort measures.

NURSING CONSIDERATIONS

Draw a blood sample early in the morning to evaluate patient PT levels, and have the laboratory fax or phone in the results to the physician as soon as possible.

Instruct the patient not to take the daily dose of Coumadin until the physician has reviewed the laboratory results. Tell the patient that either the home health nurse or physician (decide who) will call the patient to confirm the correct Coumadin dosage.

DOCUMENTATION GUIDELINES

Document the following on the visit report:

- The procedure and patient toleration
- Signs or reports of inappropriate bleeding
- Laboratory sampling for prothrombin time and designated laboratory for delivery
- Any patient/caregiver instructions and response to teaching, including adherence to recommendations
- Physician notification, if applicable
- *Standard Precautions*
- Other pertinent findings

Document medications on the medication record.

Update the plan of care.

Ear Instillation and Irrigation

PURPOSE
- To remove impacted cerumen from the auditory canal
- To improve impaired hearing caused by ear wax
- To remove purulent discharge or a foreign body
- To instill medication into the auditory canal

RELATED PROCEDURE
- Administration of Medications: General Guidelines

EQUIPMENT
1. Medication or irrigation solution as prescribed by the physician
2. Soft or small-bulb syringe
3. Sterile basin for solution
4. Emesis basin or bowl
5. Cotton balls and cotton-tipped applicators
6. Plastic sheet or garbage bag
7. Washcloth and towels

STOP 8. Disposable nonsterile gloves and an impermeable plastic trash bag (see *Infection Control*)

❖ Instillation

PROCEDURE
1. Explain the procedure to the patient/caregiver.
2. Assemble the equipment at the bedside or a convenient work area.
3. Assist the patient to a sitting or supine position. Drape a plastic sheet or towel around the patient's shoulders to prevent discomfort from dampness.
4. Instruct the patient to turn his or her head with the affected ear held upward.
5. Straighten the auditory canal by holding the auricle upward and backward (Fig. 9-1). For infants, pull the auricle down and back. Avoid excessive pressure.
6. Instill medication as ordered by the physician. Insert a small cotton ball in the external auditory canal.

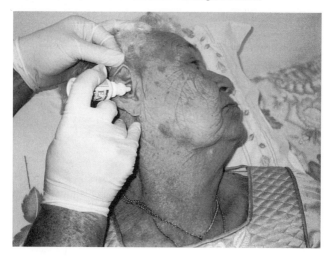

Fig. 9-1 Instillation of ear drops. (Photo courtesy Robyn Rice.)

7. Instruct the patient to remain in a position with the affected ear upward for about 10 to 15 minutes.
8. Remove the cotton ball, and assess for drainage. Dry the ear with a washcloth, as needed.
9. Provide patient comfort measures.
10. Clean and replace the equipment. Discard disposable items according to *Standard Precautions*.

❖ Irrigation

PROCEDURE

1. Follow steps *1* through *4* of the procedure for *Instillation*.
2. Warm the prescribed irrigation solution to body temperature.
3. Position the emesis basin under the patient's ear that is to be irrigated. The patient may hold the emesis basin if he or she is able.
4. Straighten the auditory canal by pulling the auricle upward and backward. For infants pull the auricle down and back. Avoid excessive pressure.
5. Fill the syringe with the prescribed irrigation solution, expel the air, and gently insert the tip of the syringe into the exter-

nal canal. Then **gently** irrigate the ear as prescribed by the physician. (Immediately stop the treatment and notify the physician if the patient complains of discomfort.)

6. Dry the external ear canal.
7. Apply a cotton ball to the external ear canal. Then position the patient on the side of his or her affected ear for 5 to 10 minutes to allow the remaining irrigation solution to drain out.
8. Follow steps *8* through *10* of the procedure for *Instillation*.

NURSING CONSIDERATIONS

Instruct the patient/caregiver in the procedure.

Instruct the patient/caregiver never to occlude the external auditory canal with the bulb syringe.

Forceful delivery of irrigation solution or medication into the ear canal can injure the eardrum.

DOCUMENTATION GUIDELINES

Document the following on the visit report:
- The procedure and patient toleration
- Color, consistency, and amount of any discharge or drainage
- Any patient/caregiver instructions and response to teaching
- Physician notification, if applicable
- *Standard Precautions*
- Other pertinent findings

Document medications on the medication record.

Update the plan of care.

Enema Administration

PURPOSE
- To remove feces
- To soften feces
- To relieve abdominal distention and discomfort
- To promote normal bowel function

RELATED PROCEDURES
- Administration of Medications: General Guidelines
- Bowel Training (see Chapter 5)
- Fecal Impaction: Manual Removal (see Chapter 5)

EQUIPMENT
1. Cleansing solution, Fleet enema, and oil retention enema as prescribed by the physician
2. Enema container with tubing and clamp
3. Water-soluble lubricant
4. Plastic trash bag or Chux pad
5. Bedpan
6. Soap and warm water, basin, tissues, washcloth, and towels
 7. Disposable nonsterile gloves and an impermeable plastic trash bag (see *Infection Control*)

❖ Cleansing Enema

PROCEDURE
1. Explain the procedure to the patient/caregiver.
2. Assemble the equipment at a convenient work area. If available, position the bedside commode next to the bed.
3. Place a plastic bag or Chux under the patient's hips.
4. Assist the patient to the left lateral Sims' position, with knees flexed. A supine position with the knees flexed and the legs separated may also be used. Drape the patient with a sheet or towel to expose the anus.
5. Prepare the cleansing enema solution in a bag. Keep at room temperature. The volume of the solution should be no greater than 1000 ml.
6. Flush the tubing with cleansing solution, then clamp.

7. Lubricate the tip of the tubing, and gently insert it into the rectum approximately 3 to 4 inches with the tip pointing toward the umbilicus.

8. Hold the enema bag about 12 to 18 inches above the patient's rectum. Unclamp the tubing, and slowly administer the solution. Instruct the patient to take slow, deep breaths. Clamp the tubing for a few minutes if the patient complains of cramps, then resume the irrigation.

9. Clamp and remove the tubing from the rectum after the solution has been administered or when the patient is unable to retain any more of the solution.

10. Instruct the patient to try to hold the solution for as long as possible (approximately 5 to 10 minutes). It may be helpful to press the patient's buttocks together for 2 to 3 minutes to prevent evacuation of the solution.

11. Offer the bedpan or assist the patient to the bedside commode or the bathroom.

12. Provide patient comfort measures.

13. Clean and replace the equipment. Discard disposable items according to *Standard Precautions.*

❖ Fleet Enema

PROCEDURE

1. Follow steps *1* through *4* of the procedure for *Cleansing Enema.*

2. Remove the plastic covering from the prelubricated tip of the Fleet Enema bottle.

3. Gently insert the tip into the rectum (approximately 2 to 3 inches).

4. Gently squeeze the bottle until the Fleet solution has been administered.

5. Gently withdraw the tip.

6. Follow steps *10* through *13* of the procedure for *Cleansing Enema.*

❖ Oil Retention Enema

PROCEDURE

1. Follow steps *1* through *4* of the procedure for *Cleansing Enema.*

2. Remove the plastic covering from the tip of the oil retention enema bottle. Lubricate the tip.

3. Gently insert the tip about 2 to 3 inches into the rectum.
4. Squeeze the bottle until the oil retention fluid is administered.
5. Gently withdraw the tip.
6. Follow steps *10* through *13* of the procedure for *Cleansing
   Enema.*

NURSING CONSIDERATIONS

Consider a bowel training program. Stress the importance of
   activity, a high-fiber diet, and adequate fluid intake to promote good bowel function.
Caution the patient/caregiver against excessive laxative, stool
   softener, or enema administration.
It is advisable to request a fecal disimpaction order when obtaining an enema order. Perform fecal disimpaction before
   administering an enema.
Warm the enema solution to room temperature (no more than
   100° C [37.8° F]) to reduce cramping and patient discomfort.

DOCUMENTATION GUIDELINES

Document the following on the visit report:
   • The procedure and patient toleration
   • Results, including the amount and color of the stool
   • Presence of flatus or abdominal distention
   • Any patient/caregiver instructions and response to teach-
     ing, including the ability to administer an enema and main-
     tain adequate bowel function
   • Physician notification, if applicable
   • *Standard Precautions*
   • Other pertinent findings
Document the type of enema and the amount of solution ad-
ministered on the medication record.
   Update the plan of care.

Eye Compresses

PURPOSE

- To reduce pain and inflammation
- To control intraocular hemorrhage and to prevent tissue damage
- To promote drainage of an infected eye

RELATED PROCEDURE

- Administration of Medications: General Guidelines

EQUIPMENT

1. Eye compress solution or medication as prescribed by the physician
2. Basin of ice water
3. Gauze eye compresses
4. Thumb forceps
5. Sterile container
6. Bath thermometer
7. Lubricant for warm compresses (petroleum jelly)
8. Washcloths and towels
9. Disposable nonsterile gloves and impermeable plastic trash bags (see *Infection Control*)

❖ Cold Compress

PROCEDURE

1. Explain the procedure to the patient/caregiver.
2. Assemble the equipment at the bedside or a convenient work area.
3. Assist the patient to a supine position, with his or her head turned toward the uninvolved side.
4. Chill the prescribed solution in a basin of ice.
5. Place the compresses in a sterile container; then pour the chilled solution over the compresses. Squeeze the compresses as dry as possible with forceps.
6. Apply the compress over the patient's lids.
7. Change the compress every 30 seconds to keep it cold for about 5 minutes. Use new compresses for each application.

8. Dry the patient's eyelids with a washcloth when the last compress is removed.
9. Provide patient comfort measures.
10. Clean and replace the equipment. Discard disposable items according to *Standard Precautions.*

❖ Warm Compress

PROCEDURE

1. Follow steps *1* through *3* of the procedure for *Cold Compresses.*
2. Apply lubricant to the area where the compresses will be applied.
3. Soak the compresses in warm water and squeeze as dry as possible with forceps; then apply the compresses over the affected eye. (The solution is not to exceed 115° F.)
4. Use new compresses for each application. Change the compresses to keep the eye warm.
5. Provide patient comfort measures.
6. Clean and replace equipment. Discard disposable items according to *Standard Precautions.*

DOCUMENTATION GUIDELINES

Document the following on the visit report:
- The procedure, including the time and duration of the treatment, as well as patient toleration
- Condition of the eyes before and after treatment
- Physician notification, if applicable
- *Standard Precautions*
- Other pertinent findings

Document medications on the medication record.

Update the plan of care.

Eye Instillation and Irrigation

PURPOSE
- To instill or apply drops or ointment into the eye
- To irrigate and clean the eyeball or eye socket
- To treat infections and relieve inflammation

RELATED PROCEDURE
- Administration of Medications: General Guidelines

EQUIPMENT
1. Medication, ointment, or irrigation solution as prescribed by the physician
2. Tissues
3. Soft-bulb syringe or eye dropper
4. Emesis basin or bowl
5. Sterile cup for irrigation solution
6. 4- × 4-inch gauze pads
7. Cotton balls
8. Plastic sheet and garbage bag
9. Washcloth and towels
 10. Disposable nonsterile gloves and an impermeable plastic trash bag (see *Infection Control*)

❖ Eye Drops

PROCEDURE
1. Review the physician's orders designating which eye requires medication:
   o.d. (oculus dexter)—right eye
   o.s. (oculus sinister)—left eye
   o.u. (oculus uterque)—both eyes
2. Explain the procedure to the patient/caregiver.
3. Assemble the equipment at a convenient work area.
4. Assist the patient to a sitting position with his or her head tilted slightly backward or supine and the neck slightly hyperextended.
5. Inspect the eye for drainage or redness, and wipe away any discharge. Gently clean any crust or drainage along the

eyelid with a damp washcloth. Always clean the eye from the inner to outer canthus.

6. Inspect the color and appearance of the noninvolved eye.
7. Using the forefinger, gently pull down the patient's lower lid. Ask the patient to look up at the ceiling.
8. Drop the prescribed number of drops into the middle of the patient's lower lid (Fig. 9-2). (Do not touch the eye with the dropper; steady your hand by resting it lightly on the patient's forehead.)
9. Instruct the patient to close his or her eyes, but not to squeeze the eyes shut.
10. Wipe off excess medication with a tissue or gauze.
11. Provide patient comfort measures.
12. Clean and replace the equipment. Discard disposable items according to *Standard Precautions.*

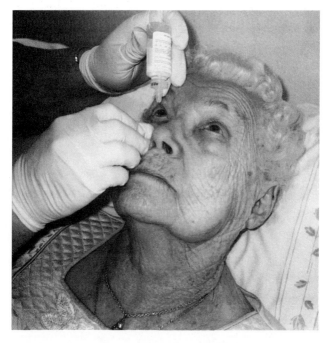

Fig. 9-2 Instillation of eye drops. (Photo courtesy Robyn Rice.)

❖ Eye Irrigation

PROCEDURE

1. Follow steps *1* through *6* of the procedure for *Eye Drops*.
2. Position and drape the patient with a plastic sheet or towel to facilitate the drainage of the fluid away from the eye.
3. Place a towel underneath the patient's face. Place an emesis basin or bowl under the patient's cheek on the side of the affected eye to collect irrigation solution.
4. Pour irrigation fluid into a sterile cup, and draw up the irrigation fluid into the bulb syringe.
5. Separate the patient's eyelids with your thumb and index finger and have the patient look up. Gently direct the fluid flow from the inner to the outer canthus. Do not touch the patient's eye area or lid with the syringe.
6. Continue irrigating as prescribed by the physician or until the secretions are cleaned from the eye.
7. Follow steps *9* through *12* of the procedure for *Eye Drops*.

❖ Eye Ointment

PROCEDURE

1. Follow steps *1* through *6* of the procedure for *Eye Drops*.
2. Squeeze a small amount of ointment from the tube into a 4- × 4-inch gauze pad, and discard.
3. Pull the patient's lower lid gently downward while having the patient look up.
4. Apply a thin line of ointment along the conjunctival surface of the retracted lower lid with the tip of the ointment tube (Fig. 9-3). (Do not touch the patient's eye with the medication tube.)
5. Instruct the patient to close his or her eye and rotate the eyeball. Rub the patient's lid lightly without traumatizing the eye to distribute the medication.
6. Wipe off the tip of the ointment tube with a 4- × 4-inch gauze pad.
7. Follow steps *9* through *12* of the procedure for *Eye Drops*.

NURSING CONSIDERATIONS

Instruct the patient/caregiver to avoid touching the eye with the applicator when administering drops or ointment.

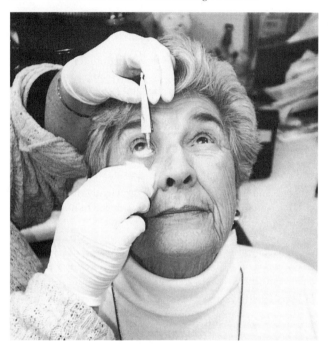

Fig. 9-3   Instillation of eye ointment. (Photo courtesy Robyn Rice.)

Temporary blurring of vision is common for certain medications, and the patient should be informed of this.

Explain that the medication is to be used only by the patient.

If the patient is receiving both eye drops and eye ointment, the
drops are to be instilled before the ointment.

DOCUMENTATION GUIDELINES

Document the following on the visit report:
- The procedure and patient toleration
- Condition and appearance of the eye, including signs of
  redness, swelling, or inflammation
- Which eye received medication or irrigation
- Any patient/caregiver instructions and response to teach-
  ing, including the ability to administer eye drops
- Physician notification, if applicable

- *Standard Precautions*
- Other pertinent findings

Document medications on the medication record.
Update the plan of care.

Gold Injection

PURPOSE

- To reduce joint/muscle pain and inflammation
- To retard the progression of bone and articular destruction

RELATED PROCEDURES

- Administration of Medications: General Guidelines
- Injections

GENERAL INFORMATION

Gold injections are usually given to treat active rheumatoid arthritis. The three most commonly used preparations are gold sodium thiomalate, aurothioglucose, and auranofin. The medication is administered by intramuscular injection.

A protein urine test and other baseline laboratory values to include a complete blood count (CBC) and platelet count are recommended before the initial dose; consult with the physician regarding blood work. Monitor laboratory blood values every 2 weeks while therapy is in progress.

Gold therapy decreases the pain, swelling, and inflammation of rheumatoid arthritis and slows the progression of the disease. However, it does not repair damaged tissue. Anticipate improvement within 3 months; otherwise the drug should be discontinued.

EQUIPMENT

1. Medication as ordered by the physician
2. 3 cc syringe
3. 1½- to 2-inch, 19- to 23-gauge needle
4. Antiseptic wipes

5. Disposable nonsterile gloves, sharps container, and an impermeable plastic trash bag (see *Infection Control*)

PROCEDURE

1. Explain the procedure to the patient/caregiver.
2. Assemble the equipment at a convenient work area.
3. Place the patient in a supine position for the injection.
4. Follow the procedure for *Intramuscular (IM) Injections.*
5. Discard the needle in a sharps container.
6. Provide patient comfort measures.
7. Observe the patient for at least 15 minutes after the procedure (watch carefully for signs of anaphylaxis).
8. Clean and replace equipment. Discard disposable items in a plastic trash bag according to *Standard Precautions* and secure.

 NURSING CONSIDERATIONS

The color of gold is pale yellow; discard if the color has darkened.

Injectable gold is one of the most toxic second-line antirheumatic drugs; many patients stop therapy because of undesired side effects. Common side effects include dermatitis, skin pigmentation with pruritus, and stomatitis. More serious side effects include renal dysfunction and hematologic reactions (e.g., anemia, leukopenia, and thrombocytopenia).

The injection should **not** be given if the patient has positive urine protein as related to potential renal side effects.

Explain to the patient that gold storage in the skin may lead to chrysiasis (a bronze or grey-blue color).

Instruct the patient/caregiver to report sore throat, fever, or bruising to physician.

 DOCUMENTATION GUIDELINES

Document the following on the visit report:
- The procedure and patient toleration; injection site
- Any patient/caregiver instructions and response to teaching
- Physician notification, if applicable
- *Standard Precautions*
- Other pertinent findings

Document medications on the medication record.
Update the plan of care.

Injections

PURPOSE

- To inject medications parenterally, either intramuscularly, subcutaneously, or by the Z-track route, depending on the action of the drug and the rate of absorption

RELATED PROCEDURE

- Administration of Medications: General Guidelines

GENERAL INFORMATION

A maximum of 3 ml may be given to adults intramuscularly (IM) in the vastus lateralis and gluteal sites. A maximum of 2 ml may be given to adults IM in the deltoid area. The physician's order for a medication to be given intramuscularly or subcutaneously implies that the standard injection sites will be used according to the state nurse practice acts.

❖ Intramuscular (IM) Injections

EQUIPMENT

1. Medication (fluid volume not to exceed 3 ml in the single adult injection) as prescribed by the physician
2. 3 cc syringe
3. 1½-inch, 18- to 20-gauge needle
4. Antiseptic wipes
 5. Nonsterile disposable gloves, sharps container, and an impermeable plastic trash bag (see *Infection Control*)

PROCEDURE

1. Explain the procedure to the patient/caregiver.
2. Assemble the equipment at a convenient work area.
3. Verify the medication with the patient's clinical record, and check the patient's identity.
4. Position the patient to expose the injection site (deltoid, vastus lateralis, or gluteal). Drape the patient for privacy.
5. Prepare an injectable medication from an ampule or a vial in the following manner:
   a. Score the neck of the ampule and break the stem, using

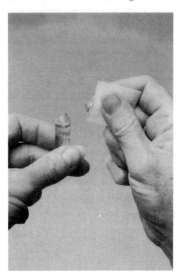

Fig. 9-4 Preparing an injectable medication from an ampule. (From Perry AG, Potter PA: *Clinical nursing skills and techniques,* ed 4, St Louis, 1998, Mosby.)

an antiseptic wipe as a protective cover to prevent cuts (Fig. 9-4); hold the ampule either inverted or right side up; insert the needle into the center of the ampule opening, without allowing the needle to touch the tip or rim of the ampule; withdraw the correct medication volume; then remove the needle from the ampule, and expel the air bubbles

b. Remove the metal cap from the vial, and clean the exposed rubber seal with an antiseptic wipe; insert air into the vial in the amount of medication to be withdrawn; invert the vial and keep the tip of the needle below the fluid level (Fig. 9-5); withdraw the correct medication volume; then remove the needle from the vial and expel the air bubbles

c. Replace the protective needle cap

d. Change the needle on the syringe if you are withdrawing medication from a vial (this may dull the needle) or if you suspect that any of the medication is on the shaft of the needle

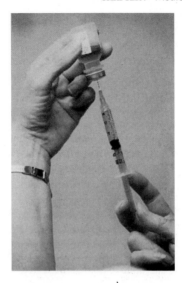

Fig. 9-5   Preparing medication from a vial. (From Perry AG, Potter PA: *Clinical nursing skills and techniques,* ed 4, St Louis, 1998, Mosby.)

6. Prepare the injection site by cleaning it with an antiseptic wipe. Begin at the center of the injection site and rotate outward in a circular motion (approximately 4 to 5 cm).
7. Remove the protective needle cap.
8. Inject the needle with a quick thrust at a 90-degree angle through the skin and into the muscle.
9. Aspirate for blood before injecting the medication. (If blood appears, withdraw the needle. Attach a new needle to the syringe, and reposition the needle to administer the injection.)
10. Inject the medication.
11. Apply pressure with an antiseptic wipe, and withdraw the needle.
12. Gently rub the site with an antiseptic wipe to distribute the medication.
13. Dispose of the needle in a sharps container.
14. Provide patient comfort measures.
15. Clean and replace the equipment. Discard disposable items according to *Standard Precautions.*

❖ Subcutaneous (SQ) Injections

EQUIPMENT

1. Medication (fluid volume not to exceed 1.5 ml in single adult injection) as prescribed by the physician
2. Syringe
3. ½- to ⅞-inch, 25- to 27-gauge needle
4. Antiseptic wipes
5. **(STOP)** Disposable nonsterile gloves, sharps container, and an impermeable plastic trash bag (see *Infection Control*)

PROCEDURE

1. Follow steps *1* through *7* of the procedure for *Intramuscular (IM) Injections.*
2. Select the site for administration (Fig. 9-6). SQ heparin is usually given in the stomach. Rotate the injection sites daily within single anatomic regions for repeated daily SQ insulin injections.

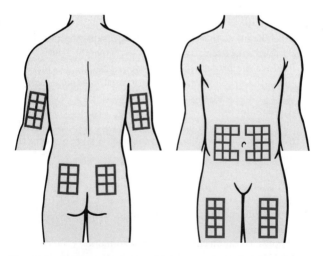

Fig. 9-6   Common sites for subcutaneous injections. (From Phipps WJ, Sands JK, Marek JF: *Medical-surgical nursing: concepts and clinical practice,* ed 6, St Louis, 1999, Mosby.)

3. Pinch the skin between the thumb and forefinger. Firmly and quickly insert the needle at a 45-degree angle.
4. Inject the medicine. Do **not** rub the injection site after SQ heparin administration because this may cause bruising or bleeding.
5. Follow steps *13* through *15* of the procedure for *Intramuscular (IM) Injections.*

❖ Z-Track Intramuscular Injections
GENERAL INFORMATION
Staining of the skin can occur with some intramuscular injections if any solution leaks into the subcutaneous tissue. Give Z-track injections in the upper-outer quadrant of the buttocks; never give Z-track injections in the arm or in other exposed areas. Subsequent injections should be made in alternating buttocks. Iron dextran *(Imferon)* is the major drug administered by the Z-track method.

EQUIPMENT
1. Medication as prescribed by the physician
2. Syringe
3. Two 1½-inch, 20-gauge needles
4. Antiseptic wipes
5. Disposable nonsterile gloves, sharps container, and an impermeable plastic trash bag (see *Infection Control*)

PROCEDURE
1. Follow steps *1* through *7* of the procedure for *Intramuscular (IM) Injections.*
2. Instill an extra 0.5 cc of air in the syringe, and replace the needle with a second sterile needle. (Injection of 0.5 cc of air after the medication will clear the needle and prevent leakage along the injection track when the needle is withdrawn; this prevents staining of the skin.)
3. Displace subcutaneous tissue laterally (approximately 1½ to 2 inches) on the upper-outer quadrant of the buttocks (Fig. 9-7). Maintain this position until the needle is withdrawn to prevent the leakage of medication into the subcutaneous tissue.
4. Insert the needle deep into the muscle at a 90-degree angle.

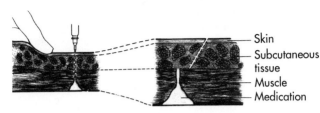

Fig. 9-7 Z-track method of injection. (From Perry AG, Potter PA: *Clinical nursing skills and techniques,* ed 4, St Louis, 1998, Mosby.)

5. Pull back on the plunger to see whether the needle is in a blood vessel. (If it is, withdraw the needle; change the needle and re-position.)
6. *Slowly* inject the medicine. Wait 10 seconds; then apply pressure with an antiseptic wipe, and withdraw the needle while releasing the displaced tissue.
7. Do not massage the injection site. Massaging the area may cause the medication to leak into the subcutaneous tissue.
8. Follow steps *13* through *15* of the procedure for *Intramuscular (IM) Injections.*

DOCUMENTATION GUIDELINES

Document the following on the visit report:
- The procedure and patient toleration; injection site
- Any patient/caregiver instructions and response to teaching
- Physician notification, if applicable
- *Standard Precautions*
- Other pertinent findings

Document medications on the medication record.

Update the plan of care.

Nose Drops

PURPOSE

- To administer medications or drops into the nose
- To alleviate inflammation and congestion of mucous membranes
- To promote self-care in the home

RELATED PROCEDURE

- Administration of Medications: General Guidelines

EQUIPMENT

1. Medication or nose drops as prescribed by the physician
2. Tissues
3. Medicine dropper
4. Disposable nonsterile gloves (optional) and an impermeable plastic trash bag (see *Infection Control*)

PROCEDURE

1. Explain the procedure to the patient/caregiver.
2. Assemble the equipment at the bedside or a convenient work area.
3. Place the patient with his or her head well back in a *sniffing* position (Fig. 9-8).
4. Instill the medication as prescribed by the physician, directing the flow toward the floor of the nasal cavity. Avoid touching the nostril with the dropper.
5. Maintain this position for approximately 5 minutes after instillation of the drops; then have the patient lower his or her head to eye level to allow the medication to flow to the lower part of the nose.
6. Provide patient comfort measures.
7. Clean and replace the equipment. Discard disposable items according to *Standard Precautions*.

DOCUMENTATION GUIDELINES

Document the following on the visit report:
- The procedure and patient toleration
- Any patient/caregiver instructions and compliance with

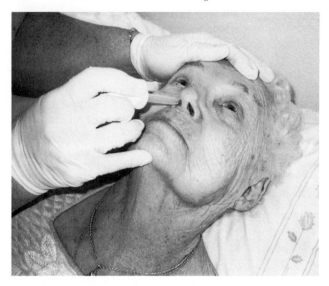

Fig. 9-8   Instillation of nose drops. (Photo courtesy Robyn Rice.)

the procedure, including the patient's ability to self-administer the nose drops
- Physician notification, if applicable
- *Standard Precautions*
- Other pertinent findings

Document medications on the medication record.

Update the plan of care.

Patient/Caregiver Self-Medication Errors at Home

PURPOSE

- To provide guidelines for potential home medication errors made by the patient/caregiver
- To safeguard the patient
- The promote self-care in the home

RELATED PROCEDURE

- Administration of Medications: General Information

GENERAL INFORMATION

Medication errors are common among the elderly because of problems with using multiple medications and compliance. Typical problems include taking medicines at the wrong times, taking medicines that are old and out of date, or not taking the medicine that has been prescribed. Follow home health agency policy and complete an incident report as needed for medication incorrectly administered by the home health nurse.

PROCEDURE

1. Explain the procedure to the patient/caregiver.
2. Assess compliance with the medication regimen and identify any prescribed medicine taken incorrectly or omitted. See the patient instruction recommendations in the procedure for *Administration of Medications: General Information.*
3. Inform the home health agency clinical supervisor and the physician of any home medication error(s).
4. Assess for side effects of medication errors; notify the physician when appropriate.
5. Identify **why** the medication error happened. Assess the patient/caregiver for the following and take corrective actions:
   a. Does he or she know the purpose of the medicine?
   b. Is he or she correctly following prescribed dosage and scheduling?

c. Does he or she know the side effects of the medicines and when to call the physician?

d. Can he or she open the medicine bottles?

e. Is he or she able to correctly administer the medication?

f. Can he or she read the medication labels?

g. Is he or she able to purchase or obtain the medications?

h. Does he or she correctly store the medications?

i. Does he or she know the difference between generic and brand name medications?

j. Is the patient taking any medications not prescribed by the primary physician, including home remedies and over-the-counter medications?

k. If the patient has difficulty with the medication regimen, is there a competent caregiver **willing and able** to assist the patient?

6. Remove inappropriate or unsafe medicines from the home as advised by the physician and home health agency.

7. Plan follow-up visits to assess the patient's status.

8. Identify problems with nonparticipation with the medication regimen, and take corrective action. Consider a learning contract and/or use of adjunct support from the caregiver, family, friends, or homemaker service.

9. Reinforce information if learning difficulties are noted.

10. Provide patient comfort measures.

NURSING CONSIDERATIONS

Be aware that mental status changes or abrupt combative behavior may be related to patient self-medication errors.

Report to the physician changes in the patient's condition or adverse side effects.

Instruct the patient/caregiver to notify the home health agency clinical supervisor and physician about any problems with medications.

Consider a social service referral if the patient cannot afford to buy his or her medications.

 ## DOCUMENTATION GUIDELINES

Document the following on the visit report:

• The procedure and patient toleration

• Medicine(s) given or taken incorrectly

• Patient's cardiopulmonary status and level of consciousness

- Why the medication error happened and corrective actions taken
- Learning difficulties or problems with comprehension, if reinforcement of medication teaching is necessary
- Any patient/caregiver instructions and response to teaching, including the ability to safely administer medications
- Physician notification, if applicable
- *Standard Precautions*
- Other pertinent findings

Complete an incident report as requested.

Update the plan of care.

Prefilling Insulin Syringes

PURPOSE

- To provide the correct amount of insulin for patients who do not have an available caregiver and who are unable to draw up the insulin dose because of functional or visual disabilities
- To instruct the patient/caregiver in storage and handling of prefilled insulin syringes
- To promote self-care in the home

RELATED PROCEDURES

- Administration of Medications: General Guidelines
- Injections

EQUIPMENT

1. Insulin as prescribed by the physician
2. Insulin syringes
3. Antiseptic and alcohol wipes

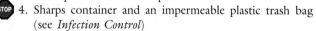 4. Sharps container and an impermeable plastic trash bag (see *Infection Control*)

PROCEDURE

1. Explain the procedure to the patient/caregiver.
2. Assemble the equipment at a convenient work area.
3. Verify the medication with the patient's clinical record.

4. Draw up the prescribed amount of insulin into the syringes. See the steps for preparing the medication from a vial in the procedure for *Injections.*

5. Instruct the patient/caregiver in the following:
   a. Keep all prefilled single or mixed insulin syringes refrigerated, and use them within 21 days
   b. Never store syringes vertically with the needle down; crystals may settle and clog the needle
   c. Re-suspend the preparation before giving the injection by rolling the syringe between the palms of your hands
   d. For consistent effect with mixtures of regular and NPH insulin, only use syringes that have been filled for at least 24 hours before injection; for example, on the day when the nurse visits and fills the syringes, use the syringe that was filled on the previous visit and not the freshly mixed syringe
   e. Administer the prefilled syringe at room temperature for optimal absorption; (take the syringe out of the refrigerator at least 1 hour before administering it)
   f. Place the used needles in a sharps container; keep the container out of the reach of children

6. Evaluate home diabetic management.

7. Clean and replace equipment. Discard disposable items according to *Standard Precautions.*

NURSING CONSIDERATIONS

Review *Fiscal Intermediary Guidelines* for Medicare reimbursement when prefilling the patient's insulin syringes.

Put prefilled syringes in the refrigerator crisper or out of sight; consider a locked box if drug abuse is a problem in the family or neighborhood.

DOCUMENTATION GUIDELINES

Document the following on the visit report:
- The procedure and patient toleration
- Number of syringes that are prefilled
- Number of syringes that the patient has used since the last visit
- Unavailability of a caregiver and visual or functional disabilities that prevent the patient from drawing up his or her own insulin
- Any patient/caregiver instructions and response to teach-

ing, including adherence with home diabetic management and the ability to administer prefilled insulin syringes
- Physician notification, if applicable
- *Standard Precautions*
- Other pertinent findings

Document medications on the medication record.

Update the plan of care.

Suppositories

PURPOSE
- To administer medications into the rectum
- To administer medications into the vagina
- To alleviate pain or discomfort
- To prevent infection
- To promote self-care in the home

RELATED PROCEDURE
- Administration of Medications: General Guidelines

EQUIPMENT
1. Medication (rectal or vaginal suppository) as prescribed by the physician
2. Water-soluble lubricant
3. Soap and warm water, basin, tissues, washcloth, and towel
 4. Disposable nonsterile glove and an impermeable plastic trash bag (see *Infection Control*)

❖ Rectal Suppositories
PROCEDURE
1. Explain the procedure to the patient/caregiver.
2. Verify the medication with the patient's clinical record.
3. Assemble the equipment at a convenient work area.
4. Position the patient in a left lateral position.
5. Perform perineal care as needed. Drape the patient for privacy.

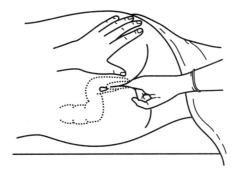

Fig. 9-9   Insertion of a rectal suppository.

6. Remove the wrapper from the suppository, and lubricate it.
7. Separate the buttocks.
8. Gently insert the suppository with the index finger of a gloved hand, until it is beyond the internal sphincter (Fig. 9-9).
9. Gently squeeze the patient's buttocks together until the urge to expel the suppository has passed.
10. Cleanse the anal area with soap and water, and dry.
11. Provide patient comfort measures.
12. Clean and replace the equipment. Discard disposable items according to *Standard Precautions.*

❖ Vaginal Suppositories

PROCEDURE

1. Explain the procedure to the patient/caregiver.
2. Verify the medication with the patient's clinical record, and check the patient's identity.
3. Position the patient in a supine position, with the knees flexed and the legs separated.
4. Perform perineal care as needed. Drape the patient for privacy.
5. Gently separate the patient's labia, and insert the vaginal suppository as far into the vagina as it can be inserted (Fig. 9-10).
6. Provide patient comfort measures.
7. Discard disposable items according to *Standard Precautions.*

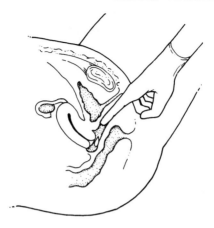

Fig. 9-10   Insertion of a vaginal suppository.

DOCUMENTATION GUIDELINES

Document the following on the visit report:
- The procedure and patient toleration
- Any signs of rectal or vaginal drainage
- Any patient/caregiver instructions and response to teaching, including the ability to administer the suppository
- Physician notification, if applicable
- *Standard Precautions*
- Other pertinent findings

Document medications on the medication record.

Update the plan of care.

Topical Medications

PURPOSE
- To apply medication to the skin
- To promote self-care in the home

RELATED PROCEDURE
- Administration of Medications: General Guidelines

GENERAL INFORMATION

A variety of medications, such as lotions, ointments, and powders, may be applied to the skin. Review and follow the manufacturer's recommendations when applying the medication to ensure maximal penetration and absorption. Avoid excessive application of topical medication; some ingredients can damage sensitive skin.

EQUIPMENT
1. Medication (cream, powder, patch, ointment, and spray) as prescribed by the physician
2. Cotton-tipped applicators or tongue blade
3. Sterile dressing and hypoallergenic tape
4. Soap and warm water, basin, washcloth, and towel
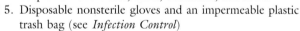 5. Disposable nonsterile gloves and an impermeable plastic trash bag (see *Infection Control*)

PROCEDURE
1. Explain the procedure to the patient/caregiver.
2. Position and drape the patient to apply topical medication.
3. Remove the old medication, and prepare the skin or tissue for the new medication in the following manner:
   a. Wash the skin with soap and water, soak the affected area, or debride the tissue; pat dry
4. Apply topical medication in the following manner:
   a. **Aerosol spray**—shake the container; spray the medication for as long as directed, and follow the manufacturer's directions for recommended distance to hold spray away from the skin (usually 6 to 12 inches); instruct the

patient to turn his or her face away from the spray to prevent inhalation of medication; spray the medication evenly over the skin or tissue

b. **Cream, lotion, or ointment**—put approximately 2 teaspoons of medication in the palm of your hand, rub it between your hands to soften and warm it, and spread the medication over the skin, using even strokes; follow the direction of hair growth to avoid causing folliculitis; repeat the procedure, until the appropriate area of skin is completely covered; if a suspension-based lotion is being used, shake the container vigorously before applying a small amount of the lotion to a pad or gauze dressing; apply with even strokes to the skin; repeat the procedure until the appropriate area of the skin is completely covered

c. **Nitroglycerin ointment**—apply the prescribed inches over a paper measuring guide; evenly spread the ointment over the paper guide to promote maximal absorption; avoid applying the ointment on hairy surfaces or over scar tissue because this inhibits absorption; record date and time of day, and initial the paper; cover the paper with plastic wrap, and secure it with tape as needed

d. **Patch**—remove the patch from its protective wrapper; hold the patch by the edge—do not touch the adhesive edges; immediately apply the patch, pressing it firmly with the palm of one hand for 10 to 15 seconds; as prescribed by the physician, remove the patch, and choose a different site to apply a new patch; record date and the time of day, and initial the patch

e. **Powder**—ensure that the skin surface is completely dry to minimize caking and crusting; completely spread apart the skin folds; lightly dust with a shake dispenser until the area is covered with a fine, thin layer of powder; powders wear off easily

5. Apply dressing as prescribed by the physician. Secure with hypoallergenic tape as needed.

6. Assist the patient to a comfortable position, and help to dress him or her as needed.

7. Clean and replace the equipment. Discard disposable items according to *Standard Precautions*.

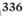 **NURSING CONSIDERATIONS**

To prevent accidental exposure to the medication, wear gloves and use applicators as appropriate.

Do not apply new medication over old medication or over encrusted areas of dead tissue; this prevents absorption and has little therapeutic effect. Always clean the skin with soap and water or debride the tissue of old medication and encrustation before applying new medication.

Instruct the patient/caregiver on how to apply topical medication.

See the patient instruction recommendations in the procedure for *Administration of Medications: General Guidelines.*

 DOCUMENTATION GUIDELINES

Document the following on the visit report:
- The procedure and patient toleration
- Site used for application of topical medication
- Condition of the skin or tissue before the application
- Any patient/caregiver instructions and response to teaching, including the ability to apply topical medication
- Physician notification, if applicable
- *Standard Precautions*
- Other pertinent findings

Document medications on the medication record.

Update the plan of care.

Tuberculin (TB) Skin Test

PURPOSE
- To identify patients with a reaction to the Mantoux antigen

RELATED PROCEDURES
- Administration of Medications: General Guidelines
- Injections

EQUIPMENT
1. Intermediate-strength purified protein derivative (PPD); 0.1 ml of 5 tuberculin units (TUs) as ordered by the physician
2. Tuberculin syringe and needle (½- to ⅞-inch, 27-gauge needle)
3. Tape measure
4. Antiseptic wipes
5. Disposable nonsterile gloves, sharps container, and an impermeable plastic trash bag (see *Infection Control*)

PROCEDURE
1. Explain the procedure to the patient/caregiver.
2. Verify the medication with the clinical record, and check the patient's identity.
3. Assemble the equipment at a convenient work area.
4. Review the steps to withdraw medication from a vial in the procedure for *Injections*.
5. Select the injection site for easy interpretation (three to four fingers width below the antecubital space and a handbreadth above the wrist).
6. Remove the cap from the needle.
7. Hold the patient's skin taut between your thumb and forefinger.
8. Insert the needle at a 15-degree angle, just under the skin (Fig. 9-11).
9. With bevel up, **slowly** inject tuberculin into the epidermis to form a wheal 6 to 10 mm in diameter (Fig. 9-12). Do **not** massage the site.

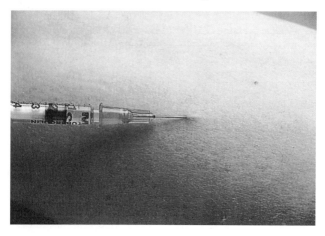

Fig. 9-11 Insertion of needle for TB test. (From Perry AG, Potter PA: *Clinical nursing skills and techniques,* ed 4, St Louis, 1998, Mosby.)

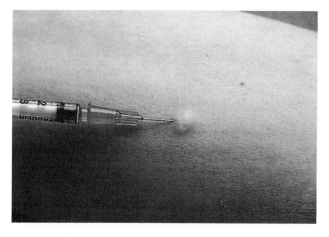

Fig. 9-12 Formation of wheal. (From Perry AG, Potter PA: *Clinical nursing skills and techniques,* ed 4, St Louis, 1998, Mosby.)

10. Provide patient comfort measures.
11. Clean and replace the equipment. Discard disposable items according to *Standard Precautions.*
12. Read the results 48 to 72 hours after the test has been administered.
13. Inspect and palpate the area for induration.
14. Measure the induration transverse to the long axis of the forearm. A significant reaction is an area of induration (not redness) of 5 mm or more.
15. Notify the patient and physician if the results are significant. The Centers for Disease Control and Prevention support the following classification of the tuberculin reaction:
    a. A tuberculin reaction of 5 mm or more is considered positive in the following groups:
       Persons who have had close, recent contact with a patient with infectious TB
       Persons who have a chest x-ray with lesions characteristic of an old healed TB lesion
       Persons who have a known human immunodeficiency virus (HIV) infection or are at risk for HIV infection
    b. A tuberculin reaction of 10 mm or more is considered positive for persons who may not meet the preceding criteria but who have other risk factors for TB, such as the following:
       Foreign-born persons from countries with a high prevalence of TB
       Intravenous drug users
       Residents of long-term care facilities
       Low-income or homeless persons with poor access to medical care, including high-risk racial and ethnic minorities
       Persons with multiple medical problems that may increase the risk of TB once infection is present
    c. A tuberculin reaction of 15 mm or more is classified as positive in all other persons

NURSING CONSIDERATIONS

Administer the skin test soon after the syringe has been filled to avoid contamination and leeching of the tuberculoprotein into the syringe.
If the first test was improperly administered, retest, selecting a site several centimeters away from the original site.

Patients with a positive PPD must have a physician verify a negative chest x-ray and sputum culture in the clinical record.

DOCUMENTATION GUIDELINES

Document the following on the visit report:
- The procedure and patient toleration
- Induration recorded in millimeters
- Physician notification, if applicable
- *Standard Precautions*
- Other pertinent findings

Document the date and time of the initial test, any retest, and the final results.

Document the following on the medication record:
- Antigen name
- Strength
- Lot number
- Dosage
- Route
- Site of administration

Update the plan of care.

CHAPTER 10

Nutrition Procedures

Medical Nutrition Therapy: Assessment of Patient's Nutrient Requirements

---

PURPOSE

- To establish parameters for calories, protein, and fluid level requirements
- To provide instruction on obtaining accurate measurements critical to the nutrition assessment of the patient

RELATED PROCEDURE

- Adult Head-to-Toe Assessment (see Chapter 2)

GENERAL INFORMATION

Medical nutrition therapy (MNT) is the process of assessing the patient, identifying treatment goals, developing the nutrition care plan, and applying specific interventions through multidisciplinary team approaches. All aspects of MNT must include input from, agreement with, and participation by the patient/caregiver. The nutrition assessment includes but is not limited to the information in Box 10-1. In this section, only establishing nutrient requirement parameters is discussed.

EQUIPMENT

1. Cloth measuring tape
2. Scales
3. Calculator
 4. Blood pressure cuff, stethoscope, and thermometer (see *Infection Control*)

PROCEDURE

1. Explain the procedure to the patient/caregiver.

Box 10-1
NUTRITION ASSESSMENT

Subjective data

- Interview with the patient to gather information about appetite, food preferences, eating pattern, weight history, reasonable weight for patient
- Physical examination to determine condition of skin, feeding and meal preparation ability, dental status, mental status, clinical manifestations of problems related to diagnosis

Objective data

- Anthropometric measurements
- Laboratory data
- Medical history to include nutrition and medication regimens

Assessment

- Interpreting and evaluating the data gathered
- Establishing nutrient requirement parameters

Planning

- Professional judgment to determine action/nursing intervention needed for each identified problem

Evaluation

- Methods to evaluate outcomes of care

---

2. Obtain the following patient measurements for nutritional care:
   a. Vital signs
   b. Weight and height; never accept a caregiver's and/or other family member's statement of height or weight of a patient; recent reports from hospital stays or from other institutions may be used as a guide, but accurate height and weight measurements at the time of assessment are preferable; obtain measurements in the following manner:

- Weight—the frequency of conducting weight measurements depends on the physician's orders but should be done at least monthly; follow correct procedures for the type of scale used; always use the same scale to weigh the patient each time; balance the scale before obtaining the patient's weight; weigh the patient at the same time of the day and have the patient wear the same type clothes, stand without support, and wear no shoes; floor scales should be placed on a solid surface, not carpet; for accurate measurements, obtain an average of two to three weight measurements
- Height—measure the patient without him or her wearing shoes; for accurate measurements, obtain an average of three measurements; measurements may be taken with a cloth measuring tape with the patient standing, lying flat in the bed, or contracted in the bed. For bilateral amputee patients, the measurement of the arm span is roughly equal (within 10%) to original height; as individuals age, height decreases
  - (1) The following are alternatives to height and weight measurements:
    - A midarm circumference (MAC) measurement may be used only to judge changes in the patient's condition (MAC does not determine weight status); use a cloth measuring tape to measure the circumference of the arm at the midpoint—between the elbow and shoulder bone; always measure the same arm; record the measurement in centimeters; measure the MAC monthly at the same time of the month
    - Knee height—use the guidelines found in Table 10-1 to estimate height and weight measurements based on knee height (KH), which is the measure of length in centimeters between the top of the knee to the bottom of the heel when the knee and heel are both positioned at right angles to the tibia
    - Frame size—measure the wrist circumference just distal to the styloid process at the wrist crease on the prominent arm using a cloth measuring tape; the "quick" method of establishing frame size is found in Table 10-2
- c. Desirable (normal or ideal) body weight (DBW)—the

Table 10-1   Estimating patient height and weight

ESTIMATING HEIGHT (CM)

Males		Formula for Calculation
White	6-18 years	[KH(cm) × 2.22] + 40.54
Black	6-18 years	[KH(cm) × 2.18] + 39.60
White	19-59 years	[KH(cm) × 1.88] + 71.85
Black	19-59 years	[KH(cm) × 1.79] + 73.42
White	60-80 years	[KH(cm) × 2.08] + 59.01
Black	60-80 years	[KH(cm) × 1.37] + 95.79

Females		Formula for Calculation
White	6-18 years	[KH(cm) × 2.15] + 43.21
Black	6-18 years	[KH(cm) × 2.02] + 46.59
White	19-59 years	[KH(cm) × 1.86] − [Age(years) × 0.05] + 70.25
Black	19-59 years	[KH(cm) × 1.86] − [Age(years) × 0.06] + 68.10
White	60-80 years	[KH(cm) × 1.91] − [Age(years) × 0.17] + 75.00
Black	60-80 years	[KH(cm) × 1.96] + 58.72

Use the following formula to convert height from centimeters to inches:

$$\text{Height in inches} = \frac{\text{Height in cm}}{2.54}$$

ESTIMATING WEIGHT (KG)

Males		Formula for Calculation
White	6-18 years	[KH(cm) × 0.68] + [MAC(cm) × 2.64] − 50.08
Black	6-18 years	[KH(cm) × 0.59] + [MAC(cm) × 2.73] − 48.32

Adapted from Ross Products Division, Abbott Laboratories, Columbus, Ohio.
KH, Knee height; *MAC,* midarm circumference.

Table 10-1   Estimating patient height and weight—cont'd

ESTIMATING WEIGHT (KG)—cont'd

Males—cont'd		Formula for Calculation—cont'd
White	19-59 years	$[KH(cm) \times 1.19] + [MAC(cm) \times 3.21] - 86.82$
Black	19-59 years	$[KH(cm) \times 1.09] + [MAC(cm) \times 3.14] - 83.72$
White	60-80 years	$[KH(cm) \times 1.10] + [MAC(cm) \times 3.07] - 75.81$
Black	60-80 years	$[KH(cm) \times 0.44] + [MAC(cm) \times 2.86] - 39.21$
Females		**Formula for Calculation**
White	6-18 years	$[KH(cm) \times 0.77] + [MAC(cm) \times 2.47] - 50.16$
Black	6-18 years	$[KH(cm) \times 0.71] + [MAC(cm) \times 2.59] - 50.43$
White	19-59 years	$[KH(cm) \times 1.01] + [MAC(cm) \times 2.81] - 66.04$
Black	19-59 years	$[KH(cm) \times 1.24] + [MAC(cm) \times 2.97] - 82.48$
White	60-80 years	$[KH(cm) \times 1.09] + [MAC(cm) \times 2.68] - 65.51$
Black	60-80 years	$[KH(cm) \times 1.50] + [MAC(cm) \times 2.58] - 84.22$

Use the following formula to convert weight in kilograms to pounds:

$$\text{Weight (lbs)} = [\text{Weight(kg)} \times 2.2]$$

Table 10-2 "Quick" method of establishing frame sizes

Males	Females	Frame size
<6 inches	<6 inches	Small
6-7 inches	6-6½ inches	Medium
≥7 inches	≥6½ inches	Large

National Institutes of Health (NIH) defines desirable weight as the midpoint of the recommended weight range at a specified height for persons of medium build, according to Metropolitan Life Insurance; the following guide may also be used to calculate DBW of medium-frame persons (subtract or add 10% for small or large frame persons, respectively):

- Women—allow 100 pounds for first 5 feet of height, plus 5 pounds for each additional inch
- Men—allow 106 pounds for first 5 feet of height, plus 6 pounds for each additional inch

d. Body mass index (BMI)—BMI is an index of a person's weight in relation to height; it is determined by dividing the weight in kilograms by the height in meters squared

Weight Status

BMI <20 = underweight
BMI 20-25 = normal
BMI 26-30 = overweight
BMI >30 = obese

e. Adjusted body weight (AjBW)—AjBW is recommended for calculating the energy requirements of persons who are 125% or more of their DBW

AjBW = [(Actual body weight −
              desirable body weight) × 0.25] + DBW

The following are methods used to estimate energy (calorie) requirements:

- The Harris-Benedict equation (Box 10-2)
- The quick method (Table 10-3)
- (1) Determine whether weight loss or gain is desirable; establish a calorie level by adding or subtracting 500

Box 10-2
HARRIS-BENEDICT EQUATION

Estimated Energy Requirement = Basal energy expenditure (BEE) × activity factor (AF) × injury factor (IF)

BEE is calculated using the Harris-Benedict formula below.

English Measurements

Males: BEE = 66.5 + 6.3W + 12.7H − 6.8A
Females: BEE = 655.1 + 4.4W + 4.6H − 4.7A

W = Weight in pounds

H = Height in inches

A = Age in years

Metric Measurements

Males: BEE = 66.5 + 13.8W + 5.0H − 6.8A
Females: BEE = 655.1 + 9.6W + 1.8H − 4.7A

W = Weight in kilograms

H = Height in centimeters

A = Age in years

Conversions

1 pound = 0.454 kilograms
1 kilogram = 2.2 pounds
1 inch = 2.54 centimeters

Once BEE is determined, energy requirements are calculated by multiplying BEE by the appropriate activity factor and injury factor as listed below.

Activity Factor (AF)

Confined to bed	1.2
Ambulatory, low activity	1.3
Average activity	1.5-1.75
High activity	2

BSA = Body surface area

Adapted from Harris JA, Benedict FG: *A biometric study of basal metabolism in man,* Washington, DC, 1989, Carnegie Institution of Washington.

Continued

Box 10-2
HARRIS-BENEDICT EQUATION—cont'd

Injury Factor (IF)

Mild starvation	0.85-1
Minor surgery	1-1.1
Major surgery	1-1.3
Mild infection	1-1.2
Moderate infection	1.2-1.4
Severe infection	1.3-1.8
Skeletal trauma	1.1-1.3
Burns (<20% BSA)	1.2-1.5
Burns (20%-40% BSA)	1.5-1.8
Burns (>40% BSA)	1.8-2

Combined AF + IF

COPD	1.75-2

BSA = Body surface area

Adapted from Harris JA, Benedict FG: *A biometric study of basal metabolism in man,* Washington, DC, 1989, Carnegie Institution of Washington.

calories from the estimated energy requirements (EER) to produce a 1-pound weight gain or loss per week, respectively; the established calorie level must be discussed with and accepted by the patient for successful diet adherence

(2) Use AjBW to calculate energy requirements of obese individuals who are 125% or more than their DBW

(3) Patients with congestive heart failure (CHF) may have 30% to 50% higher energy requirements than normal

(4) Patients with depleted protein stores (DPS) (e.g., as a result of pressure ulcers, burns, surgery, cancer, sepsis, and hospitalization) require 150 to 300 calories per gram of nitrogen ratio, depending on the severity of their condition; nitrogen grams are calculated by dividing the required protein grams by 6.25; DPS energy needs are calculated by dividing the required protein grams by 6.25, then multiplying the outcome by 150 to 300 calories

Table 10-3   Quick Method

Status	kcal/kg of ideal body weight
Basal energy needs	25-30
Ambulatory with weight maintenance	30-35
Malnutrition with mild stress	40
Severe injuries and sepsis	50-60
Extensive burns	80

      (5) Patients diagnosed with failure to thrive (FTT) require 30 to 35 calories per kilogram of actual body weight (ABW)

   f. Protein requirements—protein requirements are based on grams of protein per kilogram of ABW or DBW and are condition-specific; the following are formulas used to calculate protein requirements for specific patient statuses:

- Normal healthy adults: ABW (kg) × 0.8 g
- Geriatric patients: ABW (kg) × 0.8 to 1 g
- Patients with DPS: ABW (kg) × 1.25 to 1.5 g
- Patients diagnosed with FTT: ABW (kg) × 1 to 1.5 g
- Obese patients: DBW (kg) (used for estimated lean weight) × 1.5 g

   g. Fluid requirements—fluid requirements are based on milliliters of free water fluid per kilogram of ABW and are condition-specific; a minimum of 1500 ml is recommended unless contraindicated by patient's clinical condition; the following are fluid requirements for specific patient statuses:

- Normal health adults: ABW (kg) × 30 to 35 ml
- Geriatric patients: ABW (kg) × 30 ml
- Patients with DPS: ABW (kg) × 30 to 35 ml
- Patients diagnosed with FTT: ABW (kg) × 30 ml
- Obese patients: ABW (kg) × 25 ml
- Patients with CHF: ABW (kg) × 25 ml

3. Use the following to provide nutritional care:
   a. Food diary—use the food diary form (Fig. 10-1) to record a 24-hour recall of the patient's intake
   b. Feedback questions—Use the following list of questions

Write down *any* food you eat or *anything* you drink, the amount you ate or drank, and the time of day you ate it.

Time You Ate	What You Ate or Drank	How Much You Ate or Drank	Instructor's Comments
	Breakfast		
	Snack		
	Lunch		
	Snack		
	Dinner		
	Snack		

Fig. 10-1   Food diary. (From Dantone JJ: *Bridging the gap diet manual,* Grenada, Miss, 1997, Nutrition Education Resources.)

to determine how well the patient has understood the diet instruction; can patients do the following:
- Name three foods and portion sizes allowed on their diet?
- Identify the times of the day they are supposed to eat meals?
- Identify a 1 cup, 2 cup, 1 tablespoon, and 1 teaspoon measuring utensil from the samples you have shown them or from their own kitchen?
- Name a snack food they are allowed to eat on their diet?
- Plan a sample menu for 1 day?

- Tell you the name of their diet and the reason why it is important to follow the diet?
4. Clean and replace the equipment. Discard disposable items according to *Standard Precautions*.

NURSING CONSIDERATIONS

The procedures described throughout this chapter require the home health nurse to establish nutrient requirements for the patient. This is the cornerstone to teaching the patient/caregiver the appropriate amount of food and fluid that should be consumed. It is necessary to compare the amount of food and fluid actually consumed by the patient to this *requirement* and make meaningful constructive recommendations for modifying the diet.

DOCUMENTATION GUIDELINES

Document the following on the visit report:
- Vital signs
- Height—measure at least annually for patients 65 years or older
- Frame size—obtain the wrist measurement of the prominent arm whenever height is measured
- Weight—frequency per physician's orders or at least monthly
- Nutrient requirements—state method used and show calculations for listing calories, protein, and fluid requirements; these parameters should be re-calculated whenever the patient's condition changes
- Comparison between food intake nutrient levels and requirement of nutrients
- Modifications suggested to patient/caregiver
- Physician notification, if applicable
- *Standard Precautions*
- Other pertinent findings
Update the plan of care.

Medical Nutrition Therapy: Chronic Obstructive Pulmonary Disease

PURPOSE

- To instruct the patient/caregiver to maintain adequate intake of calories and protein
- To instruct the patient to maintain a stable, reasonable body weight
- To maintain immunocompetence
- To promote self-care in the home

RELATED PROCEDURES

- Medical Nutrition Therapy: Assessment of Patient's Nutrient Requirements
- Weight (see Chapter 2)

GENERAL INFORMATION

Chronic obstructive pulmonary disease (COPD) is defined as a variety of respiratory diseases characterized by chronic airflow obstruction, namely, chronic bronchitis, asthmatic bronchitis, and emphysema. Signs and symptoms include chronic cough and productive sputum daily for 3 or more months during at least 2 consecutive years, dyspnea, and general difficulty in breathing. COPD is also characterized by shortness of breath, in part as a result of taking in decreased amounts of oxygen and expelling inadequate amounts of carbon dioxide.

The type of foods eaten affects the amount of oxygen and carbon dioxide in the blood. Oxygen is used to change food into fuel, and during this process carbon dioxide is formed as a waste product. Patients with COPD have a lack of oxygen and an increase of carbon dioxide in the blood. This situation leads to lactic acidosis, which makes the patient feel weak.

Malnutrition is a risk factor of respiratory failure. The progression of COPD can be slowed by providing nutrients in correct proportions that place the least amount of stress on respiratory function. Nutritional status is determined by the following:

- Body weight
- Lean body mass

- Biochemical markers
- Skinfold measurements

The following are the most common symptoms of COPD that affect the patient's nutritional status:

- Early satiety
- Bloating
- Anorexia
- Dyspnea
- Fatigue
- Constipation
- Dental problems

The following are recommended calorie distributions for patients with COPD and normal healthy adults:

COPD	Normal
55% fat	30% fat
15% protein	20% protein
30% carbohydrate	50% carbohydrate

A high-fat diet places low stress on the respiratory system. Protein intake should be monitored to prevent overfeeding. The use of long-term steroids can cause protein catabolism. Low-protein intake coupled with high-carbohydrate intake decreases theophylline elimination. Some studies indicate that diets high in vitamins C and E and omega-three fatty acids provide some protection for smokers against developing COPD.

Low body weight is a common problem for patients with COPD because these patients experience the following:

1. Increased calorie expenditure from infection and increased work from breathing, which can be 10 times greater than what a healthy person requires
2. Decreased calorie intake from the following:
   - High doses of theophylline, causing nausea and/or vomiting
   - Chronic sputum, causing poor appetite
   - Full stomach, causing the diaphragm to be restricted after a large meal and resulting in difficulty in breathing
   - Shortness of breath and weakness, causing difficulty in preparing meals
   - Depression
   - Bronchodilators, which are gastric irritants

- Peptic ulcers or gastrointestinal distress (experienced by up to 25% of patients with COPD)

EQUIPMENT

1. Cloth measuring tape
2. Scales or recent weight history of patient
3. Calculator
4. Food labels
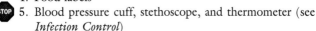 5. Blood pressure cuff, stethoscope, and thermometer (see *Infection Control*)

PROCEDURE

1. Explain the procedure to the patient/caregiver.
2. Consider implementing the following:
    a. Assessing vital signs on each visit; weigh the patient at least once weekly; report abnormal findings to the physician
    b. Setting nutritional requirements for the patient; see the procedure for *Medical Nutrition Therapy: Assessment of Patient's Nutrient Requirements*
    c. Recording a 24-hour recall of the patient's nutritional intake on the food diary form (see Fig. 10-1); analyze the calories, fat, carbohydrate, and protein content of the diet intake
    d. Instructing the patient/caregiver on the COPD diet instruction sheet and menu (Box 10-3 and Table 10-4); use food labels to demonstrate calorie, fat, carbohydrate, and protein content in various foods
    e. Comparing the patient's 24-hour diet recall to his or her prescribed diet order as instructed; make appropriate recommendations to the patient/caregiver for modifying any nutrient intake that is found to be inappropriate on the food intake record
    f. Making suggestions to improve calorie intake, keeping in mind the need to increase fat, monitor protein, and limit carbohydrate intake; use the following feeding strategies:
        - Eat high-calorie foods first, especially those high in fat
        - Use low-cholesterol fatty food sources instead of high-carbohydrate foods for snacks (e.g., eat peanut butter on whole wheat bread rather than a candy bar)
        - Eat small multiple meals
        - Drink liquid 1 hour before meals

Box 10-3
DIET FOR PATIENTS WITH COPD
(High Fat, Low Carbohydrate, Moderate Protein)

Reason for the diet

By increasing the fat and decreasing the carbohydrates (sugars and starchy foods) in the diet, the lungs are able to lower the amount of carbon dioxide in the blood, so you can breathe much better and easier.

How much and/or what to eat

BREAKFAST	LUNCH AND DINNER (SAME)
1 serving unsweetened juice	2 ounces meat with fat
1 serving cereal with fat	1 serving starch with fat
1 serving egg with fat	1 serving vegetables with fat
1 serving bacon, ham, or sausage	1 serving bread
1 serving bread	2 servings fat
2 servings fat	1 serving unsweetened fruit
Diet jelly or syrup	1 serving whole milk
1 serving whole milk	Tea or coffee
Coffee	

10 AM	2 PM	BEDTIME SNACK
1 serving meat or substitute	1 serving bread	1 serving whole milk
1 serving bread	1 serving whole milk	1 serving bread or sandwich
1 serving fruit or juice		

Modified from Dantone JJ: *Bridging the gap diet manual,* Grenada, Miss, 1997, Nutrition Education Resources. *Continued*

Box 10-3
DIET FOR PATIENTS WITH COPD—cont'd
(High Fat, Low Carbohydrate, Moderate Protein)

Do not eat these foods

Regular sugar	Pies
Syrup	Cakes
Jam	Cookies
Jelly	Doughnuts
Candy	Dried fruits
Regular soft drinks	Anything with a lot of sugar in it

Do not take medicines with sugar in them, such as cough syrups.

Special instructions

- The COPD diet listed here is approximately 2200 calories, distributed as 55% fat, 30% carbohydrate, and 15% protein.
- Eat small frequent meals, 6 meals a day if possible. This will keep you from feeling too full at one time. See Table 10-4 for sample menus.
- If you feel too full, it will seem harder to breathe. If you can't breathe you won't eat as well as you should and then you'll lose weight.
- Following the above six-meal plan will help prevent weight loss.

Modified from Dantone JJ: *Bridging the gap diet manual*, Grenada, Miss, 1997, Nutrition Education Resources.

- Do not drink a lot of fluids with meals
- Rest before meals
- Take breathing treatments before meals
- Take oxygen during the meal
- Have the patient take advantage of the times he or she feels good by eating more
- Treat food like a medication—take it seriously, sufficiently, and on time
- Avoid gas-forming foods

- Eat in a relaxed atmosphere and preferably with a companion
3. Clean and replace equipment. Discard disposable items according to *Standard Precautions.*

NURSING CONSIDERATIONS

Beneficial interventions for COPD include smoking cessation; avoiding irritants such as dust, fumes, and air pollutants; and avoiding extreme temperature changes. It is important that the patient with COPD receive influenza and pneumonia vaccines to avoid complications with infection and protect against further digression.

Medications and other therapies such as corticosteroids, antibiotics, bronchodilators, pulmonary rehabilitation, oxygen therapy, exercise, and reconditioning can help maintain functional independence, but no therapy can reverse lung damage. As previously mentioned, many of these therapies have poor nutritional side effects associated with them.

Since COPD is commonly associated with weight loss, low body weight, and calorie-protein malnutrition, prognosis is particularly poor—especially for patients who require mechanical ventilation. Because of high rates of infections and poor lung function, COPD is a common source of morbidity and mortality in older adults.

Because of the aforementioned, it is imperative that the following be done:

- Weigh the patient each visit
- Report to the physician a weight change of 2 pounds in 1 day or 5 or more pounds between visits
- Observe the patient for increased difficulty in breathing or shortness of breath
- Fill out a food intake record once a week and compare it to nutrient requirements

DOCUMENTATION GUIDELINES

Document the following on the visit report:

- The procedure and patient toleration
- Vital signs
- Weight
- Food intake/appetite
- Patient/caregiver instructions and response to teaching, including understanding of the diet and adherence to nutritional recommendations

Table 10-4 Menu for COPD diet *(High Fat, Low Carbohydrate, Moderate Protein)*

	Sunday	Monday	Tuesday
Breakfast	Juice of choice	Juice of choice	Juice of choice
	Oatmeal with margarine	Grits with margarine	Cream of wheat with margarine
	Fried eggs	Fried eggs	Fried eggs
	Sausage	Bacon	Ham
	Biscuit or toast	Biscuits or toast	Biscuit or toast
	2 tsp margarine	2 tsp margarine	2 tsp margarine
	Diet jelly	Diet Jelly	Diet jelly
	Whole milk	Whole milk	Whole milk
	Coffee	Coffee	Coffee
Lunch	Fried chicken	Cheeseburger with:	Roast turkey
	Dried beans or peas	bun	Giblet gravy
	Seasoned greens of choice	Lettuce/pickle/onion	Cornbread dressing
		Mayonnaise/mustard	English peas
	Buttered cornbread	Chips of choice	Buttered roll

	Banana	Diet apple cobbler	Diet jelly
	Unsweetened tea	Unsweetened tea	Angel food cake
	Whole milk	Whole milk	Unsweetened tea
			Whole milk
Dinner	Ham	Beef tips	Potato salad
	Potato salad	Gravy	Tuna salad sandwich
	Seasoned green beans	Rice	Sliced tomatoes
	Buttered roll	Buttered broccoli	Crackers
	Diet pineapple tidbits	Buttered biscuit	Mayonnaise/mustard
	Whole milk	Prunes	Fresh orange
		Whole milk	Whole milk

From Dantone JJ: *Bridging the gap diet manual*, Grenada, Miss, 1997, Nutrition Education Resources.

- Physician notification, if applicable
- *Standard Precautions*
- Other pertinent findings

Update the plan of care.

Medical Nutrition Therapy: Congestive Heart Failure

PURPOSE

- To provide education to the patient/caregiver about the prevention and treatment of congestive heart failure (CHF)
- To stabilize and improve the patient's body weight
- To stabilize and improve the patient's cardiac output through manipulation of sodium and fluid intake
- To promote self-care in the home

RELATED PROCEDURES

- Medical Nutrition Therapy: Assessment of Patient's Nutrient Requirements
- Edema (see Chapter 2)
- Intake and Output (see Chapter 2)
- Weight (see Chapter 2)

GENERAL INFORMATION

CHF occurs when the heart cannot circulate blood to the body tissues in a sufficient manner. This mechanical inadequacy can result in the following signs and symptoms:

- Congestion from edema, especially in the lungs, liver, legs, and bowel
- Shortness of breath
- Fatigue and poor tolerance to exercise
- Rapid pulse rate
- Abdominal fullness with discomfort and loss of appetite
- Mental confusion

Severe weight loss and malnutrition are documented with advanced CHF and are possibly a result of the following:

- Increased metabolism

- Nausea, vomiting, and/or anorexia resulting from digitalis toxicity or congestive enlargement of the liver and abdominal fullness
- Intestinal malabsorption related to venous congestion and edema of the bowel
- Protein-losing intestinal disease

EQUIPMENT

1. Scales
2. Cloth measuring tape
3. Calculator
4. Food models or packages with food labels of sodium content
5. Measuring cup and pint-size and quart-size containers or examples of common containers of the same sizes
 6. Blood pressure cuff, stethoscope, and thermometer (see *Infection Control*)

PROCEDURE

1. Explain the procedure to the patient/caregiver.
2. Consider implementing the following:
   a. Assessing vital signs and evaluating for edema each visit; pay close attention to abnormal changes in blood pressure or adventitious lung sounds; report findings to the physician as necessary
   b. Setting nutritional requirements for the patient; see the procedure for *Medical Nutrition Therapy: Assessment of Patient's Nutrient Requirements*
   c. Obtaining a measurement of the serum albumin or prealbumin level; it is recommended this be done every 3 months to assess for protein-energy malnutrition; obtain physician's orders for laboratory evaluation
   d. Obtaining a measurement of the serum sodium level, which is necessary to determine the need for a fluid restriction; obtain physician's orders for laboratory evaluation
   e. Calculating the fluid requirement for the patient; patients with CHF normally need approximately 25 ml of fluid per kilogram of actual body weight; fluids may be restricted if hyponatremia occurs; in cases of mild CHF, 1500 to 2000 ml of fluid is recommended, in severe cases of CHF, a restriction of 1000 ml or less is common; demonstrate

to the patient/caregiver the correct volume of fluid recommended for the patient to consume daily by using a measuring container familiar to the patient

f. Recording a 24-hour recall of the patient's nutritional intake on the food diary form (see Fig. 10-1); analyze the calories, sodium, and fluid content of the diet intake

g. Instructing the patient/caregiver on the low-salt diet instruction sheet and menu (Box 10-4 and Table 10-5); use food labels to demonstrate sodium content in various foods (just 1 teaspoon of common table salt contains about 2 g of sodium); use measuring cups familiar to the patient to demonstrate proper fluid amounts to consume

h. Comparing the patient's 24-hour diet recall to his or her prescribed diet order as instructed; make appropriate recommendations to the patient/caregiver for modifying any nutrients found to be inappropriate on the food intake record

3. Clean and replace equipment. Discard disposable items according to *Standard Precautions.*

NURSING CONSIDERATIONS

If the patient is taking a potassium-depleting diuretic, a potassium supplement may be necessary. If the patient is taking a potassium-sparing diuretic and an angiotensin-converting enzyme (ACE) inhibitor, the patient should be cautioned about the use of salt substitutes and light salts. Salt substitutes generally contain 2500 to 2800 mg of potassium per teaspoon. Light salt contains 1100 mg of sodium and 1500 mg of potassium per teaspoon. If salt substitutes and/or light salts are used, an increased potassium blood level may result. Make the physician aware of any salt substitute product that the patient is using. Furosemide therapy greater than 80 mg per day for more than 3 months can result in a thiamin deficiency, which causes high-output cardiac failure and impaired cardiac performance.

Studies indicate that thiamin supplementation of 200 mg per day orally for 6 weeks improves left ventricular function, diuresis, and sodium excretion in patients with CHF.

Dysrhythmias and/or increased heart rates can be caused by use of caffeine-containing beverages or medications.

Energy requirements for patients with CHF can be 30% to 50%

Box 10-4
LOW-SALT DIET
(2 g Sodium)

Reason for the diet

To lower blood pressure levels and help you lose fluid that may cause complications with blood pressure problems. To decrease ascites (fluid build up in the body cavity), which may occur if you have heart, kidney, or liver problems. Normal blood pressure in persons younger than 65 years is 120/80 mm Hg. In persons 65 years or older, blood pressure is considered high if it is greater than 160/95 mm Hg.

How much and/or what to eat

BREAKFAST	LUNCH AND DINNER (SAME)
Fruit or juice	Low-salt meat
Low-salt cereal	Low-salt starch
Egg with little salt	Low-salt vegetable
Toast or biscuit	Low-salt salad with low-salt dressing
Margarine	Bread
Jelly	Margarine
Milk	Dessert
Coffee	Coffee or tea
	Milk (at dinner only)

Do not eat these foods

- **Seasonings:** raw salt, garlic salt, onion salt, celery salt, seasoned salt, soy sauce, Worcestershire sauce, barbecue sauce
- **Beverages:** buttermilk, instant cocoa mix
- **Meats:** canned, cured, processed, or smoked meats, such as ham, bacon, sausage, salt pork, fat back, luncheon meat, bologna, Vienna sausage, potted meat

Modified from Dantone JJ: *Bridging the gap diet manual,* Grenada, Miss, 1997, Nutrition Education Resources.

Continued

Box 10-4
LOW-SALT DIET—cont'd
(2 g Sodium)

- **Snacks:** regular crackers, chips, nabs, pretzels, salted nuts, dips, olives, pickles, regular canned soups, popcorn, sauerkraut
- **Fats:** bacon drippings, fat back, regular salad dressings

You may eat these foods

- **Seasonings:** garlic powder, onion powder, herbs, spices, salt substitute (if approved by physician); it is better for you to use herbs and spices to season foods than salt substitute
- **Beverages:** whole, low-fat, or skim milk (up to 2 cups a day)
- **Meats:** fresh pork chops, pork roast, beef, chicken, turkey, fish, lamb, or veal
- **Snacks:** low-salt crackers, crackers with unsalted tops, unsalted popcorn, unsalted nuts, homemade soups with no salt added, any fresh fruits and vegetables, canned fruits and vegetables with no added salt
- **Fats:** margarine, mayonnaise, low-salt salad dressings

Special instructions

If you wish to use a salt substitute make sure it is approved by your physician first. Use fresh or frozen vegetables and meats instead of canned or cured ones. Use seasoning powders instead of seasoning salts, such as garlic powder instead of garlic salt. Read labels on foods carefully—watch for words such as sodium or salt in the ingredients list.

Modified from Dantone JJ: *Bridging the gap diet manual,* Grenada, Miss, 1997, Nutrition Education Resources.

higher than for healthy individuals because of increased metabolic rates from cardiac and pulmonary expenditures.

The following nutrition intervention guidelines should be monitored by the nurse:

- Ensure that the patient's intake of calories and protein is adequate
- Restrict sodium to 3 g daily in cases of mild CHF; if large doses of diuretics are required (greater than 80 mg of furosemide daily), restrict sodium to 2 g daily
- Limit excessive fluid intake; restrict fluids in patients with hyponatremia
- Limit alcohol intake to no more than 1 drink per day of 30 ml of liquor or the equivalent of beer or wine
- Encourage smoking cessation
- Encourage exercise as tolerated by the patient and allowed by the physician
- Recommend thiamin supplementation for patients taking large doses of diuretics
- Weigh the patient on each visit; report to the physician a weight gain of 2 pounds in 1 day or 5 pounds between visits
- Obtain vital signs
- Observe the patient for increased difficulty in breathing or shortness of breath

DOCUMENTATION GUIDELINES

Document the following on the visit report:

- The procedure and patient toleration
- Vital sign measurements
- Weight—a 3- to 5-pound weight gain may suggest fluid retention sufficient to cause heart failure; report any weight change to the physician
- Appetite—analyze the intake of calories, sodium, and fluid
- Laboratory data (serum sodium and albumin levels are of special significance)
- Observance of any changes in breathing (e.g., shortness of breath)
- Tolerance of activities such as limited exercise; level of fatigue
- Any patient/caregiver instructions and response to teaching, including answers to feedback questions

Table 10-5 Menu for low-salt diet *(2 g Sodium)*

	Sunday	Monday	Tuesday
Breakfast	Juice of choice	Juice of choice	Juice of choice
	1s cereal	1s Cereal	1s Cereal
	1s Eggs of choice	1s Eggs of choice	1s Eggs of choice
	1s Turkey sausage		1s Turkey sausage
	Biscuit or toast	Biscuits or toast	Biscuits or toast
	Margarine	Margarine	Margarine
	Jelly	Jelly	Jelly
	Milk	Milk	Milk
	Coffee	Coffee	Coffee
Lunch	1s Fried chicken	Sandwich with:	1s Roast turkey
	1s Dried beans or Peas	1s Hamburger/1s cheese	1s Giblet gravy
	1s Greens	Bun	1s Cornbread dressing

	Buttered cornbread Banana Tea	Lettuce/tomato/onion Mayonnaise ls Mustard ls oven fries Apple cobbler Tea	ls English peas Buttered roll Cranberry sauce Angel food cake Tea
Dinner	ls Pork steak ls Potato salad ls Green beans Buttered roll Pineapple tidbits Milk	ls Beef tips ls Gravy ls Rice ls Buttered broccoli Buttered biscuit Stewed prunes Milk	ls Potato stew ls Tuna salad sandwich Sliced tomatoes ls Crackers Mayonnaise Fresh orange Milk

From Dantone JJ: *Bridging the gap diet manual*, Grenada Miss, 1997, Nutrition Education Resources.
ls, low salt

- Physician notification, if applicable
- *Standard Precautions*
- Other pertinent findings

Update the plan of care.

Medical Nutrition Therapy: Coronary Heart Disease

PURPOSE

- To instruct the patient/caregiver in the prevention and treatment of coronary heart disease (CHD)
- To improve and stabilize the patient's blood levels of total cholesterol (TC), low-density lipoprotein (LDL), and high-density lipoprotein (HDL)
- To improve and stabilize the patient's body weight
- To improve and stabilize the patient's blood pressure
- To improve and stabilize the patient's blood glucose level
- To promote self-care in the home

RELATED PROCEDURE

- Medical Nutrition Therapy: Assessment of Patient's Nutritional Requirements

GENERAL INFORMATION

CHD is a disorder resulting from narrowing of the arteries that supply oxygen and nutrients directly to the heart (coronary arteries). CHD is caused by the thickening and hardening of the walls of these arteries by deposits of lipids and other compounds. This process is known as *atherosclerosis*. Atherosclerosis causes inadequate supply of blood and oxygen to the heart and can lead to heart muscle damage, chest pain, heart attack, and death. The following are risk factors associated with CHD:

- Age—men, 45 or older; women, 55 or older or premature menopausal women who do not receive estrogen replacement therapy
- Family history of premature CHD—father or brother

younger than 55 years; mother or sister younger than 65 years
- Smoking—accounts of one-fifth of all CHD deaths
- Estrogen replacement therapy in postmenopausal women
- Obesity—20% or more over desirable body weight
- Hypertension—blood pressure of 140/90 mm Hg or more or medicine for hypertension (HTN)
- Diabetes—80% of patients with diabetes have some degree of heart disease
- Lack of exercise—60% of the U.S. population does not get 30 minutes of exercise per day
- High TC—200 mg/dl or greater
- High LDL—160 mg/dl or greater with two or more risk factors, 130 mg/dl with fewer than two risk factors, or 100 mg/dl with no other risk factor
- Low HDL—less than or equal to 35 mg/dl
- Inadequate consumption of B-complex vitamins (proposed)
- Hyperinsulinemia (proposed)
- Psychosocial factors—poverty, isolation, depression, hostility

The following are dietary guidelines for individuals at risk for CHD:
- Achieve and maintain a reasonable body weight
- Increase physical activity
- Adhere to a diet that is less than or equal to 30% total fat, 10% saturated fat, and 300 mg of cholesterol per day; (for patients with documented CHD, more strict limits are encouraged: 30% total fat, 7% saturated fat, 200 mg cholesterol per day)
- Increase dietary intake of B-complex vitamins (folate, B6, B12) and vitamin E
- Moderate alcohol consumption of about 1 ounce per day
- Smoking cessation
- For patients with diabetes, promote intensive control of blood glucose levels to prevent the requirement of high insulin levels, therefore preventing hyperinsulinemia

EQUIPMENT

1. Scales
2. Cloth measuring tape

3. Calculator
4. Food models or packages with food labels of calories, cholesterol, saturated fat, and sodium content
STOP 5. Stethoscope, blood pressure cuff, and thermometer (see *Infection Control*)

PROCEDURE

1. Explain the procedure to the patient/caregiver.
2. Consider implementing the following:
   a. Setting nutritional requirements for the patient; see the procedure for *Medical Nutrition Therapy: Assessment of Patient's Nutrient Requirements.*
   b. Assessing vital signs on each visit; weigh patient at least monthly; report abnormal findings to the physician
   c. Recording a 24-hour recall of the patient's nutritional intake on the food diary form (see Fig. 10-1); analyze the total calories, cholesterol, saturated fat, and sodium content of foods eaten
   d. Instructing the patient/caregiver on the low-cholesterol, high-fiber, no-added–salt diet instruction sheet and menu (Box 10-5 and Table 10-6); use food labels to demonstrate sodium, total fat, and saturated fat content in various foods
   e. Comparing the patient's 24-hour diet recall to his or her prescribed diet order as instructed; make appropriate recommendations to the patient/caregiver for modifying any nutrients found to be inappropriate on the food intake record
   f. Instructing the patient/caregiver to limit total fat intake to no more than 30% of his or her calorie intake per day (e.g., in a 2000 calorie diet, 30% fat = 600 calories; 600 calories of fat = about 65 g of fat a day; of that 65 g of total fat, only about 20 g should be from a saturated fat source); use food labels to add up grams of fat and milligrams of cholesterol in foods eaten daily
3. Clean and replace equipment. Discard disposable items according to *Standard Precautions.*

NURSING CONSIDERATIONS

If the patient is more than 10% over ideal body weight, a weight loss of 10 pounds can make a significant reduction in blood pressure and CHD management.

Continued on p. 376

Box 10-5
LOW-CHOLESTEROL, HIGH-FIBER, NO-ADDED–SALT DIET (AMERICAN HEART ASSOCIATION DIET)

(4 g Sodium)

Reason for the diet

To lower blood cholesterol and help prevent hardening of the arteries. To control bowel movement, to lose fluid, or to help lower blood pressure. Normal total blood cholesterol level is 150-200 mg/100 ml for persons younger than 70 years. For females 70 and older, normal total blood cholesterol level may be 240-300 mg/100 ml. For males 70 years or older, normal blood cholesterol levels may be 240-260 mg/100 ml. A cholesterol level less than 160 mg/100 ml in an elderly person might indicate that the person is malnourished.

How much and/or what to eat

BREAKFAST	LUNCH AND DINNER (SAME)	BEDTIME SNACK
Fruit or juice	Lean meat or substitute	2 cups prune juice or 4 prunes
Whole grain cereal	Starch	2 graham crackers
Egg substitute	Vegetable and/or salad	
Whole wheat toast	Whole wheat bread	
Margarine	Margarine	
Jelly	Dessert (usually fruit)	
Skim milk	Skim milk	
Coffee	Coffee or tea	

Modified from Dantone JJ: *Bridging the gap diet manual,* Grenada, Miss, 1997, Nutrition Education Resources. *Continued*

Box 10-5
LOW-CHOLESTEROL, HIGH-FIBER, NO-ADDED–SALT DIET (AMERICAN HEART ASSOCIATION DIET)—CONT'D
(4 g Sodium)

Do not eat these foods
- **Milk:** Whole milk (3.5%), low-fat milk (2%), cream
- **Meats:** Meats fried in animal fat (saturated fat), fats on meats, bacon, sausage, hot dogs, bologna, liver, heart, kidney, skin of chicken or turkey, duck, deer meat sausage
- **Fats:** Real butter, lard, fat back, salt pork, regular margarine, bacon drippings, gravies, sweet cream, sour cream, coconut or coconut oil, chocolate
- **Other:** Regular cheeses, egg yolks

You may eat these foods
- **Milk:** Skim milk (.5%)
- **Meats:** Baked, broiled, or boiled lean meats; beef, pork, chicken, fish, lamb, or veal; most wild game (except duck and deer meat sausage); cut off all fat on meat that you can see; take skin off of chicken and turkey before eating it; use low-fat meats with very little fat marbling; use 100% vegetable oil (unsaturated fat) when frying meats
- **Fats:** 100% vegetable oils, low-cholesterol margarine, cocoa powder
- **Other:** Low-fat cheese, egg whites, egg substitutes such as Egg Beaters (two whole eggs are allowed per week), peanut butter

Special instructions
- Cholesterol is found mostly in meats and other animal food sources, such as milk and eggs. If you do not eat a lot of fats from animals (saturated fats), you will lower your total blood cholesterol level.

Modified from Dantone JJ: *Bridging the gap diet manual,* Grenada, Miss, 1997, Nutrition Education Resources.

Box 10-5

LOW-CHOLESTEROL, HIGH-FIBER, NO-ADDED–SALT DIET (AMERICAN HEART ASSOCIATION DIET)—CONT'D

(4 g Sodium)

Special instructions—cont'd

- Increasing the amount of 100% vegetable oils (unsaturated fats) will lower your total blood cholesterol level.
- There are many fat-free, cholesterol-free products available now. Read labels carefully when shopping.
- Increase the amount of water or other fluids you drink to six to eight glasses daily

Add fiber to your diet

- Eat only whole wheat breads (brown breads) and cereals, such as all bran, bran flakes, oat bran, and unprocessed wheat bread
- Eat brown or wild rice
- Eat raw fruits and vegetables daily
- Eat cooked vegetables such as greens, dried beans and peas, potatoes with skins, fresh beans and peas
- Drink prune juice or eat prunes daily

Decrease salt intake

- Use salt very lightly when preparing foods (do not use more than a total of 2 teaspoons of salt in **all** foods prepared for one meal), and never use any salt at the table when eating meals
- Avoid foods high in salt, such as cured or canned meats (e.g., bacon, ham, sausage, fat back, salt pork, Vienna sausage, potted meat, cold cuts, luncheon meats)
- Do not eat salted crackers; snack foods such as potato chips or other chips; nuts; nabs; regular cheeses; or seasonings with salt in them, such as garlic salt, onion salt, Worcestershire sauce or soy sauce.

Table 10-6 American Heart Association diet

	Sunday	Monday	Tuesday
Breakfast	Prune juice	Orange juice	Apple juice
	ff All bran cereal	ff Oatmeal	ff Raisin bread
	ff Egg substitute	ff Egg substitute	ff Egg substitute
	ff Whole wheat toast	Bran muffin	ff Turkey sausage
	Margarine	Margarine	ff Whole wheat toast
	Jelly	Jelly	Margarine
	Skim milk	Skim milk	Jelly
	Coffee	Coffee	Skim milk
			Coffee
Lunch	ff Baked chicken	Sandwich:	ff Roast turkey
	ff Dried beans	ff Hamburger	Giblet gravy (1 tbsp)
	ff Greens	Whole wheat bun	ff Cornbread dressing
	1 slice whole wheat bread	Lettuce/pickle/onion	ff English peas

Margarine (1 tsp) Banana Tea	ff Mayonnaise (1 tsp) Mustard ff Oven fries ff Stewed apples Tea	ff Roll Cranberry sauce Angel food cake Tea
Dinner		
ff Ham Potato salad with 1 tsp ff Mayonnaise ff Green beans ff Roll Pineapple tidbits Skim milk	ff Beef tips Gravy ff Rice ff Broccoli 1 Slice whole wheat toast Margarine (1 tsp) Stewed prunes Skim milk	ff Potato stew Tuna salad on whole wheat bread Sliced tomatoes Crackers ff Mayonnaise (1 tsp) Fresh orange Skim milk

From Dantone JJ: *Bridging the gap diet manual*, Grenada, Miss, 1997, Nutrition Education Resources.
ff, fat free.
Do not add salt to foods at the table.

One of the functions of insulin is to deposit fat. When there is an increase in insulin requirement related to diabetes or insulin resistance, there is also a likelihood that more fat will be deposited, possibly leading to atherosclerosis. The best practice is tight control of blood glucose and use of as little exogenous insulin as possible. A low-glycemic–index diet has shown to be beneficial for this purpose.

If the patient is taking a potassium-depleting diuretic, a potassium supplement may be necessary. Adequate potassium intake of 3500 mg (90 mEq) per day is recommended. If the patient is taking a potassium-sparing diuretic and an ACE inhibitor, he or she should be cautioned about the use of salt substitutes and light salts. Salt substitutes generally contain 2500 to 2800 mg of potassium per teaspoon. Light salt contains 1100 mg of sodium and 1500 mg of potassium per teaspoon. If salt substitutes/and or light salt are used in excess, an increased potassium blood level may result. Make the physician aware of any salt substitute product the patient is using.

The following nutrition intervention guidelines should be monitored by the nurse:

- Total calorie intake to promote weight loss or maintenance
- Intake of cholesterol, total fats, and saturated fats
- Sodium intake—limit to 4 to 5 g daily
- Alcohol intake—limit to no more than 1 drink per day of 30 cc of liquor or the equivalent of beer or wine for women; men may have no more than 2 drinks daily
- Smoking frequency or cessation
- Exercise—regular minimum of 20 to 30 minutes daily; nonvigorous; exercise program should be initiated after blood pressure is under control and with the physician's approval; encourage chair/bed exercise when appropriate
- Intake of low-fat dairy products—twice daily; if the patient refuses to or cannot drink or eat dairy products, recommend a calcium supplement of 800 to 1200 mg per day and a magnesium supplement of 280 to 350 mg per day to meet recommended daily allowances (RDAs) (higher doses of magnesium have been known to cause diarrhea)
- Intake of foods rich in B-complex vitamins (folate, B6, B12); this includes orange juice, green leafy vegetables, milk, eggs, and lean meats—especially liver and other organ meats

DOCUMENTATION GUIDELINES

Document the following on the visit report:

- The procedure and patient toleration
- Vital signs
- Serum lipid and glucose levels
- Weight—report any weight change to the physician
- Food intake—analyze the intake of calories, sodium, potassium, calcium, and alcohol; document any suggestions for modifications in the diet
- Physical fitness level and amount of routine allowed exercise the patient gets
- Smoking frequency or cessation
- Evaluation of current medications
- Any patient/caregiver instructions and response to teaching, including answers to feedback questions
- *Standard Precautions*
- Physician notification, if applicable
- Other pertinent findings

Update the plan of care.

Medical Nutrition Therapy: Diabetes Mellitus

PURPOSE

- To achieve and maintain normal blood glucose levels
- To achieve and maintain optimal blood lipid levels
- To achieve and maintain healthy body weight
- To prevent, delay, or treat nutrition-related complications
- To promote self-care in the home

RELATED PROCEDURES

- Medical Nutrition Therapy: Assessment of Patient's Nutrient Requirements
- Blood Glucose Testing (see Chapter 12)

GENERAL INFORMATION

In 1994 the American Diabetes Association (ADA) revised the nutrition principles for diabetes according to the results of the Diabetes Control and Complications Trial (DCCT). In the past, the health care industry held to the belief that sugars, both added and naturally occurring, are rapidly absorbed and lead to hyperglycemia and an increased need for insulin. However, more recent scientific research has indicated that sucrose and other sugars do not create a more harmful effect on blood glucose levels and are not absorbed more rapidly than starches. The ADA's revision, which was based on this research, sets forth the principle that "a carbohydrate is a carbohydrate is a carbohydrate."

The ADA's current position is that sucrose can be used as part of the total amount of carbohydrate in a meal plan, but not as added carbohydrate. An overall healthy diet based on the Food Guide Pyramid should be followed. The total amount of food, as well as the total amount of carbohydrate, eaten will have more of an effect on blood glucose levels than the source of the carbohydrate. Overeating of any food, not just carbohydrates, will affect blood glucose control.

EQUIPMENT

1. Cloth measuring tape
2. Scales
3. Calculator
4. Measuring cups and spoons
5. Food models

6. Blood pressure cuff, stethoscope, thermometer, and glucose meter (see *Infection Control*)

PROCEDURE

1. Explain the procedure to the patient/caregiver.
2. Consider implementing the following:
   a. Assessing vital signs on each visit; weigh the patient at least weekly; obtain the blood glucose value; have the patient perform self-monitoring of blood glucose (SMBG) before eating breakfast; report abnormal findings to the physician
   b. Setting nutritional requirements for the patient; see the procedure for *Medical Nutrition Therapy: Assessment of Patient's Nutrient Requirements;* establish a reasonable body weight that is agreeable with the patient to set as a goal
   c. Recording a 24-hour recall of the patient's nutritional in-

Here is a simple chart you should use to keep up with the food you eat, carbohydrate choices you make, and to record your blood glucose level. You should write down everything you eat and how much you eat every day. This will help you get used to the amount of food you should eat. Keeping a food record along with a blood glucose record will help you see how different amounts of foods affect your blood glucose level.

TIME	WHAT I ATE OR DRANK	HOW MUCH I ATE OR DRANK	NUMBER OF CARBOHYDRATE CHOICES	BLOOD GLUCOSE LEVEL

Instructor's signature: _____ Date: _____

Patient's signature: _____

Patient's name: _____ Pt./Room#: _____

Fig. 10-2   Daily food and blood glucose record.
(From Dantone JJ: *Bridging the gap diet manual*, Grenada, Miss, 1997, Nutrition Education Resources.)

take and any available blood glucose data on the daily food and blood glucose record form (Fig. 10-2); analyze the carbohydrate and total calorie content of the diet intake

d. Instructing the patient/caregiver on carbohydrate counting for patients with diabetes (Box 10-6, Table 10-7, and Fig. 10-2)

e. Comparing the patient's 24-hour diet recall to his or her prescribed diet order as instructed; make appropriate recommendations to the patient/caregiver for modifying any nutrients found to be inappropriate on the food intake record

f. Discussing with the patient the importance of accurately

Text continued on p. 386

Box 10-6
CARBOHYDRATE COUNTING
FOR PATIENTS WITH DIABETES

Reason for the diet

To help prevent high or low blood glucose levels. Eating a constant equal amount of carbohydrate at each meal and at snacks can help control weight and maintain a normal blood glucose level.

Carbohydrates are either:

1. Sugars (e.g., sugar, syrup, hard candy, fruits, fruit juices, or the sugar in milk [lactose])

or

2. Starches (e.g., bread, cereal, rice, pasta, or starchy vegetables such as potatoes or corn)

After either sugars or starches are eaten, all of it turns into sugar in the stomach and goes into the blood stream at the same speed. The total amount of carbohydrate you eat will affect your blood glucose level more than the kind of carbohydrate you eat. In other words, one carbohydrate is equal to another carbohydrate in how fast it enters the blood stream. Eating the same amount of carbohydrate at each meal and at snacks will help your blood glucose level to stay normal at all times.

How much and/or what to eat

Carbohydrate counting is adding up the number of "carbohydrate choices" you eat at each meal or snacks. One "carbohydrate choice" has about 15 g of carbohydrate. A gram is the weight of the carbohydrate in the food.

Foods that contain carbohydrates

1. **Starches:** breads; crackers; cereals; pasta such as spaghetti, noodles, or macaroni; rice; grains; starchy vegetables such as potatoes or corn; and fresh, dried, or canned beans or peas (except green beans or wax beans)
2. **Fruits:** fruits and juices
3. **Milk:** milk, yogurt

Modified from Dantone JJ: *Bridging the gap diet manual,* Grenada, Miss, 1997, Nutrition Education Resources.

Box 10-6

CARBOHYDRATE COUNTING FOR PATIENTS WITH DIABETES—CONT'D

Foods that contain carbohydrates—cont'd

4. **Other:** sugar—white granulated, powdered, or brown; honey; syrup; jam; jelly; molasses; ice cream; cookies; doughnuts; cake; or pie (many of these "other" foods have fat in them that makes the calorie level in the diet too high)

Reading the nutrition facts food label

The number of grams of carbohydrate in each food can be found on the nutrition facts label on all packages of food you buy in the store. Look at the illustration below

This label is from a loaf of whole wheat bread. Read the label and find the following information:

- Serving size = 1 slice
- Calories per serving (1 slice) = 60 calories
- Fat per serving = 1 g
- Carbohydrate per serving = 12 g

A one-slice serving of this bread would be counted as 1 carbohydrate choice. You will not usually find foods that have exactly 15 g of carbohydrate per serving. You may allow 7 to 22 g of carbohydrate per serving as equal to 1 carbohydrate choice.

The nutrition facts label is very helpful for other information, such as how much fat, cholesterol, sodium, fiber, and protein is in each serving. To manage your blood glucose level more effectively select foods with no more than 3 to 5 g of fat per carbohydrate choice. For example, this bread has only 1 g of fat per serving (per carbohydrate choice). That is very good.

Continued

Box 10-6
CARBOHYDRATE COUNTING
FOR PATIENTS WITH DIABETES—cont'd

When the food is not labeled

Some foods do not have nutrition facts labels, such as fresh fruits and vegetables. The following is a quick and simple food group list to tell you how much of a food counts as 1 carbohydrate choice. All foods listed in this chart count as 1 carbohydrate choice for each serving.

GOOD GROUP LISTS	SERVING SIZE (1 CARBOHYDRATE CHOICE, OR 15 G)
1. Starches	
Cereal, starchy vegetable (potato), or pasta	½ cup
Bread, biscuit, or roll	1 slice or small piece
2. Fruits	
Fresh fruit, fruit canned in light syrup or its own juice, fruit juice	½ cup
Dried fruit	¼ cup
3. Milk	
Skim, low-fat, whole milk, or buttermilk	1 cup
Nonfat yogurt	¾ cup (6 oz)
4. Other	
Regular syrup, honey, jam, or jelly	1 tbsp
Sugar-free pudding or nonfat, sugar-free ice cream	2 cups
Fat-free cookies	2 small cookies

Modified from Dantone JJ: *Bridging the gap diet manual,* Grenada, Miss, 1997, Nutrition Education Resources.

Box 10-6
CARBOHYDRATE COUNTING
FOR PATIENTS WITH DIABETES—cont'd

Examples of carbohydrate choices (each equals 1 choice, or 15 g, of carbohydrate)

- 1 slice of bread
- ½ cup of pasta
- ½ cup of corn

1 medium apple
1 cup of low-fat milk
1 tbsp regular syrup
½ cup nonfat, sugar-free ice cream

Special instructions

The Food Guide Pyramid, p. 384, shows the number of servings from each food group that you should eat every day to remain healthy. The fats, sweets, and alcohol list is at the top of the pyramid; you should only eat very small amounts of these foods and no alcohol at all if possible (ask your physician, dietitian, or nurse about how much you are allowed to eat). The meat and others list on the pyramid tells you to eat 2 to 3 servings each day. Meat is very important—it has protein in it but has little or no carbohydrate. Protein will keep your skin healthy and your blood rich. There is no limit on meat, but eating less is best. Vegetables that are not starchy, such as green beans, tomatoes, lettuce, and greens, have a small amount of carbohydrate. If you eat 3 servings of these vegetables at one meal, you must count them as a carbohydrate choice.

Continued

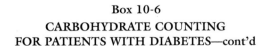

Box 10-6
CARBOHYDRATE COUNTING
FOR PATIENTS WITH DIABETES—cont'd

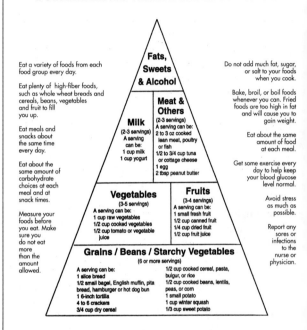

Eat a variety of foods from each food group every day.

Eat plenty of high-fiber foods, such as whole wheat breads and cereals, beans, vegetables and fruit to fill you up.

Eat meals and snacks about the same time every day.

Eat about the same amount of carbohydrate choices at each meal and at snack times.

Measure your foods before you eat. Make sure you do not eat more than the amount allowed.

Do not add much fat, sugar, or salt to your foods when you cook.

Bake, broil, or boil foods whenever you can. Fried foods are too high in fat and will cause you to gain weight.

Eat about the same amount of food at each meal.

Get some exercise every day to help keep your blood glucose level normal.

Avoid stress as much as possible.

Report any sores or infections to the nurse or physician.

Fats, Sweets & Alcohol

Meat & Others (2-3 servings)
A serving can be:
2 to 3 oz cooked lean meat, poultry or fish
1/2 to 3/4 cup tuna or cottage cheese
1 egg
2 tbsp peanut butter

Milk (2-3 servings)
A serving can be:
1 cup milk
1 cup yogurt

Vegetables (3-5 servings)
A serving can be:
1 cup raw vegetables
1/2 cup cooked vegetables
1/2 cup tomato or vegetable juice

Fruits (3-4 servings)
A serving can be:
1 small fresh fruit
1/2 cup canned fruit
1/4 cup dried fruit
1/2 cup fruit juice

Grains / Beans / Starchy Vegetables (6 or more servings)
A serving can be:
1 slice bread
1/2 small bagel, English muffin, pita bread, hamburger or hot dog bun
1 6-inch tortilla
4 to 6 crackers
3/4 cup dry cereal
1/2 cup cooked cereal, pasta, bulgur, or rice
1/2 cup cooked beans, lentils, peas, or corn
1 small potato
1 cup winter squash
1/3 cup sweet potato

How many carbohydrate choices to eat

The physician, dietitian, or nurse will help you decide which of the following amounts of calories and carbohydrate choices allowed each day or at each meal is best for you. This amount will be based on your height, weight, amount of exercise you get on a routine basis, blood glucose level, and diabetic condition at this time. The following chart shows how carbohydrate grams and carbohydrate choices are allowed for each calorie level.

Modified from Dantone JJ: *Bridging the gap diet manual,* Grenad Miss, 1997, Nutrition Education Resources.

Box 10-6
CARBOHYDRATE COUNTING
FOR PATIENTS WITH DIABETES—cont'd

CALORIES/ DAY	CARBOHY- DRATE TOTAL GRAMS/ DAY	CARBOHY- DRATE CHOICES/ DAY	CARBOHY- DRATE CHOICES/ SIX-MEAL PLAN
1200	150	10	1½
1500	188	12	2
1800	225	15	2½
2000	250	17	3
2200	275	18	3
2500	313	21	3½
2800	350	23	4
3000	375	25	4

For example if you should eat 1800 calories per day, you are allowed to have a total of 225 g of carbohydrate per day, which would be the same as 15 carbohydrate choices per day, or 2½ carbohydrate choices at each meal and at snacks. The "six-meal plan" listed in the far right column means you can eat three regular meals and have three snacks between meals.

Calories and carbohydrate choices patients should have daily

(The instructor should complete the following information, working with the patient to fit the meal pattern into his or her lifestyle.)

_____ Total calories every day
_____ Total grams of carbohydrate every day
_____ Total carbohydrate choices every day
_____ Carbohydrate choices at each of three meals and three snacks every day

Continued

Box 10-6
CARBOHYDRATE COUNTING
FOR PATIENTS WITH DIABETES—cont'd

Break down carbohydrate choices for meals

Take the number of carbohydrate choices allowed and decide which foods to eat each time.

_____ Carbohydrate choices at breakfast:
____ starch, ____ fruit, ____ milk, ____ other.
_____ Carbohydrate choices at midmorning:
____ starch, ____ fruit, ____ milk, ____ other.
_____ Carbohydrate choices at lunch:
____ starch, ____ fruit, ____ milk, ____ other.
_____ Carbohydrate choices at midafternoon:
____ starch, ____ fruit, ____ milk, ____ other.
_____ Carbohydrate choices at dinner:
____ starch, ____ fruit, ____ milk, ____ other.
_____ Carbohydrate choices at bedtime snack:
____ starch, ____ fruit, ____ milk, ____ other.

You may want to have your carbohydrate choices at different times than listed above, but remember that your blood glucose level will stay more normal if the carbohydrate choices are eaten in equal amounts and about the same time every day.

Modified from Dantone JJ: *Bridging the gap diet manual,* Grenada, Miss, 1997, Nutrition Education Resources.

measuring the foods as listed on the diet instruction sheet; illustrate correct measurement using standard measuring cups and spoons; in the home setting, identify utensils commonly used to measure foods

g. Discussing with the patient the times of the day he or she usually eats meals; compare those times to the times indicated on the diet instruction sheet; work with the patient to establish a regular eating pattern, due to the importance of food and medication timing in controlling his or her disease process

3. Clean and replace equipment. Discard disposable items according to *Standard Precautions.*

NURSING CONSIDERATIONS

Carbohydrate counting is not applicable to all patients. The historical ADA exchange lists meal planning system is still available. It is of utmost importance when deciding between these two methods of diet counseling that the patient be treated in a way to incorporate diabetic management into his or her lifestyle, not his or her lifestyle into the diabetic regimen. To assist in this process, it is important to have a team of health care professionals working with the patient. This team should include a registered dietitian, physician, registered nurse, and other health care professionals to bring a continuum of care to the patient.

Carbohydrate counting can be done successfully if the patient is instructed in a very simple manner. Carbohydrate counting will be difficult for patients who have always been told "do not eat sugar." If the blood glucose level of such patients is under good control, these patients should remain on their current regimen. The carbohydrate counting system can be used by patients in any age group.

The carbohydrate counting diet is not to be attempted without the full cooperation of the multidisciplinary team. All parameters of the patient's care should be taken into consideration before beginning any new therapy. Mental status, stress—both physical and emotional—exercise or activity level, blood glucose levels, and the medication regimen all are a part of this new diet therapy.

DOCUMENTATION GUIDELINES

To monitor the patient's adherence to his or her diet, have him or her record the times he or she eats, the foods and beverages consumed, and his or her daily blood glucose level if available on the daily food and blood glucose record forms. Evaluate the data by comparing the information to the patient's actual meal plan. Counsel the patient on any modifications he or she needs to make.

Document the following in the visit report:
- The procedure and patient toleration
- Vital signs, including blood glucose values and/or SMBG
- Height, frame size, desirable body weight, body weight goal, and established calorie level
- Data from the daily food and blood glucose record forms completed by the patient

Table 10-7 Menu for carbohydrate counting for patients with diabetes

	Day 1	Day 2	Day 3
Breakfast	½ cup Orange juice*	1 Banana	1 cup Cantaloupe cubes*
	1 Egg (cooked any way)	¾ cup Corn flakes*	½ cup Cream of Wheat*
	1 Slice bacon	1 Slice ham	1 Cheese toast* or 1 sausage
	1 Slice whole wheat toast*	1 Slice whole wheat toast*	and biscuit
	1 tsp margarine	1 tsp Margarine	1 tsp Margarine
	1 tbsp Jelly or jam*	1 tbsp Jelly or jam*	Coffee/tea/water
	Coffee/tea/water	1 cup Low-fat milk*	
		Coffee/tea/water	
Midmorning snack	¼ cup Low-fat granola*	Bagel*: ½ large or 1 small	¾ cup Raisin bran*
	1 cup Low-fat yogurt* (custard	1 tbsp Cream cheese	1 cup Low-fat milk*
	or frozen style)	1 tbsp Jelly or jam*	
		½ cup Grapefruit juice	
Lunch	3 oz Baked chicken	6 oz Vegetable soup	3 oz Roast beef
	½ cup Dried beans/peas*	1 Hamburger on bun†	½ cup Rice*
	½ cup Turnip or mustard	20 French fries*	½ cup Carrots
	greens	Lettuce/pickle/onion	½ cup Green salad
	½ cup Tomato/cucumber salad	1 tsp Mayonnaise	2 tbsp Fat-free dressing*
	1 piece Cornbread*	1 tsp Mustard	1 Roll*

	1 tsp Margarine 12 Fresh cherries* Coffee/tea/water	1 tsp Catsup ½ cup Diet gelatin/fruit cocktail Coffee/tea/water	1 tsp Margarine ½ cup Sliced peaches* Coffee/tea/water
Midafternoon snack	3 cups Popcorn* 1 Diet soft drink	½ cup Low-fat ice cream* 4 Vanilla wafers*	1 Apple* 1 oz Low-fat cheese
Dinner	3 oz Barbecue pork ½ cup Pasta salad* ½ cup Green beans 1 piece French bread* 1 tsp Margarine ½ cup Pineapple tidbits* Coffee/tea/water	3 oz Fried or baked fish 1 Corn on the cob* ½ cup Coleslaw 3 Hushpuppies* 1 tbsp Low-fat tartar sauce ⅛th Lemmon custard pie* Coffee/tea/water	3 oz Roast turkey 1 tbsp Giblet gravy ½ cup Cornbread dressing* ½ cup Summer squash 1 Roll* 1 tsp Margarine 1 tsp Cranberry sauce 1 piece Angel food cake* Coffee/tea/water
Bedtime snack	¾ cup Dry cereal of choice* 1 cup Low-fat milk*	3 Graham crackers* 1 cup Nonfat yogurt* (custard or frozen style)	2 tbsp Peanut butter 4 Whole wheat crackers* 1 cup Low-fat milk*

From Dantone JJ: *Bridging the gap diet manual*, Grenada, Miss, 1997, Nutrition Education Resources.
*1 carbohydrate choice (15 g of carbohydrates)
†2 carbohydrate choices (30 g of carbohydrates)

- Analysis of the patient's food intake and the modifications suggested
- Patient/caregiver instructions and response to teaching, including understanding of the diet and adherence to nutritional recommendations
- Physician notification, if applicable
- *Standard Precautions*
- Other pertinent findings

Update the plan of care.

Medical Nutrition Therapy: Enteral Nutrition Support

PURPOSE

- To provide liquid nourishment to the patient who is unable to maintain sufficient oral intake because of anatomic or mental disease processes
- To provide adequate nutrients for support, maintenance, or restoration of nutritional status
- To instruct the patient/caregiver on tube feeding procedures and schedule
- To promote self-care in the home

RELATED PROCEDURES

- Medical Nutrition Therapy: Assessment of Patient's Nutrient Requirements
- Gastrostomy Tube Feeding (see Chapter 5)
- Enteral Feeding (see Chapter 5)

GENERAL INFORMATION

Indications for enteral nutrition support include the following:
- Malnutrition risk or presence
- Inadequate intestinal digestion and absorption
- Absence of bowel obstruction
- Accessibility of tube site
- Adequate tolerance to formula

The following are common conditions that warrant enteral nutrition support:

- Dysphagia
- Cerebral vascular accident
- Cancer
- Gastrointestinal disease
- Coma
- Cardiac failure
- Respiratory failure
- Depression

Determine the optimal feeding route by using the following guidelines:

- Parenteral nutrition—if the patient's gastrointestinal tract is nonfunctional
- Nasogastric tube—if the patient requires tube feeding for less than 6 weeks
- Gastrostomy tube—if the patient requires tube feeding for more than 6 weeks
- Jejunostomy tube—if the patient is at risk for aspiration or has severe esophageal reflux, obstruction, stricture, fistulae, or ileus of the upper gastrointestinal tract

EQUIPMENT

1. Cloth measuring tape
2. Scales
3. Measuring cups, syringes
4. Calculator
5. Tube feeding formula
6. Administration system specified for the patient (e.g., pump, gravity bags, syringes)

 7. Blood pressure cuff, stethoscope, thermometer, and glucose meter (see *Infection Control*)

PROCEDURE

1. Explain the procedure to the patient/caregiver.
2. Consider implementing the following:
   a. Assessing vital signs on each visit; weigh the patient at least weekly; report abnormal findings to the physician
   b. Obtaining a physician's order for the patient's enteral nutrition support
   c. Setting nutritional requirements for the patient; see the

procedure for *Medical Nutrition Therapy: Assessment of Patient's Nutrient Requirements*.

d. Calculating the calories, protein, and fluid volume in the patient's current physician's order using the calorie, protein, and fluid information on the can of formula or other reference guides

e. Comparing the patient's nutrient requirements to the nutrients in the current order; if the patient's order is inadequate, refer the patient to the registered dietitian for a thorough assessment and/or contact the physician regarding the deficit

f. Discussing the enteral nutrition procedure and schedule with the patient/caregiver (Box 10-7); establish an agreeable schedule that enables the patient/caregiver to have some amount of freedom; when the patient's enteral nutrition support order is adequate and agreeable with the patient/caregiver, write down the schedule on the form (see Box 10-7) and review it with the patient/caregiver; specify water flushes before and after feedings and medications to ensure adequate volume for the patient

3. Clean and replace equipment. Discard disposable items according to *Standard Precautions*.

NURSING CONSIDERATIONS

Administration techniques vary according to location of the feeding tube, tolerance of the formula, and nutrition goals. The three methods of administration are bolus, intermittent, and continuous. Monitoring for complication resulting from any administration method is essential. Bolus feedings are more likely to result in nausea, diarrhea, vomiting, distention, cramps, or aspiration than other methods. Bolus or intermittent feedings can be scheduled for daytime hours so that the patient/caregiver does not have to be disturbed at night. Continuous pump feedings are usually tolerated the best. Position the patient up (at least 45 degrees during and 30 minutes after feedings). See the procedures for *Gastrostomy Care* and *Enteral Feedings* in Chapter 5.

DOCUMENTATION GUIDELINES

Document the following on the visit report:
• The procedure and patient toleration
• Vital signs

Box 10-7
CANNED TUBE FEEDING SCHEDULE

Name and amount of formula and flush ordered by the physician:_____

_____

_____

_____

Time	Water Flush cc	Formula Amount (cc) or Pump Rate	Water Flush cc	Time	Water Flush cc	Medicine Type Amount	Water Flush cc

Directions

1. Make sure to wash your hands before handling the tube or formula.
2. Keep the formula stored at room temperature. Shake the can of formula well before pouring it into the tube.
3. Use a measuring cup or syringe to measure the formula and water accurately. Follow the preceding schedule carefully. If any formula in the can is left over, cover and store in the refrigerator for the next feeding.

Modified from Dantone JJ: *Bridging the gap diet manual,* Grenada, Miss, 1997, Nutrition Education Resources. *Continued*

Box 10-7
CANNED TUBE FEEDING SCHEDULE—cont'd

4. Always flush the tube with 30-60 ml of water before and after putting the formula or medicines into the tube.
5. Do not put juices into the tube unless ordered by physician. They will cause the formula to clabber or curdle and stop up the tube. If juices are ordered, make sure that the tube is flushed with 60 cc of water before and after putting juices into the tube.
6. If all flushes are followed correctly and the tube still gets stopped up, flush the tube with 2-3 ounces of soft drink (e.g., Coke, Diet Coke, Pepsi) 2-3 times a week to keep the tube open. If the patient has diabetes, make sure that the soft drink is sugar-free.
7. When a tube-fed patient has diarrhea it is usually **not** a result of the tube feeding or the formula. Problems that may result from a certain formula usually occur within the first 24 to 48 hours of administration. If diarrhea occurs after the patient has been using a formula for a long time, do the following:
   • Stop the formula feedings, and for 24-48 hours give clear liquids, such as water; Gatorade; and glucose electrolyte solutions (GES), such as Pedialyte, until bowel movements stop. If the occurrence of diarrhea does not slow down or stop, then it is not caused by the formula.
   • If the diarrhea is caused by antibiotic use, the patient's guts may now be sterile. Give the patient 4 ounces of buttermilk or plain yogurt, with live and active cultures, diluted half strength 4 times a day to help restore the intestinal bacteria.

Modified from Dantone JJ: *Bridging the gap diet manual,* Grenada, Miss, 1997, Nutrition Education Resources.

Box 10-7
CANNED TUBE FEEDING SCHEDULE—cont'd

- See whether the patient is taking any medicines containing sorbitol, such as syrup forms of acetaminophen (Tylenol), theophylline, cough medicines, codeine, cimetidine, isoniazid, lithium, and vitamins; magnesium or aluminum antacids, such as Mylanta or Maalox; or an antibiotic.
- Change or stop giving the patient these medicines to see whether they are the cause of the diarrhea. It is usually not necessary to give tube-fed patients an antacid.
- Consider consulting with the dietitian about having the patient try a formula containing fiber, such as Jevity, Fibersource, or Sustacal with Fiber. Changing the formula to one that is not as rich (lower in osmolality) has not been shown to be helpful. If there is no improvement, the physician should be informed to diagnose other possible causes.

8. Continuous around-the-clock tube feedings delivered by pump can affect the absorption of some medicines, such as phenytoin (Dilantin), or affect some laboratory values, such as albumin. If this occurs, it is suggested that the patient be placed on bolus or gravity feedings and that medications be given 1-2 hours after feeding.

- Type, rate/quantity, frequency, and administration method of formula feedings
- Total calories, grams, protein, and volume that the patient receives daily
- Who administers the formula
- Infection control measures taken by patient/caregiver
- Positioning of the patient during administration of the formula
- Patient tolerance of the formula; type of intolerance, if any
- Patient/caregiver instructions and response to teaching, including understanding of the diet and adherence to nutritional recommendations
- Physician notification, if applicable
- *Standard Precautions*
- Other pertinent findings

Update the plan of care.

Medical Nutrition Therapy: Failure to Thrive

PURPOSE

- To provide education to the patient/caregiver about the prevention and treatment of failure to thrive (FTT) in the dependent elder adult
- To increase intake of nutrient-dense foods
- To increase, maintain a reasonable, or prevent a decrease in body weight
- To prevent complications resulting from a low body weight
- To promote self-care in the home

RELATED PROCEDURES

- Medical Nutrition Therapy: Assessment of Patient's Nutrient Requirements
- Skin Care (see Chapter 4)

GENERAL INFORMATION

FTT is defined as a gradual decline in physical and/or cognitive function that occurs in the elderly near the end of life. FTT is characterized by decline in independence, social withdrawal, unexplained weight loss, and otherwise poor nutritional status.

It is important to consider FTT on first contact with an elderly patient. Since most elderly patients have a wide range of overlapping diagnoses, FTT is often overlooked and can remain untreated. The following are nutrition-related factors related to FTT:

- Decreased shopping ability
- Diminished meal preparation ability
- Decreased appetite
- Weight loss
- Chronic anemia
- Dehydration
- Dysphagia
- Skin condition leading to pressure ulcers
- Alcohol use leading to abuse
- Constipation

The following are nutrition guidelines for patients with FTT:

- Maintenance of a reasonable body weight
- Increased food, fluid, and other nutrients intake to meet requirements
- Serum albumin level of 3.5 g/dl or greater
- Serum cholesterol level of 160 to 200 mg/dl
- Moderation or elimination of alcohol use
- Stabilization of other diseases or conditions that contribute to FTT

EQUIPMENT

1. Cloth measuring tape
2. Scales
3. Calculator
4. Measuring cups and spoons
5. Food models
6. Food labels

 7. Blood pressure cuff, stethoscope, thermometer, and glucose meter (see *Infection Control*)

PROCEDURE

1. Explain the procedure to the patient/caregiver.
2. Consider implementing the following:
   a. Assessing vital signs on each visit; weigh the patient at least weekly; pay attention to the patient's skin and over-

all physical appearance; report abnormal findings to the physician

b. Setting nutritional requirements for the patient; see the procedure for *Medical Nutrition Therapy: Assessment of Patient's Nutrient Requirements*
   or
   Identifying the calorie, protein, and fluid intake required by the patient, using the following guidelines (discuss with the patient/caregiver the importance of the patient meeting the following nutrient requirements):
   - **Calories:** minimum of 30 to 35 kcal/kg body weight
   - **Protein:** 1 to 1.5 g of protein/kg body weight
   - **Fluids:** minimum of 1500 ml (unless medically contra-indicated) or 30 ml/kg body weight per day

c. Recording a 24-hour recall of the patient's nutritional intake on the food diary form (see Fig. 10-1); analyze the total calories and protein content of the diet intake

d. Instructing the patient/caregiver on the high-calorie diet for weight gain instruction sheet and menu (Boxes 10-8 and 10-9 and Table 10-8); use food models, measuring utensils, and food labels to demonstrate calorie and protein content of different foods

e. Comparing the patient's 24-hour diet recall to his or her prescribed diet order as instructed; make appropriate recommendations to the patient/caregiver for modifying any nutrients found to be inappropriate on the food intake record

f. Discussing with the patient the importance of accurately measuring the foods as listed on the diet instruction sheet; illustrate correct measurements using standard measuring cups and spoons; in the home setting, identify utensils that can be used to measure foods

g. Discussing with the patient the times of the day he or she usually eats meals; compare those times to the times indicated on the diet instruction sheet; work with the patient to establish a regular eating pattern, due to the importance of food and medication timing in controlling his or her disease process

h. Discussing the following nutrition risk factors for FTT with the patient/caregiver:
   - Significant weight loss
   - Significantly low weight for height

Text continued on p. 406

Box 10-8
HIGH-CALORIE DIET
(About 2500-3000 Calories)

Reason for the diet

To teach you which foods are high in calories and protein. This diet will help you gain weight, prevent weight loss, and make you healthier. These foods are common and readily available, eliminating the need to purchase expensive canned supplements.

How much and/or what to eat

BREAKFAST	LUNCH AND DINNER (SAME)	BEDTIME SNACK
1 serving juice	3 oz meat	1 serving bread or cereal
1 serving cereal	1 serving starch	1 serving whole milk
2 eggs	1 serving vegetable	
2 servings bacon, sausage, or ham	1 serving bread 3 servings fat	
2 servings bread	1 serving dessert	
Jelly or syrup	1 serving whole milk	
1 serving whole milk Coffee	Water	

Modified from Dantone JJ: *Bridging the gap diet manual,* Grenada, Miss, 1997, Nutrition Education Resources.   *Continued*

Box 10-8

HIGH-CALORIE DIET—cont'd

(About 2500-3000 Calories)

Do not eat these foods

Do not drink coffee or soft drinks—these items contain a lot of sugar and caffeine, which decrease appetite.

Special instructions

(Instructors should give the patient a copy of the Nourishment List, also [see Box 10-9])

- To help you gain weight, it is best to eat at regular meal times. If you cannot hold all the foods listed at one time, divide your meals into 6 meals a day.
- If your appetite is poor, ask your physician for an appetite stimulant, such as cyproheptadine (Periactin), or permission to drink one glass of wine before meals.

The following foods are high in calories:

- Fats such as mayonnaise, oils, margarine, and fats on meats
- Any kind of meat such as beef, pork, chicken, or fish
- Peanut butter
- Eggs
- Whole milk
- Ice cream, pudding, regular yogurt with fruit, custards
- Honey, syrup, jelly
- Cakes, candy, cookies, pies.

Modified from Dantone JJ: *Bridging the gap diet manual,* Grenada, Miss, 1997, Nutrition Education Resources.

Box 10-9
NOURISHMENT LIST

The following is a list of foods that are high in calories and protein. These foods can be used for patients who are underweight or who are losing weight related to problems that cause poor appetite, swallowing problems, or diseases that cause the patient to require more calories or protein than normal. The list provides several choices so that the need to buy more expensive pharmaceutical supplements is not as necessary.

Helpful tips to add calories and/or protein to meals:

1. Use melted margarine on all hot foods at each meal. Eat fried foods if tolerated. Use gravy on meats and potatoes.
2. Make "double milk" by adding 3 tbsp nonfat dry milk to 8 ounces of whole milk. Use double milk in cooked cereals, cream soups, mashed potatoes, cream sauces, dry cereal, hot chocolate mixes, eggnog, and milkshakes, or as a coffee creamer.
3. Use mayonnaise instead of salad dressing—mayonnaise has twice the calories.
4. Eat ice cream or whipped cream on pies, pudding, hot chocolate, gelatin, or other desserts.
5. Add nonfat dry milk to casseroles such as meat loaf; croquettes; and cooked cereals such as oatmeal, cream of wheat, grits, and farina.
6. Use sour cream on potatoes or as a dip with vegetables.
7. Add half and half cream instead of milk or water to soups or dry cereal.
8. Eat six small meals per day instead of three large ones.
9. Drink plenty of water. Depending on your size, drink about six to eight 8-ounce glasses of beverages a day.

Modified from Dantone JJ: *Bridging the gap diet manual,* Grenada, Miss., 1997, Nutrition Education Resources. *Continued*

Box 10-9
NOURISHMENT LIST—cont'd

NOURISHMENTS	CALORIES	PROTEIN
Whole milk (8 oz)	150	8
Double milk (8 oz whole milk with 3 tbsp dry milk)	200	13
Evaporated whole milk (4 oz)	170	9
Skim milk or cultured buttermilk (8 oz)	90	8
Nonfat dry milk (3 tbsp or ¼ cup)	50	5
Half and half (4 oz)	160	1
Sour cream (1 tbsp)	25	1
Homemade milkshake (12 oz)	275	10
Vanilla ice cream, regular (10% fat)(4 oz)	130	2
Peanut butter (2 tbsp)	190	8
Peanut butter/jelly sandwich	340	12
Cottage cheese, creamy (½ cup)	130	15
Cheese (1 oz)	100	7
Cheese sandwich	240	11
Eggs (1)	80	7
Meat (high fat) (1 oz)	100	7
Raisins (1 dozen)	100	0
Honey, corn syrup (1 tbsp)	60	0
Sherbet (4 oz)	135	1
Instant breakfast mix (9 oz) (mixed with whole milk)	280	15
Diet instant breakfast mix (9 oz) (mixed with low-fat milk)	190	15
Fat: oil, margarine, gravy, mayonnaise, salad dressing (1 tbsp)	100	0

Modified from Dantone JJ: *Bridging the gap diet manual,* Grenada, Miss., 1997, Nutrition Education Resources.

Box 10-9
NOURISHMENT LIST—cont'd

PHARMACEUTICAL SUPPLEMENTS	CALORIES	PROTEIN
Advera (8 oz)	303	14
Boost (8 oz)	240	10
Choice DM (8 oz)	250	11
Deliver 2.0 (8 oz)	480	18
Ensure (8 oz)	250	9
Ensure Plus (8 oz)	360	13
Equate (8 oz)	250	9
Equate Plus (8 oz)	360	14
Glucerna (8 oz)	240	10
Kroger Complete Nutritional Drink (8 oz)	250	9
Kroger Plus Complete Nutritional Drink (8 oz)	360	13
Resource Standard (8 oz)	260	9
Resource Diabetic (8 oz)	250	15
Resource Plus (8 oz)	355	13
Suplena (8 oz)	480	7
Sustacal (8 oz)	240	15
Sustacal Plus (8 oz)	360	14
Two Cal HN (8 oz)	480	20

Table 10-8 Menu for high-calorie diet for weight gain

	Sunday	Monday	Tuesday
Breakfast	Juice of choice	Juice of choice	Juice of choice
	Cereal of choice	Cereal of choice	Cereal of choice
	2 Eggs of choice	2 Eggs of choice	2 Eggs of choice
	2 Sausages	2 Pieces of bacon	2 Sausages
	2 Biscuits or pieces of toast	2 Biscuits or pieces of toast	2 Biscuits or pieces of toast
	Margarine	Margarine	Margarine
	Jelly	Jelly	Jelly
	Whole milk	Whole milk	Whole milk
	Coffee	Coffee	Coffee
Lunch	3 oz Fried chicken	Sandwich with:	3 oz Roast turkey
	Black eyed peas	3 oz Cheeseburger	2 tbsp Giblet gravy
	Seasoned greens	Bun	Cornbread dressing
	2 tsp Margarine	Lettuce/pickle/onion	English peas

	Buttered cornbread	2 tsp Mayonnaise	2 tsp Margarine
	Banana	Mustard	Buttered roll
	Tea	Chips of choice	Cranberry sauce
	Whole milk	Apple cobbler	Coconut cake
		Tea	Tea
		Whole milk	Whole milk
Dinner	3 oz Ham	3 oz Beef tips	Potato stew
	Potato salad	Gravy	3 oz Tuna salad with:
	Seasoned green beans	Rice	Bread
	2 tsp Margarine	Buttered broccoli	Sliced tomatoes
	Buttered roll	2 tsp Margarine	2 tsp Mayonnaise
	Pineapple tidbits	Buttered biscuit	Crackers
	Whole milk	Stewed prunes	Fresh orange
		Whole milk	Whole milk

From Dantone JJ: *Bridging the gap diet manual*, Grenada, Miss, 1997. Reprinted with permission Nutrition Education Resources.

- Poor appetite, not meeting nutritional requirements
- Significant change in functional status (activities of daily living)
- Depression or recent loss
- Deficient biochemical markers—albumin, prealbumin, hemoglobin, hematocrit, cholesterol
- Vitamin/mineral deficiency
- Dehydration

3. Clean and replace equipment. Discard disposable items according to *Standard Precautions.*

NURSING CONSIDERATIONS

The home health nurse should initiate the following interventions in patients with FTT:

- Maintenance of reasonable body weight
- Maintenance of serum albumin ≥ 3.5 g/dl
- Maintenance of serum cholesterol 160 to 200 mg/dl
- Chewing/swallowing evaluation if necessary
- Access to food or funds if necessary
- Prevention of isolation/potential abuse or neglect
- Improvement of hydration status
- Improvement of oral health
- Improvement of cognitive and functional status

Be aware that nutrition interventions do not have to be expensive or out of the ordinary.

Food thickener can be added to pureed foods to add texture and improve the patient's acceptance of the product. Non-pharmaceutical nutritional supplements are available through the use of common foods found in local stores. Refer to the nourishment list (see Box 10-8). Just adding extra margarine to foods or serving the patient whole milk can increase calories and protein substantially.

Ask the patient about any signs and symptoms of abuse or neglect. Report to the physician as necessary.

DOCUMENTATION GUIDELINES

Document the following on the visit report:

- The procedure and patient toleration
- Vital signs and functional, cognitive, and emotional status
- Weight—report any weight change to the physician
- Food intake—analyze the intake of calories, protein, and fluid; document any suggestions for modifications in the diet

- Serum albumin and cholesterol levels
- Condition of oral health
- Use of alcohol
- Patient/caregiver instructions and response to teaching, including understanding of the diet and adherence to nutritional recommendations
- Physician notification, if applicable
- *Standard Precautions*
- Other pertinent findings

Update the plan of care.

Medical Nutrition Therapy: Hypertension

PURPOSE

- To provide education to the patient/caregiver about the prevention and treatment of hypertension (HTN)
- To improve and stabilize blood pressure to less than 140/90 mm Hg
- To improve blood pressure through manipulation of sodium intake
- To improve the diet-related diseases associated with HTN
- To promote self-care in the home

RELATED PROCEDURE

- Medical Nutrition Therapy: Assessment of Patient's Nutrient Requirements

GENERAL INFORMATION

HTN is diagnosed when there is a sustained blood pressure of 140/90 mm Hg or greater. Essential or primary HTN lacks an identifiable cause. Secondary HTN is diagnosed when a cause can be identified. Unrecognized, untreated, or uncontrolled HTN can lead to damage of target organs and possibly cause the following conditions:

- Congestive heart failure
- Cardiovascular disease
- Renal disease

- Cerebrovascular disease
- Peripheral vascular disease
- Retinal disease

The following are diet-related diseases associated with HTN:

- Overweight/obesity
- Diabetes
- Dyslipidemia

The following are inappropriate dietary intake and lifestyle factors associated with HTN:

- High-calorie intake, especially saturated fats
- High-sodium intake
- High-alcohol intake
- Low-potassium intake
- Low-calcium intake
- Poor fitness level and low physical activity
- Smoking

Nonpharmacologic treatment of HTN includes the following (best results have been documented with multifaceted interventions):

- Weight reduction—a 10-pound weight loss in one study equaled a 5.4/2.4 mm Hg decrease in blood pressure; results were even greater when weight loss was combined with sodium restriction
- Salt restriction—studies show greater decrease in HTN related to sodium restriction in the elderly, African-Americans, and patients with chronic renal disease or familial HTN
- Exercise—regular minimum of 20 to 30 minutes daily; nonvigorous; exercise program should be initiated after blood pressure is under control and with the physician's approval; encourage chair/bed exercise when appropriate
- Increased potassium and calcium consumption—population groups with diets high in potassium and calcium have been shown to have lower incidence of HTN; high-calcium foods include dairy products, spinach, shrimp, sardines, greens (remember that cheese and buttermilk are high in sodium)
- Reduced saturated fat
- Decreased alcohol consumption—increased alcohol consumption accounts for 5% to 30% of all cases of HTN

EQUIPMENT

1. Scales
2. Cloth measuring tape
3. Calculator
4. Food models or packages with food labels of sodium content
 5. Blood pressure cuff, stethoscope, thermometer, and glucose meter (see *Infection Control*)

PROCEDURE

1. Explain the procedure to the patient/caregiver.
2. Consider implementing the following:
   a. Assessing vital signs on each visit; weigh the patient at least weekly; pay close attention to blood pressure; report abnormal findings to the physician
   b. Setting nutritional requirements for the patient; see the procedure for *Medical Nutrition Therapy: Assessment of Patient's Nutrient Requirements*
   c. Recording a 24-hour recall of the patient's nutritional intake on the food diary form (see Fig. 10-1); analyze the total calories and sodium content of foods eaten
   d. Instructing the patient/caregiver on the low-salt diet instruction sheet and menu (see Box 10-4 and Table 10-5); use food labels to demonstrate sodium content in various foods; just 1 teaspoon of common table salt contains about 2 g of sodium; use measuring cups common to the patient to demonstrate proper fluid amounts to consume
   e. Comparing the patient's 24-hour diet recall to his or her prescribed diet order as instructed; make appropriate recommendations to the patient/caregiver for modifying any nutrients found to be inappropriate on food intake record
   f. Instructing the patient/caregiver on the dietary approaches to stop hypertension (DASH), which are the following:
      • Increase in fruits
      • Increase in vegetables
      • Increase in low-fat dairy products
      • Reduction in sodium to no more than 2 g daily
   g. Instructing the patient/caregiver to limit total fat intake to no more than 30% of his or her calories per day (e.g., in a 2000 calorie diet, 30% = 600 calories; 600 calories

of fat equals about 65 g of fat a day; of that 65 g of total fat, only about 20 g should be from a saturated fat source); use food labels to add up fat grams of foods eaten daily

3. Clean and replace equipment. Discard disposable items according to *Standard Precautions.*

NURSING CONSIDERATIONS

If the patient is more than 10% of ideal body weight, a weight loss of 10 pounds can make a significant reduction in blood pressure.

If the patient is taking a potassium-depleting diuretic, a potassium supplement may be necessary. Adequate potassium intake of 3500 mg (90 mEq) per day is recommended. If the patient is taking a potassium-sparing diuretic and an ACE inhibitor, he or she should be cautioned about the use of salt substitutes and light salts. Salt substitutes generally contain 2500 to 2800 mg of potassium per teaspoon. Light salt contains 1100 mg of sodium and 1500 mg of potassium per teaspoon. If salt substitutes and/or light salt are used in excess, an increased potassium blood level may result. Make the physician aware of any salt substitute product that the patient is using.

The following nutrition intervention guidelines should be assessed by the home health nurse:
- Calorie intake—limit intake of saturated fats
- Sodium intake—limit to 2 g daily
- Alcohol intake—limit to no more than 1 drink per day of 30 ml of liquor or the equivalent of beer or wine
- Smoking cessation
- Exercise as tolerated and allowed by the physician

Encourage low-fat milk or milk products twice daily. If the patient refuses to or cannot drink or eat milk or milk products, recommend a calcium supplement of 800 to 1200 mg per day and a magnesium supplement of 280 to 350 mg per day to meet RDAs. Higher doses of magnesium have been known to cause diarrhea.

DOCUMENTATION GUIDELINES

Document the following on the visit report:
- The procedure and patient toleration
- Vital signs
- Weight—report any weight change to the physician

- Food intake—analyze the intake of calories, sodium, potassium, calcium and alcohol; document any suggestions for modifications in the diet
- Physical fitness level and amount of routine allowed exercise the patient gets
- Smoking frequency or cessation
- Patient/caregiver instruction and response to teaching, including understanding of the diet and adherence to nutritional recommendations
- Physician notification, if applicable
- *Standard Precautions*
- Other pertinent findings

Update the plan of care.

Medical Nutrition Therapy: Pressure Ulcers

PURPOSE
- To educate individuals who are at risk of developing pressure ulcers (PUs) by identifying nutrition risk factors and biochemical markers
- To provide instruction on appropriate nutritional measures to prevent PUs
- To offer nutritional interventions for treatment of existing PUs
- To promote self-care in the home

RELATED PROCEDURES
- Medical Nutrition Therapy: Assessment of Patient's Nutrient Requirements
- Blood Glucose Testing (see Chapter 12)
- Skin Care (see Chapter 4)
- Wound Assessment (see Chapter 2)

GENERAL INFORMATION
The following factors are associated with PU development:
- Progressive dependency on others to meet activities of daily living (ADLs)

- Low body weight, low body mass index, or small triceps skinfolds
- Low serum albumin level
- Low serum cholesterol level
- Low hemoglobin and hematocrit levels

Extrinsic variables include shearing forces and friction. Intrinsic variables include malnutrition; anemia; reduced oxygen delivery to tissue, which already may be ischemic; both increased and decreased body weight; elevation of temperature; skin moisture—particularly incontinence and dehydration—either from low fluid intake or high fluid loss from excessive wound drainage; diuretic therapy; diarrhea and vomiting; acute blood loss; or uncontrolled diabetes. The etiology of pressure ulcers appears to be multifactorial and often the result of multiple pathologies. The common thread of treatment of all of these conditions is improvement of the patient's nutritional status. With the use of the proper MNT, clinical and functional outcomes will be positively affected.

EQUIPMENT

1. Cloth measuring tape
2. Scales or recent weight history
3. Calculator
4. Food labels
5. Food models
6. Measuring cups and spoons commonly used by the patient
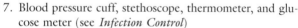 7. Blood pressure cuff, stethoscope, thermometer, and glucose meter (see *Infection Control*)

PROCEDURE

1. Explain the procedure to the patient/caregiver.
2. Consider implementing the following:
   a. Assessing vital signs on each visit; weigh the patient at least weekly; report abnormal findings to the physician
   b. Assessing the patient's skin and wound; report abnormal findings to the physician
   c. Setting nutritional requirements for patient; see the procedure for *Medical Nutrition Therapy: Assessment of Patient's Nutrient Requirements*
      or
      Identifying the calorie, protein, and fluids required by the patient, using the following guidelines (discuss with

the patient/caregiver the importance of the patient meeting the following nutrient requirements):

- **Calories**—minimum of 30 to 35 kcal/kg body weight
- **Protein**—1.2 to 1.5 g protein/kg body weight
- **Fluids**—minimum of 1500 ml (unless medically contraindicated) or 30 ml/kg body weight per day

d. Recording a 24-hour recall of the patient's nutritional intake on the food diary form (see Fig. 10-1); analyze the total calories and protein content of the diet intake

e. Instructing the patient/caregiver on the diet instruction sheet and menu for wound healing (Box 10-10 and Table 10-9); use food models, measuring utensils, and food labels to demonstrate calorie and protein content of different foods

f. Comparing the patient's 24-hour diet recall to his or her prescribed diet order as instructed; make appropriate recommendations to the patient/caregiver for modifying any nutrients found to be inappropriate on the food intake record

g. Discussing with the patient the importance of accurately measuring the foods as listed on the diet instruction sheet; illustrate correct measurement using standard measuring cups and spoons; in the home setting, identify utensils that can be used to measure foods

h. Discussing with the patient the times of the day he or she usually eats meals; compare those times to the times indicated on the diet instruction sheet; work with the patient to establish a regular eating pattern, due to the importance of food and medication timing in controlling the patient's disease process

i. Discussing the following nutrition risk factors for PUs with the patient/caregiver:
- Significant weight loss
- Significantly low weight for height
- Poor appetite, not meeting nutritional requirements
- Significant change in functional status (ADLs)
- Deficient biochemical markers—albumin, prealbumin, hemoglobin, hematocrit, cholesterol
- Vitamin/mineral deficiency
- Dehydration
- Presence of disease management processes (e.g., diabetes, Alzheimer's)

Box 10-10
WOUND HEALING DIET
(High Protein, High Iron, High Vitamin C)

Reason for the diet

To help you learn which foods are needed to correct iron deficiency and anemia and to heal skin problems, pressure sores, surgery, broken bones, and/or burns.

How much and/or what to eat

BREAKFAST	LUNCH AND DINNER (SAME)
Orange, grapefruit, or tomato juice	3-4 oz meat or meat substitute
Cereal	Starch
2 eggs	Vegetable
Bacon, ham, or sausage	Salad with dressing
Toast, biscuit, or muffin	Bread
Margarine	Margarine
Jelly, syrup, or gravy	Dessert
Milk	Milk (both meals)
Coffee or tea	

Do not eat these foods

There are no foods you cannot eat on this diet. But if your appetite is poor, do not drink a lot of coffee, tea, or soft drinks with caffeine, which will make your appetite even worse.

Special instructions

It is important that you eat at least one serving from each of the basic four food groups at each meal. This combination of foods will increase the iron in your blood and keep it normal. The basic four food groups are listed on p. 415. The foods high in protein, iron, or vitamin C are listed for each food group. The foods in italic type and followed by an asterisk are highest in iron.

Modified from Dantone JJ: *Bridging the gap diet manual*, Grenada, Miss, 1997, Nutrition Education Resources.

Box 10-10
WOUND HEALING DIET—cont'd
(High Protein, High Iron, High Vitamin C)

Meat or meat substitutes

beef*	oysters*	turkey	peanut butter
pork*	dried beans, peas*	lamb	nuts
liver*	red meats*	veal	
eggs*	chicken	fish	

Milk

whole milk	nonfat instant milk	cheese	pudding
buttermilk	milk shakes	yogurt	chocolate milk
ice cream	cottage cheese		

Breads and cereals

"instant" cream of wheat*   bran cereal*
"Total" dry cereal*   fortified or enriched cereal*

Fruits and vegetables

Dried fruits (e.g., prunes, raisins, apricots, apples, dates, figs) *		Greens (e.g., turnips, mustards, collard, chard, kale) *	
spinach*	oranges	orange juice	grapefruit
grapefruit juice	tomatoes	tomato juice	V-8 juice
broccoli	white potatoes		

Continued

Box 10-10
WOUND HEALING DIET—cont'd
(High Protein, High Iron, High Vitamin C)

Other

Molasses* (the darker the better)

For wound healing, it is suggested that your diet intake include zinc and vitamin C. The recommended amounts to heal a wound is zinc sulfate 220 mg (or zinc 50 mg) once a day and vitamin C 500 mg twice a day. Zinc should be taken only if a deficiency exists. Your physician will notify you of such a deficiency, based on the results of a blood test. Any vitamin/mineral supplement should be approved by the physician first. Also drink plenty of water—1 to 2 quarts per day as tolerated, according to your weight. A vitamin or mineral supplement pill should be taken with a citrus juice, such as orange juice, to increase the absorption of iron.

Modified from Dantone JJ: *Bridging the gap diet manual,* Grenada, Miss, 1997, Nutrition Education Resources.

- Presence of factors that reduce dietary intake (e.g., dysphagia, depression)
j. Discussing with the patient/caregiver the importance of prevention of PUs; the key in preventing PUs is routine assessment of the patient's nutritional status and estimation of nutritional intake; food preference and consistency tolerances must be individualized to each patient; instruct the patient/caregiver how to be creative with food preparation methods, seasonings, types of foods to keep the menu selections appetizing and yet sufficient in nutrients; continual reassessment of the patient's food intake through logging of a food intake diary is helpful
k. Supplementing vitamins/minerals; the importance of each should be instructed to the patient/caregiver; because of possible toxicity and nutrient interactions, vitamin/mineral supplementation in high doses is not recommended unless the patient is suspected of being

Table 10-9 Menu for wound diet *(High Protein, High Iron, High Vitamin C)*

	Sunday	Monday	Tuesday
Breakfast	Orange juice Total cereal 2 Eggs of choice Sausage Biscuit or toast Margarine Dark molasses Milk Coffee	Grapefruit juice Instant cream of wheat 2 Eggs of choice Bacon Biscuits or toast Margarine Dark molasses Milk Coffee	Tomato juice Total cereal 2 Eggs of choice Sausage Biscuit or toast Margarine Dark molasses Milk Coffee

Lunch	Fried chicken livers
	Dried black eyed peas
	Seasoned greens of choice
	Buttered cornbread
	Banana
	Coffee
		Sandwich with:
		  Cheeseburger
		  Bun
		  Lettuce/ pickle/ onion
		  Mayonnaise/ mustard
		Baked potato
		Margarine/sour cream
		Apple cobbler
		Milk
			Roast turkey
			Giblet gravy
			Cornbread dressing
			English peas
			Cranberry sauce
			Coconut cake
			Milk

Dinner	Ham Potato salad Seasoned green beans Buttered roll Pineapple tidbits Milk	Beef tips Gravy Rice Buttered broccoli Buttered biscuit Stewed prunes Milk	Potato salad Tuna salad sandwich Sliced tomatoes Crackers Mayonnaise Fresh orange Milk

From Dantone JJ: *Bridging the gap diet manual,* Grenada, Miss, 1997. Nutrition Education Resources.

deficient; the physician should order any vitamin/mineral; consider the following:

- Vitamin C—helps make collagen, promotes healing, helps build resistance to infection; requirements are increased in acute stress, malnutrition, and with smoking
- Stage I to II: patients may require 100 to 200 mg vitamin C daily
- Stage III to IV: patients may require 1000 to 2000 vitamin C daily
- Vitamin A—helps body make new skin cells
- RDA is 800 to 1000 μg RE for adults
- Zinc—promotes wound healing, improves immunity; assess the patient's serum zinc level for deficiency before administering a zinc supplement; 15 to 25 mg of zinc per day may be beneficial in healing PUs; zinc is not recommended in quantities of more than 50 mg per day because of the possibility of causing a copper deficiency, leading to anemia
- Iron—helps carry oxygen to nourish cells
- RDA is 10 to 15 mg for adults

3. Clean and replace equipment. Discard disposable items according to *Standard Precautions*.

NURSING CONSIDERATIONS

Treatment depends on the stage of the pressure ulcer. Pressure ulcers are classified, or staged, according to the degree of tissue damage. (See the procedures for *Skin Care* in Chapter 4 and *Wound Assessment* in Chapter 2.)

The literature on treating pressure ulcers with MNT emphasizes increasing protein intake. Before increasing protein intake, assess total energy intake first. The body's first priority is adequate energy intake.

DOCUMENTATION GUIDELINES

Document the following on the visit report:
- The procedure and patient toleration
- Vital signs
- Calorie, protein, and fluid requirements of the patient
- Medical treatment used for PUs
- Nutrition interventions/treatments used for PUs
- Analysis of the patient's food intake and the modifications suggested
- Patient/caregiver instruction and response to teaching, in-

cluding understanding of the diet and adherence to nutritional recommendations
- Answers to feedback questions
- Physician notification, if applicable
- *Standard Precautions*
- Other pertinent findings

Update the plan of care.

Medical Nutrition Therapy: Weight Management

PURPOSE

- To provide education to the patient/caregiver about the prevention and treatment of weight management for overweight or obese conditions
- To decrease weight, total body fat, and risk factors associated with obesity
- To promote self-care in the home

RELATED PROCEDURES

- Medical Nutrition Therapy: Assessment of Patient's Nutrient Requirements
- Weight (see Chapter 2)

GENERAL INFORMATION

Obesity refers to a condition of excess body fat. Overweight refers to excess body weight, which means increases in body fat or lean body mass. The National Institutes of Health specifies the following definitions:

Term of Weight	% Desirable Body Weight	Body Mass Index (Male/Female)
Desirable	100	22/21.5
Overweight/mild obesity	>120	27.2/26.9
Severe overweight/ moderate obesity	>140	31.1/32.3
Severe obesity	141-200	
Morbid obesity	>200	

A reduction in caloric intake of 3500 kcal is required to produce a weight loss of 1 pound of body fat. For example, subtract 500 a day from the amount of calories required to maintain current weight to produce a weight loss of 1 pound in 1 week: $500 \times 7 = 3500$ calories.

There is some evidence that repetitive weight loss followed by weight gain and reloss progressively lowers the resting metabolic rate. A 10% weight loss will significantly improve blood pressure, glucose tolerance, sleep disorders, respiratory function, and lipid profiles. Weight loss decreases production of very low–density lipoprotein (VLDL) and therefore lowers serum triglycerides; one study showed an increase in HDL.

The following are chronic conditions that are exacerbated or have increased severity in the presence of obesity:

- Cancer
- Coronary heart disease
- Degenerative arthritis
- Diabetes
- Dyslipidemia
- Gallbladder disease
- Hypertension
- Lung disease
- Bone and joint disease
- Embolus or thrombus

A reasonable goal is a moderate weight loss of 5% to 10 % of body weight to achieve a healthier weight that helps to control signs and symptoms of these chronic diseases. This weight loss can be accomplished by setting individual goals for a gradual, yet sustained weight loss. If attempts are made to reduce weight to "ideal levels" too quickly, nonadherence to the prescribed regimen is usually the result.

EQUIPMENT

1. Cloth measuring tape
2. Scales
3. Calculator
4. Measuring cups and spoons
5. Food models
6. Food labels
7. Blood pressure cuff, stethoscope, thermometer, and glucose meter (see *Infection Control*)

PROCEDURE

1. Explain the procedure to the patient/caregiver.
2. Consider implementing the following:
   a. Assessing vital signs on each visit; weigh the patient at least weekly; report abnormal findings to the physician
   b. Setting nutritional requirements for the patient; see the procedure for *Medical Nutrition Therapy: Assessment of Patient's Nutrient Requirements;* use an appropriate table to determine desirable body weight from height and frame size; establish a reasonable body weight that is agreeable with the patient to set as a goal; assuming that weight loss is necessary, establish a daily caloric level by subtracting 500 calories from the estimated energy requirements to produce a 1-pound weight loss per week; the calorie level set must be discussed with and accepted by the patient for successful diet adherence
   c. Recording a 24-hour recall of the patient's nutritional intake on the food diary form (see Fig. 10-1); analyze the carbohydrate and total calorie content of the diet intake
   d. Instructing the patient/caregiver on the 1500-calorie diet instruction sheet and menu (Box 10-11 and Table 10-10); this 1500-calorie diet is offered in general—a diet with the correct calorie level (formulated using the calculation in step *b*) should be reviewed with the patient
   e. Comparing the patient's 24-hour diet recall to his or her prescribed diet order as instructed; make appropriate recommendations to the patient/caregiver for modifying any nutrients found to be inappropriate on the food intake record
   f. Discussing with the patient the importance of accurately measuring the foods as listed on the diet instruction sheet; illustrate correct measurement using standard measuring cups and spoons; in the home setting, identify utensils commonly used to measure foods
   g. Discussing with the patient the times of the day he or she usually eats meals; compare those times to the times indicated on the diet instruction sheet; work with the patient to establish a regular eating pattern, due to the importance of food and medication timing in controlling his or her disease process
3. Clean and replace equipment. Discard disposable items according to *Standard Precautions.*

Text continued on p. 427

Box 10-11
1500-CALORIE DIET
FOR WEIGHT CONTROL

Reason for the diet

To help control your weight.

How much and/or what to eat

BREAKFAST	LUNCH
1 serving unsweetened juice	2 ounces low-fat meat
2 servings fat-free starch/bread	2 servings fat-free starch/bread
1 fat-free egg or meat	1 serving fat-free vegetable
1 serving fat	1 serving fat-free salad
1 serving low-fat milk (2%)	1 serving fat
Coffee	1 serving unsweetened fruit
Unsweetened tea	
Water	

DINNER	BEDTIME SNACK
2 ounces low-fat meat	1 serving low-fat milk (2%)
2 servings fat-free starch/bread	1 serving starch/bread
1 serving fat-free vegetable	
1 serving fat-free salad	
1 serving unsweetened fruit	
Unsweetened tea	
Water	

Modified from Dantone JJ: *Bridging the gap diet manual,* Grenada, Miss, 1997, Nutrition Education Resources.

Box 10-11
1500-CALORIE DIET
FOR WEIGHT CONTROL—cont'd

Serving sizes

FOOD GROUP	1 SERVING SIZE
1. Starches/bread	½ cup of cereal, starchy vegetable, or pasta or 1 slice or small piece bread
2. Meats	Number of ounces listed
3. Vegetables	½ cup of cooked vegetable or vegetable juice or 1 cup of raw vegetables
4. Fruits	½ cup of fresh or unsweetened canned fruit or juice or, cup of dried fruit
5. Milk	1 cup of fluid milk
6. Fat	1 tsp of margarine, oil, or mayonnaise or 1 tbsp of gravy, diet margarine, or diet mayonnaise

For additional information on serving sizes refer to the food lists for patients with diabetes (Box 10-6 and Table 10-7)

Do not eat these foods or beverages

sugar	ice cream	doughnuts
syrup	sherbet	fried foods
jam	ice milk	whiskey
jelly	pies	beer
candy	cakes	Gatorade
regular	soft drinks	cookies

Continued

Box 10-11
1500-CALORIE DIET
FOR WEIGHT CONTROL—cont'd

Special instructions
- You *must* eat meals at a regular meal times daily. Eat breakfast, lunch, and dinner about 4 or 5 hours apart and always have a bedtime snack.
- All foods on this diet should be cooked as fat free. Do not add any fat (e.g., margarine, butter, oil, mayonnaise) to the food before or during cooking. The amount of fat listed in the "How Much and/or What to Eat" section may be added to foods before eating.
- When a food is listed as diet, it has been prepared without added sugar or has been bought fresh, canned without sugar or syrup, or canned in its own juices.
- Eat high-fiber foods such as whole wheat bread and cereals or fresh fruits and vegetables daily.

Additional instructions for low-cholesterol diets
(Note to instructor: Cross this section out if not ordered by patient.)
- Use egg whites or egg substitutes (e.g., Egg Beaters instead of regular eggs) whenever eggs are needed
- Trim all fat you can see off of all meats
- Use only 100% vegetable margarines and oils

Do not eat

liver	heart	lunch meat	lard
brains	bacon	hot dogs	real butter
kidney	sausage	chicken skin	whole milk

egg yolks
(more than
twice/week)

This combination of diabetic and low-cholesterol diets will also help lower blood triglyceride levels.

Modified from Dantone JJ: *Bridging the gap diet manual,* Grenada, Miss, 1997, Nutrition Education Resources.

Table 10-10 Menu for 1500-calorie diet for weight loss

	Sunday	Monday	Tuesday
Breakfast	4 oz **uns** orange juice ½ cup **ff** Cereal 1 oz Sausage 1 Biscuit (1 fat) 1 tsp Diet jelly 8 oz Milk (2%) 1 cup Coffee	3 oz **uns** Cranberry juice cocktail ½ cup **ff** Cereal 1 **ff** Egg 1 slice Bacon 1 **ff** Toast 1 tsp Diet jelly 8 oz Milk (2%) 1 cup Coffee	4 oz **uns** Grapefruit juice ½ cup **ff** Cereal 1 oz Sausage 1 Biscuit (1 fat) 1 tsp Diet jelly 8 oz Milk (2%) 1 cup Coffee
Lunch	2 oz **ff** Baked chicken ⅓ cup **ff** Dried beans or peas ½ cup **ff** Greens 1 square Cornbread (1 fat) ½ Banana 8 oz Unsweetened Tea	Sandwich with: 2 oz **ff** Hamburger ½ Bun 2 slices Lettuce/onion 1 slice dill pickle 1 tsp Mayonnaise 1 tsp Mustard 10 ea Chips of choice ½ cup **dt ff** Stewed apple 8 oz Unsweetened tea	2 oz **ff** Roast turkey 1 tbsp Giblet gravy ½ cup **ff** Cornbread dressing ½ cup **ff** Green beans 1 ea **ff** Roll 1 tbsp Diet jelly 2 halves Diet pears 8 oz **uns** tea

Continued

From Dantone JJ: *Bridging the gap diet manual,* Grenada, Miss, 1997, Nutrition Education Resources.
uns, unsweetened; *ff,* fat free; *dt,* diet; *wp,* water-packed.

Table 10-10 Menu for 1500-calorie diet for weight loss—cont'd

	Sunday	Monday	Tuesday
Dinner	2 oz Ham	2 oz **ff** Beef rice	4 oz **ff** Vegetable soup
	½ cup **ff** Potato salad	½ cup **ff** Rice	½ Sandwich
	½ cup **ff** Green beans	½ cup **ff** Broccoli	2 oz **ff** Tuna on 1 slice bread
	1 ea **ff** Roll	1 slice bread	4 slices Tomato
	½ cup **dt** Pineapple tidbits	3 **wp** Prunes	6 crackers
	8 oz Water or **uns** tea	8 oz Water or **uns** tea	1 Orange
			8 oz Water or **uns** Tea
Bedtime snack	8 oz Milk (2%)	8 oz Milk (2%)	8 oz Milk (2%)
	3 Graham crackers	6 Vanilla wafers	6 Saltines

From Dantone JJ: *Bridging the gap diet manual,* Grenada, Miss, 1997, Nutrition Education Resources.
uns, unsweetened; *ff,* fat free; *dt,* diet; *wp,* water-packed.

NURSING CONSIDERATIONS

For older patients for whom weight reduction is inappropriate, the goal should be to prevent further weight gain, which can exacerbate more severe problems, and to improve quality of life. If weight loss can alleviate acute symptoms of a co-morbid–related condition, then aggressive weight management may be a viable option.

Several studies have documented shorter life expectancy with physical inactivity. A program of regular, nonvigorous exercise for a minimum of 20 to 30 minutes daily is beneficial. No exercise program should be initiated until after the physician's approval has been obtained. Encourage chair/bed exercise when appropriate.

Be aware that "diet" and "weight" are very personal issues with patients. Like certain diseases, obesity may "run" in families with patient genetic predisposition toward being overweight. Approach the topic in a sensitive manner. Suggest healthy substitutes instead of telling patients to eliminate favorite foods from their diet.

DOCUMENTATION GUIDELINES

To monitor the patients' adherence to their diet, have them record the times they eat and all foods and beverages they consume on a daily food diary form (see Fig. 10-1). Evaluate this by comparing it to the patient's calorie meal plan. Counsel patients on any modifications they need to make.

Document the following on the visit report:
- The procedure and patient toleration
- Vital signs
- Height, frame size, ideal body weight, desirable body weight, estimated energy requirement, and established calorie level
- The daily food diary completed by the patient
- Analysis of the patient's food intake and the modifications suggested
- Patient/caregiver instructions and response to teaching, including understanding of the diet and adherence to nutritional recommendations
- Answers to feedback questions
- Physician notification, if applicable
- *Standard Precautions*
- Other pertinent findings

Update the plan of care.

CHAPTER 11

Rehabilitative and Palliative Care Procedures

Aphasia Care

PURPOSE

- To assist patients to communicate their needs
- To promote the recovery of language
- To promote self-care in the home

EQUIPMENT

1. Blackboard, chalk, eraser, paper, pen and pencil
2. Magazines
3. Pictures and paintings
4. Flash cards
5. Games
6. Money

PROCEDURE

1. Explain the procedure to the patient/caregiver.
2. Assemble the equipment at a convenient work area.
3. Assess the extent of the communication limitations, the degree of comprehension, and the ability to respond with understandable speech patterns. Evaluate the patient's ability to swallow.
4. Approach the patient in a calm and unhurried manner.
5. Establish eye contact, and talk to the patient while you perform the nursing procedures.
6. Speak slowly and distinctly in a normal volume. Use simple words or short sentences, depending on the patient's ability to comprehend.

7. Use gestures and pointing as references of communication.
8. Provide realistic support that is considerate of the individual's limitations.
9. Encourage the patient in social interaction and involvement.
10. Use the blackboard, pictures, magazines, cards, paper, pencil, and money to stimulate communication and comprehension.
11. Allow the patient/caregiver to ventilate his or her feelings and concerns.
12. Encourage a working and trusting relationship with the patient/caregiver.
13. Provide patient comfort measures.

NURSING CONSIDERATIONS

It may take a long time for the patient to relearn speech and communication.

The patient may feel depressed or frustrated.

Work within the patient's individual limitations in a caring and humanistic manner.

Consult with the physician for speech and occupational therapy referrals.

DOCUMENTATION GUIDELINES

Document the following on the visit report:
• The patient's progress in reading, verbalization, and comprehension
• Any patient/caregiver instructions and response to teaching, including the ability to communicate needs during emergencies, such as fires or chest pain
• Physician notification, if applicable
• Other pertinent findings
Update the plan of care.

Arm Sling

PURPOSE
- To elevate and support the upper extremities with correct body alignment
- To promote self-care in the home

EQUIPMENT
1. Arm sling (triangle or manufactured)
2. Safety pins

PROCEDURE
1. Explain the procedure to the patient/caregiver.
2. Assemble the equipment at a convenient work area.
3. Place the patient in a sitting position.
4. Position the sling so that the point of the triangle is beyond the patient's elbow, with the sides of the triangle or strap of the sling over the injured shoulder.
5. Place the patient's elbow at a right angle, and apply the sling.
6. Bring ends of the sling over the shoulder. The patient's hand should be raised approximately 5 inches above the elbow when the knot is tied.
7. Tie and knot the two ends of the sling at the side of the patient's neck. (Many slings have buckles or Velcro straps for a correct fit; follow the manufacturer's recommendations for adjustment.)
8. Avoid putting pressure of the knot and straps over the spine. Evaluate for comfort, and adjust as necessary.
9. Bring the apex of the sling forward, and secure it with safety pins.
10. Provide patient comfort measures.

DOCUMENTATION GUIDELINES
Document the following on the visit report:
- The procedure and patient toleration
- Time of application
- Temperature and color of fingers
- Physician notification, if applicable

- *Standard Precautions*
- Other pertinent findings

Update the plan of care.

Cane

PURPOSE

- To promote patient balance and support when walking
- To instruct the patient how to ambulate with a cane
- To promote self-care in the home

EQUIPMENT

1. Rubber-tipped cane, quad cane
2. Transfer belt as needed

PROCEDURE

1. Explain the procedure to the patient/caregiver.
2. Assemble the equipment at a convenient work area.
3. Place the transfer belt around the patient's waist.
4. To ambulate, instruct the patient to do the following:
   a. Hold the cane on the uninvolved side, close to the body; walk with a steady, even gait using the cane as support
5. To ascend the stairs, instruct the patient to do the following:
   a. Ascend stairs that have a railing by stepping up with the uninvolved leg and then follow with the involved leg
   b. Ascend stairs without a railing by holding the cane on the uninvolved side, close to the body; lead with the cane; step up, using the uninvolved leg and then follow with the involved leg
6. To descend stairs, instruct patient to do the following:
   a. Descend stairs that have a railing by stepping down using the involved leg and then follow with the uninvolved leg
   b. Descend stairs without a railing by holding cane on uninvolved side, close to the body; lead with the cane; step

down using the involved leg and then follow with the uninvolved leg

7. To sit down, instruct patient to do the following:
   a. Place the cane near or against a chair for easy reach when standing; stand with the back of the legs against the edge of the seat of the chair; grasp the chair armrests with both hands; slowly lower self into the chair

8. To stand up, instruct patient to do the following:
   a. Grasp the armrests of the chair; place the involved foot/ leg slightly forward; using the armrests for support, push up to rise from chair; ambulate with the cane as previously instructed

9. Remove the transfer belt from around the patient's waist.
10. Provide patient comfort measures.
11. Clean and replace equipment. Discard disposable items according to *Standard Precautions.*

DOCUMENTATION GUIDELINES

Document the following on the visit report:
- The procedure and patient toleration
- Any patient/caregiver instructions and response to teaching, including the ability to ambulate with a cane
- Physician notification, if applicable
- *Standard Precautions*
- Other pertinent findings

Update the plan of care.

Cast Care

PURPOSE
- To maintain the integrity of the cast
- To provide the patient/caregiver with guidelines for cast care at home
- To promote self-care in the home

RELATED PROCEDURE
- Arm Sling

EQUIPMENT
1. Arm sling
2. Silk or adhesive tape
3. Damp cloth, scouring powder or Woolite as needed
4. Lotion
5. Disposable nonsterile gloves and an impermeable plastic trash bag (see *Infection Control*)

PROCEDURE
1. Explain the procedure to the patient/caregiver.
2. Instruct the patient how to perform isometric exercise. Instruct the patient to move all joints above and below the cast.
3. Instruct the patient not to walk on a leg cast for the first 48 hours.
4. When walking is permitted by the physician, instruct the patient to walk on the walking heel portion of the cast.
5. Position the upper-extremity casts with the fingers raised above the elbow; place a pillow under the elbow.
6. Use an arm sling to support an arm cast.
7. Position the lower-extremity cast with the foot raised above the hip; place a pillow under the ankle.
8. Every 2 hours turn the patient who is in a large spica cast, and give meticulous hygienic care. (Additional help will be required to turn the patient. Move the patient as a unit. Do not grasp the bar of the spica cast to move the patient.)
9. Inspect the patient's fingers and toes for adequate circulation; assess for swelling, coldness, blanching, and excessive

pain. Notify the physician if signs of inadequate circulation are apparent.

10. Observe the cast for areas of pressure and for constriction of circulation. Petal the rough edges of the cast with silk or adhesive tape to prevent skin irritation. (The physician is responsible for trimming the cast.)

11. Do not let a plaster cast get wet because it weakens the cast. Instruct the patient/caregiver to cover the plaster cast with a plastic trash bag during baths to keep the cast dry. Use a towel or a hair dryer to dry the cast if it should become damp.

12. Clean spots off the cast with a damp cloth and scouring powder.

13. Consult with the physician regarding recommendations for skin care when the cast is removed. Consider the following suggestions:

    a. Once the cast is off, soften and remove flakes of skin with a damp cloth and Woolite (Woolite contains enzymes that loosen the dead cells, and they wash off without injuring healthy tissue)

    b. Wash the area with warm water and Woolite

    c. Leave the Woolite-soaked washcloth on the skin for 5 minutes; rinse thoroughly, and pat dry

    d. Apply moisturizing lotion to the area

    e. Wash the area with warm water and Woolite the next day; the skin should look nearly normal

14. Provide patient comfort measures.

15. Clean and replace the equipment. Discard disposable items according to *Standard Precautions.*

NURSING CONSIDERATIONS

Instruct the patient not to insert objects under the cast to avoid damaging the skin or causing an infection.

Use powders and lotions on the skin outside the cast to keep the skin clean, soft, and supple.

DOCUMENTATION GUIDELINES

Document the following on the visit report:
- The procedure and patient toleration
- Condition of the cast
- Patient toleration, color, and temperature of the extremities

- Any swelling or discomfort
- Any patient/caregiver instructions and response to teaching
- Physician notification, if applicable
- *Standard Precautions*
- Other pertinent findings

Update the plan of care.

Elastic Bandage

PURPOSE

- To limit movement and provide support
- To secure dressings and splints
- To alleviate edema in the lower extremities
- To promote self-care in the home

GENERAL INFORMATION

Apply the elastic bandage or Ace wrap over a clean area with the extremity and the body in good alignment. If applying the bandage over a wound, aseptically dress the wound before applying the bandage. Apply the elastic bandage from the distal to the proximal part of the body to aid in the return of venous blood to the heart. Leave the toes and fingers visible. Elastic bandages should be applied evenly, overlapping one half to two thirds of the width of each bandage. The distal portion of the bandage should be left exposed so that any restriction in circulation can be detected.

The free roller end of the bandage is called the *initial portion,* the rolled portion is called the *body,* and the opposing end of the bandage is called the *terminal end.* The following describes the two common turns used in bandaging:

1. The *circular turn* is used to bandage a cylindrical part of the body or to secure a bandage at its initial and terminal ends. The bandage should be wrapped about the extremity in such a way that each turn exactly covers the previous one. Two circular turns are usually used to initiate and to terminate a bandage (Fig. 11-1).

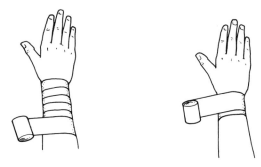

Fig. 11-1 Circular turn of Ace bandage.

2. The *figure-of-eight* turn is commonly used at a joint, but it may also be used to bandage the entire length of an arm or a leg; it consists of repeated oblique turns that are made alternately above and below a joint in the form of a figure-of-eight (Fig. 11-2).

EQUIPMENT
1. Two to four Ace bandages, 3 inches or 4 inches wide
2. Fasteners or safety pins
3. Supplies to clean/dress around the wound if applicable
4. Disposable sterile and nonsterile gloves and an impermeable plastic trash bag (see *Infection Control*)

PROCEDURE
1. Explain the procedure to the patient/caregiver.
2. Assemble the equipment at a convenient work area.
3. Place the patient in a sitting or supine position, and expose the extremity to be wrapped.
4. Make sure that the extremity is clean and aligned with the body. Dress the wound as required.
5. Begin bandaging by holding the *initial portion* in place with one hand, while the other hand passes the roll around the area being wrapped. If the patient is ambulatory, do not start the initial portion of the bandage on the sole of the foot.
6. Bandage from the distal to the proximal and from the medial to the lateral, overlapping one half to two thirds of the width of each wrap.

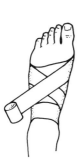
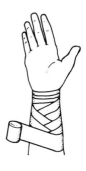

Fig. 11-2 Figure-of-eight turn of Ace bandage.

7. Once the bandage is anchored, pass the body of the bandage from hand to hand, being careful to exert equal tension. Secure the *terminal end* of the bandage with fasteners.
8. Launder bandages with soap and water when they become soiled; air dry. Reapply clean bandages.
9. Provide patient comfort measures.
10. Clean and replace the equipment. Discard disposable items according to *Standard Precautions.*

NURSING CONSIDERATIONS

Assess for signs or symptoms of impaired circulation, such as pulses, pallor, erythema, cyanosis, or numbness; remove the bandage and report to the physician as needed.

Instruct the patient/caregiver to remove, rewrap, and reapply clean bandages daily.

Ideally, bandages should be put on before getting out of bed in the morning because edema begins as soon as the lower extremities are dependent.

Always check the condition of the skin before reapplying the bandage.

DOCUMENTATION GUIDELINES

Document the following on the visit report:
• Area bandaged
• Time of application and size of bandage
• Skin condition

- Color and temperature of skin
- Any patient/caregiver instructions and response to teaching, including the ability to apply bandages
- Physician notification, if applicable
- *Standard Precautions*
- Other pertinent findings

Update the plan of care.

Hoyer Lift

PURPOSE

- To assist the patient out of the bed using a Hoyer lift
- To instruct the caregiver how to use the Hoyer lift
- To promote self-care in the home

EQUIPMENT

1. Hoyer lift, including sling and chains
2. Wheelchair or chair

PROCEDURE

1. Explain the procedure to the patient/caregiver.
2. Assemble the equipment at a convenient work area. Position the Hoyer lift and wheelchair/chair for smooth transfer of the patient.
3. Position the patient in the center of the bed.
4. Roll the patient toward you.
5. Fold the Hoyer lift sling half-way under the patient so that the lower edge of the sling is slightly below the patient's knees.
6. Go to the opposite side of the bed.
7. Roll the patient over the sling and pull the sling out flat.
8. Position the Hoyer lift with the arms perpendicular to and directly over the patient. The Hoyer lift base legs should be spread wide apart.
9. Connect the Hoyer lift chains to the sling. Connect the other ends of the Hoyer lift chains to side arms of the lift.

10. Instruct the patient to keep his or her arms inside the chains with the arms folded across the chest.
11. Slowly pump the Hoyer lift hydraulic handle to raise the patient from the bed.
12. As soon as the patient is clear of the bed, swing him or her away from the bed.
13. Immediately position the patient over the wheelchair/chair.
14. Press the Hoyer lift hydraulic release valve, and stabilize the patient while slowly lowering him or her into the wheelchair/chair.
15. Remove the Hoyer lift hooks and chains; keep the patient seated on the Hoyer lift sling.
16. Provide patient comfort measures.
17. Clean and replace equipment. Discard disposable items according to *Standard Precautions.*

NURSING CONSIDERATIONS

Instruct the caregiver in the procedure. Instruct the caregiver to never leave the patient while the patient is in the Hoyer lift.

Reverse the procedure to return the patient back to the bed.

DOCUMENTATION GUIDELINES

Document the following on the visit report:
- The procedure and patient toleration
- Any patient/caregiver instructions, including the caregiver's ability to safely use the Hoyer lift
- Physician notification, if applicable
- *Standard Precautions*
- Other pertinent findings

Update the plan of care.

Pain Management

PURPOSE
- To provide effective pain relief

RELATED PROCEDURES
- Intravenous Therapy (see Chapter 7)
- Medications (see Chapter 9)
- Pain Assessment (see Chapter 2)
- Positioning and Seating the Immobilized Patient (see Chapter 2)
- Range of Motion Exercises: Passive
- Skin Care (see Chapter 4)
- Transcutaneous Electrical Nerve Stimulation (TENS)

GENERAL INFORMATION

Pain is usually a result of anoxia, inflammation, or tearing or stretching of bone or soft tissue. To be successful, pain management must be tailored to the individual patient's needs, which vary with diagnosis, stage of disease or type of disability, response to pain, and personal preference as well as cultural considerations for control of pain. See the procedure for *Pain Assessment* in Chapter 2; a thorough pain assessment must precede intervention strategies. Review specific intravenous (IV) therapy procedures in Chapter 7 for administration of parenteral therapies. Review the procedures for other medication administration techniques in Chapter 9.

NOTE: Pain management guidelines are currently under review by the Agency for Health Care Policy and Research; revised recommendations should be available by 2001.

PROCEDURE

1. Take part in a case conference with the physician and multidisciplinary team. Mutually identify pain intervention strategies and techniques acceptable to the patient/caregiver.
2. Consider the following intervention strategies for nonpharmacologic management of pain:
   a. Provide cutaneous stimulation therapy (e.g., applications of superficial heat and cold, pressure or vibration to relieve muscle pain or tension)

b. Encourage patients to remain active and participate in self-care when possible

c. Avoid prolonged immobilization to prevent joint contracture, muscle atrophy, decubitus, etc; provide range of motion exercises, and reposition the bedbound patient on a scheduled basis

d. Instruct in relaxation therapy or guided-imagery exercises

e. Provide counter stimulation therapy (e.g., acupuncture or transcutaneous electrical nerve stimulation [TENS])

f. Provide good skin care to prevent breakdown and decubitus formation

g. Correctly position and seat the chairbound patient to promote comfort and to prevent skin breakdown

h. Provide therapeutic touch

i. Offer information about community resources that provide spiritual care and support of the patient/caregiver

3. Consider the following guidelines for pharmacologic pain management:

a. Individualize the pain medication regimen according to the patient's needs

b. Plan to use the simplest dosage schedules and least invasive pain management modalities first

c. The oral route is the preferred route of analgesic administration because it is the most convenient and cost-effective method of administration; when patients cannot take medications orally, transdermal and rectal routes should be considered because they are also relatively noninvasive; avoid intramuscular administration of pain medication because this route can be painful and inconvenient, and absorption is not reliable; intravenous or subcutaneous routes are effective alternatives; analgesics may be administered intraspinally or by an intraventricular route when pain cannot be controlled by other methods

d. Pharmacologic management of mild to moderate pain should include a nonsteroidal antiinflammatory drug (NSAID) or acetaminophen (unless contraindicated); if pain persists, add an opioid; treatment of persistent or moderate to severe pain should be based on increasing the opioid potency or dose (Tables 11-1, 11-2, and 11-3)

4. Instruct the patient/caregiver in pain management intervention strategies.

Text continued on p. 450

Table 11-1 Dosing data for acetaminophen (APAP) and nonsteroidal antiinflammatory drugs (NSAIDs)

Drug	Usual dose for adults and children ≥50 kg body weight	Usual dose for children[1] and adults[2] ≤50 kg body weight
ACETAMINOPHEN AND OVER-THE-COUNTER NSAIDs		
Acetaminophen[3]	650 mg q 4 h	10-15 mg/kg q 4h
	975 mg q 6h	15-20 mg/kg q 4 h (rectal)
Aspirin[4]	650 mg q 4 h	10-15 mg/kg q 4 h
	975 mg q 6 h	15-20 mg/kg q 4 h (rectal)
Ibuprofen (Motrin, others)	400-600 mg q 6 h	10 mg/kg q 6-8 h[5]
PRESCRIPTION NSAIDs		
Carprofen (Rimadyl)	100 mg tid	
Choline salicylate[6] (Trilisate)	1000-1500 mg tid	25 mg/kg tid
Choline salicylate (Arthropan)[6]	870 mg q 3-4 h	
Diflunisal (Dolobid)[7]	500 mg q 12 h	
Etodolac (Lodine)	200-400 mg q 6-8 h	
Fenoprofen (Nalfon)	300-600 mg q 6 h	
Ketoprofen (Orudis)	25-60 mg q 6-8 h	
Ketorolac tromethamine[8] (Toradol)	10 mg q 4-6 h to a maximum of 40 mg/day	
Magnesium salicylate (Doan's, Magan, Mobidin, others)	650 mg q 4 h	

Meclofenamate (Meclomen)[9]	50-100 mg q 6 h	
Mefenamic acid (Ponstel)	250 mg q 6 h	
Naproxen (Naprosyn)	250-275 mg q 6-8 h	
Naproxen (Anaprox DS)	275 mg q 6-8 h	
Sodium salicylate (generic)	325-650 mg q 3-4 h	5 mg/kg q 8 h

PARENTERAL NSAIDs

Ketorolac[8,10] (Toradol)	60 mg initially, then 30 mg q 6 h	
	Intramuscular dose not to exceed 5 days	

SOURCE: Management of Cancer Pain Panel: *Management of cancer pain. Clinical Practice Guideline. ACHPR Pub. No. 94-0502*, 1994 Rockville, Md, Agency for Health Care Policy and Research, Public Health Service, U.S. Department of Health and Human Services.

q, every; *tid*, three times daily.

[f] Only drugs that are FDA approved as an analgesic for use in children are included.

[2] Acetaminophen and NSAID dosages for adults weighing less than 50 kg should be adjusted for weight.

[3] APAP lacks the peripheral anti-inflammatory and antiplatelet activities of the other NSAIDs.

[4] The standard against which other NSAIDs are compared. May inhibit platelet aggregation for $\geq$ 1 week and may cause bleeding. Aspirin is contraindicated in children with fever or other viral disease because of its association with Reye's syndrome.

[5] Not FDA approved for use in children as an over-the-counter drug; has FDA approval for use in children as a prescription drug for fever. However, clinicians have experience in prescribing ibuprofen for pain in children.

[6] May have minimal antiplatelet activity.

[7] Administration with antacids may decrease absorption.

[8] For short-term use only.

[9] Coombs-positive autoimmune hemolytic anemia has been associated with prolonged use.

[10] Has the same gastrointestinal toxicities as oral NSAIDs.

NOTE: Only the above NSAIDs have FDA approval for use as simple analgesics, but clinical experience has been gained with other drugs as well.

Table 11-2 Dose equivalents for opioid analgesics in opioid-naive adults and children ≥50 kg body weight[1]

Drug	Approximate equianalgesic dose		Usual starting dose for moderate-to-severe pain	
	Oral	Parenteral	Oral	Parenteral
OPIOID AGONIST[2]				
Morphine[3]	30 mg q 3-4 h (repeat around-the-clock dosing) 60 mg q 3-4 h (single dose or intermittent dosing)	10 mg q 3-4 h	30 mg q 3-4 h	10 mg q 3-4 h
Morphine, controlled-release[3,4] (MS Contin, Oramorph SR)	90-120 mg q 12 h	N/A	90-120 mg q 12 h	N/A
Hydromorphone[3] (Dilaudid)	7.5 mg q 3-4 h	1.5 mg q 3-4 h	6 mg q 3-4 h	1.5 mg q 3-4 h
Levorphanol (Levo-Dromoran)	4 mg q 6-8 h	2 mg q 6-8 h	4 mg q 6-8 h	2 mg q 6-8 h
Meperidine (Demerol)	300 mg q 2-3 h	100 mg q 3 h	N/R	100 mg q 3 h

Methadone (Dolophine, others)	20 mg q 6-8 h	10 mg q 6-8 h	20 mg q 6-8 h	10 mg q 6-8 h
Oxymorphone[3] (Numorphan)	N/A	1 mg q 3-4 h	N/A	1 mg q 3-4 h

SOURCE: Management of Cancer Pain Panel: *Management of cancer pain. Clinical Practice Guideline. ACHPR Pub. No. 94-0592,* 1994, Rockville, Md, Agency for Health Care Policy and Research, Public Health Service, U.S. Department of Health and Human Services.

q, every; *N/A,* not available, *N/R,* not recommended; *NSAID,* nonsteroidal antiinflammatory drug; *IM,* intramuscular; *SC,* subcutaneous.

[1]Caution: Recommended doses do not apply for adult patients with body weight <50 kg. For recommended starting doses for children and adults <50 kg body weight, see Table 11-3.

[2]Caution: Recommended doses do not apply to patients with renal or hepatic insufficiency or other conditions affecting drug metabolism and kinetics.

[3]Caution: For morphine, hydromorphone, and oxymorphone, rectal administration is an alternative route for patients unable to take oral medications. Equianalgesic doses may differ from oral and parenteral doses because of pharmacokinetic differences.

[4]Transdermal fentanyl (Duragesic) is an alternative option. Transdermal fentanyl dosage is not calculated as equianalgesic to a single morphine dose. See the package insert for dosing calculations. Doses greater than 25 μg/h should not be used in opioid-naive patients.

NOTE: Published tables vary in the suggested doses that are equianalgesic to morphine. Clinical response to the criterion that must be applied for each patient; titration to clinical responses is necessary. Because there is no complete cross-tolerance among these drugs, it is usually necessary to use a lower-than-equianalgesic dose when changing drugs and to retitrate to response.

Continued

Table 11-2 Dose equivalents for opioid analgesics in opioid-naive adults and children ≥50 kg body weight[1]—cont'd

Drug	Approximate equianalgesic dose		Usual starting dose for moderate-to-severe pain	
	Oral	Parenteral	Oral	Parenteral
COMBINATION OPIOID/NSAID PREPARATIONS[5]				
Codeine[6] (with aspirin or acetaminophen)	180-200 mg q 3-4 h	130 mg q 3-4 h	60 mg q 3-4 h	60 mg q 2 h (IM/SC)
Hydrocodone (in Lorcet, Lortab, Vicodin, others)	30 mg q 3-4 h	N/A	10 mg q 3-4 h	N/A
Oxycodone (Roxicodone, also in Percocet, Percodan, Tylox, others)	30 mg q 3-4 h	N/A	10 mg q 3-4 h	N/A

[5]Caution: Doses of aspirin and acetaminophen in combination opioid/NSAID preparations must also be adjusted to the patient's body weight. Aspirin is contraindicated in children in the presence of fever or other viral disease because of its association with Reye's syndrome.

[6]Caution: Codeine doses greater than 65 mg often are not appropriate because of diminishing incremental analgesia with increasing doses but continually increasing nausea, constipation, and other side effects.

Table 11-3 Dose equivalent for opioid analgesics in opioid-naive children and adults <50 kg body weight[1]

Drug	Approximate equianalgesic dose		Usual starting dose for moderate-to-severe pain	
	Oral	Parenteral	Oral	Parenteral
OPIOID AGONIST[2]				
Morphine[3]	30 mg q 3-4 h (repeat around-the-clock dosing) 60 mg q 3-4 h (single dose or intermittent dosing)	10 mg q 3-4 h	0.3 mg/kg q 3-4 h	0.1 mg/kg q 3-4 h

SOURCE: Management of Cancer Pain Panel: *Management of cancer pain. Clinical Practice Guideline. AHCPR Pub. No. 94-0592,* 1994, Rockville, Md, Agency for Health Care Policy and Research, Public Health Service, U.S. Department of Health and Human Services.

q, every; *N/A,* not available; *NSAID,* nonsteroidal inflammatory drug; *N/R,* not recommended.

[1] Caution: doses listed for patients with body weight <50 kg cannot be used as initial starting doses in infants younger than 6 months.

[2] Caution: Recommended doses do not apply to patients with renal or hepatic insufficiency or other conditions affecting drug metabolism and kinetics.

[3] Caution: For morphine, hydromorphone, and oxymorphone, rectal administration is an alternate route for patients unable to take oral medications. Equianalgesic doses may differ from oral and parenteral doses because of pharmacokinetic differences.

NOTE: Published tables vary in the suggested doses that are equianalgesic to morphine. Clinical response is the criterion that must be applied for each patient; titration to clinical responses is necessary. Because there is not complete cross-tolerance among these drugs, it is usually necessary to use a lower-than-equianalgesic dose when changing drugs and to retitrate to response.

Continued

Table 11-3 Dose equivalent for opioid analgesics in opioid-naive children and adults <50 kg body weight[1]—cont'd

Drug	Approximate equianalgesic dose		Usual starting dose for moderate-to-severe pain	
	Oral	Parenteral	Oral	Parenteral
OPIOID AGONIST[2]—cont'd				
Morphine controlled-release[3,4] (MS Contin, Oramorph)	90-120 mg q 12 h	N/A	N/A	N/A
Hydromorphone[3] (Dilaudid)	7.5 mg q 3-4 h	1.5 mg q 3-4 h	0.06 mg/kg q 3-4 h	0.015 mg/kg q 3-4 h
Levorphanol (Levo-Dromoran)	4 mg q 6-8 h	2 mg q 6-8 h	0.04 mg/kg q 6-8 h	0.02 mg/kg q 6-8 h
Meperidine (Demerol)	300 mg q 2-3 h	100 mg q 3 h	N/R	0.75 mg/kg q 2-3 h
Methadone (Dolophine, others)	20 mg q 6-8 h	10 mg q 6-8 h	0.2 mg/kg q 6-8 h	0.1 mg/kg q 6-8 h

COMBINATION OPIOID/NSAID PREPARATIONS[5]

Codeine[6] (with aspirin or acetaminophen)	180-200 mg q 3-4 h	130 mg q 3-4 h	0.5-1 mg/kg q 3-4 h	N/R
Hydrocodone (in Lorcet, Lortab, Vicodin, others)	30 mg q 3-4 h	N/A	0.2 mg/kg q 3-4 h	N/A
Oxycodone (Roxicodone, also in Percocet, Percodan, Tylox, others)	30 mg q 3-4 h	N/A	0.2 mg/kg q 3-4 h	N/A

SOURCE: Management of Cancer Pain Panel: *Management of cancer pain. Clinical Practice Guideline. ACHPR Pub. No. 94-0592*, 1994, Rockville, Md, Agency for Health Care Policy and Research, Public Health Service, U.S. Department of Health and Human Services.

q, every; *N/A*, not available; *NSAID*, nonsteroidal inflammatory drug; *N/R*, not recommended.

[4]Transdermal fentanyl (Duragesic) is an alternative option. Transdermal fentanyl dosage is not calculated as equianalgesic to a single morphine dosage. See the package insert for dosing calculations. Doses greater than 25 μg/h should not be used in opioid-naive patients.

[5]Caution: Doses of aspirin and acetaminophen in combination opioid/NSAID preparations must also be adjusted to the patient's body weight. Aspirin is contraindicated in children in the presence of fever or other viral disease because of its association with Reye's syndrome.

[6]Caution: Some clinicians recommend not exceeding 1.5 mg/kg of codeine because of an increased incidence of side effects with higher doses.

NURSING CONSIDERATIONS

Be aware that respiratory depression and constipation are common side effects of opioid administration.

When administering pain medication, identify whether the patient has any concurrent medical condition(s) that may place him or her at risk for liver or renal failure. Patients with respiratory disease are more vulnerable to the respiratory depressant effect of opioids. Neurologic disorders can influence pain management if they produce weakness of the respiratory muscles or impair alertness so that the sedative effect of opioids are exaggerated. Patients with psychiatric illnesses must be carefully evaluated for drug interactions between any psychotropic drug and pain medication that they may take.

Consult with the physician and treat anticipated procedure-related pain prophylactically. When possible, administer pharmacologic agents by a painless route.

Opioid tolerance and physical dependence are expected with long-term opioid treatment and should not be confused with psychologic dependence (addiction), manifested as a drug-abuse behavior.

Specific drug-abuse behavior in the postoperative patient or his or her caregiver should be recognized and dealt with as quickly as possible. Opioid medications should be prescribed by only one physician, and attempts to circumvent this restriction or to falsify prescriptions should not be tolerated. The claim of needing additional medication to make up for lost or stolen controlled substances should be accompanied by documentation that the patient/caregiver has reported this to the police.

DOCUMENTATION GUIDELINES

See the documentation guidelines for *Pain Assessment* in Chapter 2.

Range of Motion Exercises: Passive

PURPOSE

- To maximize muscle tone
- To increase or maintain joint flexibility
- To increase peripheral circulation
- To improve functional mobility
- To prevent skin breakdown
- To promote self-care in the home

RELATED PROCEDURE

- Skin Care (see Chapter 4)

PROCEDURE

1. Assess the need for range of motion (ROM) exercises:
   a. Presence of contracture
   b. Unsteady gait
   c. Limited movement
   d. Poor endurance or strength
2. Explain the procedure to the patient/caregiver.
3. Perform ROM using caution:
   a. Keep movements pain-free
   b. Do not use force to go beyond the patient's point of resistance
   c. Handle the patient gently because osteoporosis may be present
   d. Avoid extremes of internal rotation, flexion, and adduction status after hip repair or when hip prothesis is present
4. Perform ROM in a slow, rhythmic fashion:
   a. *Head and neck*—flex, extend, and rotate the neck; if passive, support the head and gently move it (Fig. 11-3)
   b. *Shoulder*—stabilize the shoulder girdle, and move the arm; perform flexion, extension, abduction, adduction, internal and external rotation, hyperextension, and circumduction (Fig. 11-4)
   c. *Elbow*—stabilize the upper arm, and move the forearm; perform flexion, extension, supination, and pronation (Fig. 11-5)

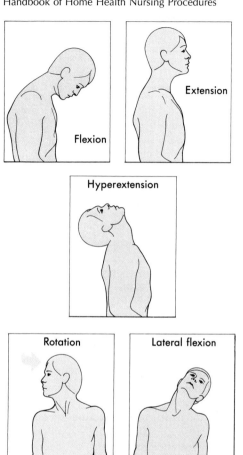

Fig. 11-3 Range of motion exercises for the head and neck. (From Beare PG, Myers JL: *Principles and practice of adult health nursing*, ed 2, St Louis, 1994, Mosby.)

d. *Wrist*—stabilize the forearm, and move the hand; perform flexion, extension, and hyperextension, (Fig. 11-6)
e. *Joints of fingers*—stabilize the hand, and move the fingers; perform flexion, hyperextension, abduction, and adduction (Fig. 11-7)

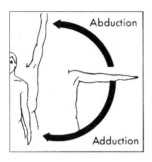
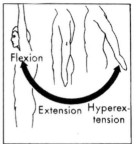

Fig. 11-4 Range of motion exercises for the shoulder. (From Beare PG, Myers JL: *Principles and practice of adult health nursing,* ed 2, St Louis, 1994, Mosby.)

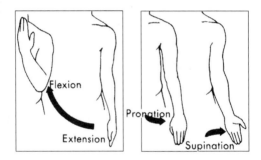

Fig. 11-5 Range of motion exercises for the elbow. (From Beare PG, Myers JL: *Principles and practice of adult health nursing,* ed 2, St Louis, 1994, Mosby.)

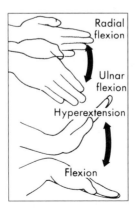

Fig. 11-6 Range of motion exercises for the wrist. (From Beare PG, Myers JL: *Principles and practice of adult health nursing,* ed 2, St Louis, 1994, Mosby.)

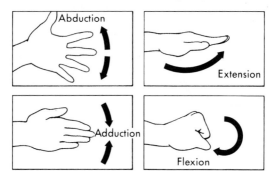

Fig. 11-7 Range of motion exercises for the fingers. (From Beare PG, Myers JL: *Principles and practice of adult health nursing,* ed 2, St Louis, 1994, Mosby.)

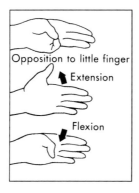

Fig. 11-8 Range of motion exercises for the thumb. (From Beare PG, Myers JL: *Principles and practice of adult health nursing,* ed 2, St Louis, 1994, Mosby.)

    f. *Thumb*—stabilize the fingers and wrist; flex, extend, adduct, abduct, and bring the thumb to the finger (opposition) (Fig. 11-8)

    g. *Hip*—with the patient in the prone position stabilize the pelvis, and move the thigh; perform abduction, adduction, internal and external rotation, extension, hyperextension, flexion, and circumduction (Fig. 11-9)

    h. *Knee*—with the patient in the prone position stabilize the

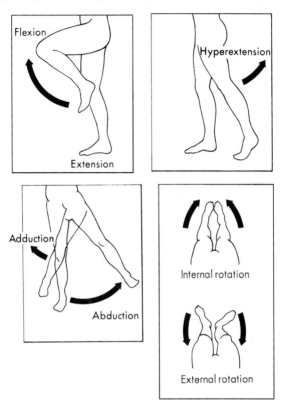

Fig. 11-9   Range of motion exercises for the hips. (From Beare PG, Myers JL: *Principles and practice of adult health nursing,* ed 2, St Louis, 1994, Mosby.)

thigh, and move the leg; perform flexion and extension (Fig. 11-10)

   i. *Ankle and foot*—stabilize the leg, and move the foot; perform dorsiflexion, plantar flexion, eversion, and inversion (Fig. 11-11)

   j. *Toes*—stabilize the foot, and move the toes; perform adduction and abduction (Fig 11-12)

5. Evaluate patient response to the ROM exercise regimen; does the patient exhibit increased mobility and flexibility of joints? Is the patient's activity level improved?

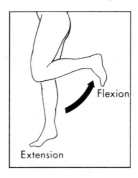

Fig. 11-10 Range of motion exercises for the knee. (From Beare PG, Myers JL: *Principles and practice of adult health nursing,* ed 2, St Louis, 1994, Mosby.)

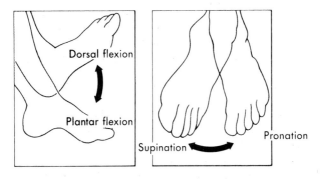

Fig. 11-11 Range of motion exercises for the ankle and foot. (From Beare PG, Myers JL: *Principles and practice of adult health nursing,* ed 2, St Louis, 1994, Mosby.)

NURSING CONSIDERATIONS

If pain or resistance occurs, discontinue the exercise and notify the patient's physician.

Consult with the physician for a physical therapy or occupational therapy referral for problems with functional limitations.

Institute a skin-care regimen for problems with immobility.

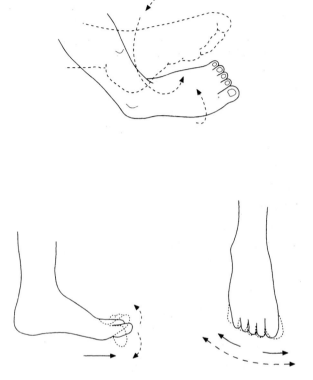

Fig. 11-12 Range of motion exercises for the toes. (From Beare PG, Myers JL: *Principles and practice of adult health nursing*, ed 2, St Louis, 1994, Mosby.)

DOCUMENTATION GUIDELINES

Document the following on the visit report:
- The procedure, including ROM exercises performed, and patient toleration
- Condition of the patient's skin
- Any patient/caregiver instructions and response to teaching, including the ability to perform range of motion exercises and the ability to perform activities of daily living (ADLs)
- Physician notification, if applicable

- *Standard Precautions*
- Other pertinent findings

Update the plan of care.

Stump Wrapping

PURPOSE

- To prevent flexion deformities and shrinkage of the stump
- To protect the stump
- To promote self-care in the home

EQUIPMENT

1. 3- or 4-inch elastic bandage or wraps
2. Fasteners or safety pins

PROCEDURE

1. Explain the procedure to the patient/caregiver.
2. Assemble the equipment at a convenient work area.
3. Assist the patient to a comfortable sitting or supine position, and examine the stump.
4. Evaluate the stump for signs of healing and intact skin integrity.
5. Wrap the stump with elastic bandages in the following manner:
   a. Start recurrent vertical turns on the anterior surface of the stump; pass the bandage distally to the gluteal crease (Fig. 11-13, *step 1*)
   b. Anchor the recurrent turns beginning at lateral side, running posterior to medial (Fig. 11-13, *step 2*)
   c. Bring the bandage down and around the stump and then up again, using the oblique or figure-of-eight (Fig. 11-13, *step 3*)
   d. Keep the pressure of the bandage always up and out at the distal portion of the stump (Fig. 11-13, *step 4*)
   e. Start at the hip spica from the anterior medial aspect and run the bandage laterally across the anterior surface of the inguinal region (Fig. 11-13, *step 5*)

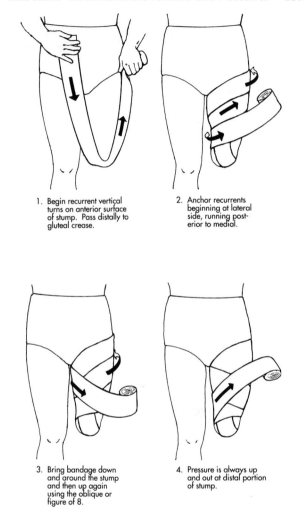

1. Begin recurrent vertical turns on anterior surface of stump. Pass distally to gluteal crease.

2. Anchor recurrents beginning at lateral side, running posterior to medial.

3. Bring bandage down and around the stump and then up again using the oblique or figure of 8.

4. Pressure is always up and out at distal portion of stump.

Continued

Fig. 11-13 Wrapping the stump after an above-the-knee amputation. (From Mourad LA: *Orthopedic disorders,* St Louis, 1991, Mosby.)

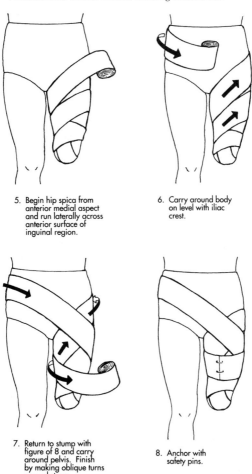

5. Begin hip spica from anterior medial aspect and run laterally across anterior surface of inguinal region.

6. Carry around body on level with iliac crest.

7. Return to stump with figure of 8 and carry around pelvis. Finish by making oblique turns around stump.

8. Anchor with safety pins.

Fig. 11-13—cont'd Wrapping the stump after an above-the-knee amputation. (From Mourad LA: *Orthopedic disorders,* St Louis, 1991, Mosby.)

  f. Draw the bandage around the patient's body on a level with the iliac crest (Fig. 11-3, *step 6*)
  g. Return the bandage to the stump with a figure-of-eight wrap, and draw it around the pelvis; finish by making oblique turns around the stump (Fig. 11-13, *step 7*)

h. Anchor with safety pins (Fig. 11-13, *step 8*)
6. Launder the stump bandages with soap and water when they are soiled; air dry.
7. Reapply clean elastic bandages.
8. Provide patient comfort measures.
9. Clean and replace the equipment. Discard disposable items according to *Standard Precautions.*

NURSING CONSIDERATIONS

Instruct the patient/caregiver to keep the stump hyperextended when the bandage is applied.

Apply moderate tension to the entire stump, being careful to guard against any tourniquet action at the proximal end of the stump.

Do not use circular turns because they tend to be constricting.

DOCUMENTATION GUIDELINES

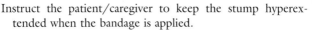

Document the following on the visit report:
- The procedure and patient toleration
- Condition of the stump and surrounding skin
- Any patient/caregiver instructions and response to teaching, including the ability to wrap the stump
- Physician notification, if applicable
- *Standard Precautions*
- Other pertinent findings

Update the plan of care.

Support Devices: Care of Immobilized Patients

PURPOSE
- To prevent contractures and skin breakdown
- To promote self-care in the home

RELATED PROCEDURES
- Skin Care (see Chapter 4)

❖ Bedboard

PURPOSE
- To provide back support and body alignment

EQUIPMENT
1. Bedboard

PROCEDURE
1. Explain the procedure to the patient/caregiver.
2. Assemble the equipment at a convenient work area.
3. Position patient in a chair, maintaining proper body alignment.
4. Remove the mattress from the bed, and place the bedboard on top of the box springs.
5. Put the mattress back on the bed, and remake the bed.
6. Assist the patient to return to bed as desired.
7. Provide patient comfort measures.
8. Return the bedboard to the equipment company when it is no longer needed.

❖ Bed Cradle

PURPOSE
- To keep linen pressure off affected extremity

EQUIPMENT
1. Bed cradle
2. Sheet

PROCEDURE

1. Explain the procedure to the patient/caregiver.
2. Assemble the equipment at a convenient work area.
3. Position the bed cradle directly over the area that needs the pressure alleviated.
4. Adjust the room temperature as the patient requests if the cradle covers a large area of the body.
5. Provide patient comfort measures.

❖ Footboard

PURPOSE

• To provide correct body alignment and to prevent footdrop

GENERAL INFORMATION

Pad the footboard with a towel, sheet, or bath blanket if it is not padded.

EQUIPMENT

1. Footboard
2. Towel, sheet, or bath blanket for padding as needed

PROCEDURE

1. Explain the procedure to the patient/caregiver.
2. Assemble the equipment at a convenient work area.
3. Secure the footboard to the end of the bed.
4. Position the patient's heels over the mattress edge when possible.
5. If the patient is in a supine position, position the patient so that the soles of the feet are flat against the footboard to prevent footdrop (Fig. 11-14).
6. Encourage the patient to flex his or her toes against the footboard. (Consider the use of high top tennis shoes to prevent footdrop as an alternative or a supplement to the footboard.)
7. Inspect the patient's feet every visit for pressure sores and for evidence of skin breakdown.
8. Provide patient comfort measures.

❖ Hand Roll

PURPOSE

• To maintain the hand in the correct anatomic position

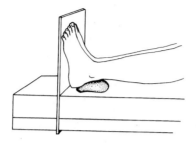

Fig. 11-14   Footboard.

- To prevent contractures
- To prevent skin breakdown

EQUIPMENT
1. Hand roll (may improvise with a washcloth)
2. Hypoallergenic tape as needed

PROCEDURE
1. Explain the procedure to the patient/caregiver.
2. Assemble the equipment at a convenient work area.
3. Instruct the patient/caregiver in the importance of daily hand care to prevent skin breakdown and odor.
4. Improvise a hand roll by using a rolled washcloth if the ready-made hand roll is not available.
5. Make sure that the hand roll is large enough to prevent finger flexion and to keep the thumb in a position of opposition.
6. If the hand roll slides out of place, anchor it to the patient's hand with a gauze wrap. Secure with tape.
7. Replace the homemade hand roll daily.
8. Inspect the hand every visit for evidence of skin breakdown.
9. Provide patient comfort measures

❖ Heel/Elbow Protector
PURPOSE
- To prevent friction and skin breakdown

EQUIPMENT

1. Heel or elbow protectors

PROCEDURE

1. Explain the procedure to the patient/caregiver.
2. Assemble the equipment at a convenient work area.
3. Apply heel and/or elbow protectors. Keep the seams straight, and smooth out any wrinkles.
   a. *Heel protector*—slip on over the foot and ankle; make sure that the padded side is against the heel
   b. *Elbow protector*—slip on over the arm and onto elbow; make sure that the padded side is against the elbow
4. Instruct the patient/caregiver to remove the protectors once every 4 hours to check pressure areas and to correct placement.
5. Wash the protectors with soap and water as needed to keep clean.
6. Provide patient comfort measures.

❖ Pillows

PURPOSE

- To elevate an extremity
- To support the patient in a constant position
- To prevent pressure sores and skin breakdown
- To prevent aspiration during tube feedings

EQUIPMENT

1. Pillows

PROCEDURE

1. Explain the procedure to the patient/caregiver.
2. Assemble the equipment at a convenient work area.
3. Use pillows with a fabric cover.
4. Place the pillows to support, elevate, and prevent pressure sores as needed. (Placing the patient in a 30-degree oblique position when at rest will prevent pressure over bony prominences.)
5. Change the pillow cases when they are soiled.
6. Provide patient comfort measures.

❖ Sheepskin

PURPOSE

- To reduce pressure to bony prominences
- To prevent skin breakdown

EQUIPMENT

1. Sheepskin

PROCEDURE

1. Explain the procedure to the patient/caregiver.
2. Assemble the equipment at a convenient work area.
3. Place a sheepskin under the area to be protected from skin breakdown. (Do **not** cover the sheepskin with multiple Chux pads or with a bedpan because this defeats the purpose of the sheepskin.)
4. Remove the sheepskin and launder if it becomes soiled.
5. Place a clean sheepskin under the patient.
6. Provide patient comfort measures.

❖ Trochanter Roll

PURPOSE

- To control external rotation of the hip

EQUIPMENT

1. Trochanter roll
2. Rolled towel, bath blanket, or pillow for improvised trochanter roll as needed

PROCEDURE

1. Explain the procedure to the patient/caregiver.
2. Assemble the equipment at a convenient work area.
3. Ensure that the trochanter roll extends from the patient's iliac crests to midthigh.
4. The leg must be in the correct anatomic position: slightly abducted.
5. Provide patient comfort measures.

NURSING CONSIDERATIONS

Consult with the physician for rehabilitation referral for problems with functional limitations.

Instruct the patient/caregiver in the purpose, use, and correct application of all support devices.

Institute a skin-care regimen for problems with immobility.

DOCUMENTATION GUIDELINES

Document the following on the visit report:

- The procedure and patient toleration
- Condition of the patient's skin
- Any patient/caregiver instructions and response to teaching, including the ability to use support devices
- Physician notification, if applicable
- *Standard Precautions*
- Other pertinent findings

Update the plan of care.

Thromboembolitic (TED) Hose

PURPOSE

- To reduce edema and swelling of the extremities
- To promote venous return
- To prevent thrombophlebitis and pulmonary embolism
- To promote self-care in the home

GENERAL INFORMATION

TED hose are usually indicated for patients at risk for deep vein thrombosis (e.g., patients who are elderly or bedridden or who have suffered stroke or undergone surgery).

EQUIPMENT

1. TED hose
2. Tape measure

PROCEDURE

1. Explain the procedure to the patient/caregiver.
2. Assemble the equipment at a convenient work area.
3. Assist the patient to a sitting or supine position.

4. Measure the patient for TED hose:
   a. *For calf or knee length*—measure around the circumference of the patient's calf at the widest point; measure the length of the patient's leg from the bottom of the heel to the back of the knee
   b. *For thigh length*—measure around the circumference of the patient's calf at the widest point; measure the patient's leg length from the bottom of the heel to the gluteal fold
   c. *For waist length*—measure around the circumference of the patient's calf and thigh at the widest points; measure the length of the patient's leg from the bottom of the heel to the waist from the side
5. Insert your hand into the stocking as far as the heel pocket. Grasp the center of the heel pocket and turn the stocking inside out to the heel area (Fig. 11-15, *A*). Carefully position the stocking over the foot and heel (Fig. 11-15, *B*). Be sure that the patient's heel is centered in the heel pocket. Put the stocking on in the following manner:
   a. *For calf or knee length*—pull the stocking up, and fit it around the ankle and calf, working to the final position; the top of the stocking is positioned approximately 1 inch below the knee caps (Fig. 11-15, *C*); make sure that the heel and toe sections are positioned correctly; as needed, pull the toe section forward (or instep, in case of open toe to eliminate wrinkles and to allow for the patient's comfort).
   b. *For thigh length*—begin pulling the body of the stocking up around the ankle and calf; the stitch change (change in fabric sheerness) should fall between 1 and 2 inches below the popliteal fossa; the final position of the gusset should center over the femoral artery; the top band rests in the gluteal folds; smooth out excess material; pull the toe section forward to smooth the ankle and instep areas and to allow for the patient's comfort
   c. *For waist length*—follow the previous procedures to pull the stocking up over the thigh, until the top band of the hose fits in the patient's gluteal folds; adjust the belt that comes with the waist-length stockings for a comfortable fit
6. Launder the TED hose with soap and water. Dry on a flat towel to prevent stretching. Reapply clean stockings.
7. Provide patient comfort measures.

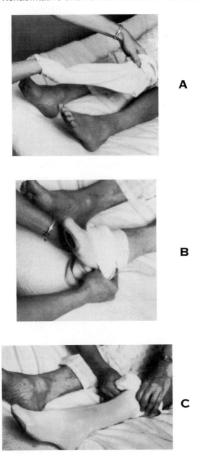

Fig. 11-15 Application of thromboembolitic (TED) hose. (From Perry AG, Potter PA: *Clinical nursing skills and techniques,* ed 3, St Louis, 1994, Mosby.)

NURSING CONSIDERATIONS

Instruct the patient/caregiver to apply the stockings in the morning before the patient gets out of bed and edema develops.

Instruct the patient/caregiver not to turn down or roll down the top of the stocking because this may impair circulation.

Keep the patient's legs in a nondependent position.

Check the color and temperature of the patient's skin when the stockings are removed. Assess for signs of impaired circulation (discoloration, swelling, loss of sensation, or coolness of extremity); report to the physician as appropriate.

Hose should be replaced when they lose their elasticity or if the patient has significant weight fluctuations.

DOCUMENTATION GUIDELINES

Document the following on the visit report:

- The procedure and patient toleration
- The time the TED hose are put on and removed
- Type of stocking applied (stocking length and size)
- Condition of the skin and extremities before and after treatment
- Any patient/caregiver instruction and response to teaching
- Physician notification, if applicable
- *Standard Precautions*
- Other pertinent findings

Update the plan of care.

Transcutaneous Electrical Nerve Stimulation (TENS) Unit

PURPOSE

- To provide pain relief
- To promote self-care in the home

RELATED PROCEDURES

- Pain Assessment (see Chapter 2)
- Pain Management

GENERAL INFORMATION

The TENS unit is a pocket-sized, battery-operated device that provides mild, continuous electric current through the skin, using two to four electrodes. The TENS unit is used for pain control. The electrodes are taped to the skin with lead wires that connect the electrodes to the device. The mild electric current blocks or modifies the pain messages and replaces them with a buzzing sensation. It is also thought that the TENS unit may stimulate the body's production of endorphin, a natural pain reliever.

EQUIPMENT

1. TENS unit
2. Electrodes
3. Hypoallergenic tape
4. Soap and water, lotion
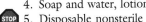 5. Disposable nonsterile gloves and an impermeable plastic trash bag (see *Infection Control*)

PROCEDURE

1. Explain the procedure to the patient/caregiver.
2. Assemble the equipment at a convenient work area.
3. Assess the quality, duration, and location of the patient's pain.
4. Apply the TENS unit in the following manner:
   a. Apply a thin coat of gel over the electrodes
   b. Secure the electrodes to the skin (place the electrodes close to the site of the pain)
   c. Tape the electrodes to the skin for a secure fit
   d. Slowly turn on the output knob of the TENS unit, until the patient feels a slight tingling or buzzing on the skin; adjust the intensity of the unit for patient comfort
5. Remove the TENS unit in the following manner:
   a. Turn off the TENS unit before removing it
   b. Replace the electrodes if the adhesive surfaces separate from the backing or if they no longer stay firmly on the skin; otherwise clean the electrodes with an alcohol wipe
   c. Recharge the TENS unit battery pack as needed
6. Clean the skin with soap and water, and apply lotion to the electrode placement sites after each TENS treatment.
7. Assess patient toleration of the TENS unit and the patient's relief from pain.
8. Provide patient comfort measures.
9. Clean and replace equipment. Discard disposable items according to *Standard Precautions*.

NURSING CONSIDERATIONS

Instruct the patient/caregiver to apply electrodes on different
   sites of the skin with each treatment to prevent redness or irritation.

DOCUMENTATION GUIDELINES

Document the following on the visit report:
 * The procedure and patient toleration, including pain relief
 * Any patient/caregiver instructions and response to teach-
   ing, including the ability to use TENS unit
 * Physician notification, if applicable
 * *Standard Precautions*
 * Other pertinent findings
Update the plan of care.

Walker

PURPOSE

 * To provide mobility
 * To promote self-care activities
 * To maximize home independence

EQUIPMENT

1. Walker
2. Gait belt

PROCEDURE

1. Explain the procedure to the patient/caregiver.
2. Bring the walker to the bedside.
3. Assist the patient to dress.
4. Assist the patient to a sitting position.
5. Instruct the patient to dangle his or her legs.
6. Evaluate the patient's strength and ability to bear weight.
   Consider using a gait belt for patients with poor strength
   or unsteady gait.
7. Place your hands under the patient's axilla, and help the
   patient to stand as straight as possible.

8. Measure the height of the walker, and adjust it accordingly.
9. Instruct the patient to move the walker forward and then to move the right foot followed by the left foot.
10. Caution the patient not to put the entire body weight on the walker.
11. Do not allow the patient to use the walker alone until he or she feels steady and secure.
12. Provide patient comfort measures.

NURSING CONSIDERATIONS

Use walkers with wheels only with patients who have sufficient strength and flexibility to handle them because the risk of falling is greater.

DOCUMENTATION GUIDELINES

Document the following on the visit report:
- The procedure and patient toleration
- Length of walking time
- Frequency of walker use
- Any patient/caregiver instructions regarding home safety when ambulating and response to teaching, including the ability to safely use the walker
- Physician notification, if applicable
- *Standard Precautions*
- Other pertinent findings

Update the plan of care.

Wheelchair

PURPOSE
- To provide safe transportation
- To promote self-care in the home

RELATED PROCEDURE
- Skin Care (see Chapter 4)

EQUIPMENT
1. Wheelchair
2. Blanket
3. Pad and pillow or cushion

PROCEDURE
1. Explain the procedure to the patient/caregiver.
2. Assemble the equipment at the bedside.
3. Adjust the foot pieces. (They can be folded and swung to the side for easy access to the bed, toilet, or tub.)
4. Lock the brakes.
5. As needed, place a pad in the bottom of the wheelchair for patient comfort.
6. Instruct the patient to dangle his or her legs.
7. Evaluate the patient's strength and ability to bear weight. Consider the use of a gait belt for patients with poor strength or unsteady gait.
8. Place your hands under the patient's axilla; help the patient to stand facing you.
9. Gently lower the patient into the wheelchair.
10. Cover the patient's legs with a blanket.
11. Instruct the patient/caregiver to check for discoloration and swelling of the patient's feet every 2 hours.
12. Return the patient to bed if he or she complains of feeling tired or ill, if swelling occurs in the lower extremities, or if the physician orders it.
13. Store the wheelchair in its designated place when it is not in use.
14. Provide patient comfort measures.

NURSING CONSIDERATIONS

Instruct the patient/caregiver on the importance of locking the wheelchair brakes before assisting the patient into the wheelchair.

Institute a skin-care regimen for the bedbound or wheelchair-bound patient.

DOCUMENTATION GUIDELINES

Document the following on the visit report:
- The procedure and patient toleration
- Length of time in the wheelchair
- Type of activity
- Any patient/caregiver instructions and response to teaching, including the patient's ability to safely use the wheelchair
- Condition of the patient's skin
- Physician notification, if applicable
- *Standard Precautions*
- Other pertinent findings

Update the plan of care.

CHAPTER 12

Specimen Collection and Transport

Blood Glucose Monitoring

PURPOSE
- To obtain an accurate, objective blood glucose reading
- To assess patterns of glucose control that can be used to evaluate and modify the treatment for diabetic patients
- To instruct the patient/caregiver in home diabetic management, including how to use a glucose meter
- To promote self-care in the home

RELATED PROCEDURES
- Administration of Medications: General Guidelines (see Chapter 9)
- Glucose and Ketone Urine Testing: Reagent Strip

GENERAL INFORMATION
When you are purchasing a blood glucose meter, the following should be considered:
1. *Accuracy and precision*—The American Diabetic Association allows a 10% variance between a meter's reading and a laboratory test.
2. *Range*—The meter must be capable of measuring glucose within a range of 0 to 500 mg/dl.
3. *Infection control*—The meter must meet the Occupational Safety and Health Administration's (OSHA) standards and the home health agency's standards to prevent staff and patient contamination when cleaning and operating the meter.
4. *Memory*—The meter must be able to recall the previous test result.

5. *User friendly*—The simplest meters are the best. The size of the readout display is important to consider, especially when you are recommending meters to patients with poor vision. A number of talking meters are available for blind patients.

6. *Manufacturer support*—The supplier should provide an 800 number that is available for 24-hour technical services and assistance.

7. *Cost*—Cost is a serious consideration for the patient. Many insurance companies and Medicare will pay for the meter and the ongoing cost of glucose monitoring if the patient is taking insulin as prescribed by a physician.

A variety of excellent glucose meters are currently on the market; review individual manufacturer recommendations for operation of any glucose meter. The following procedure discusses how to obtain a blood glucose reading using the SureStep (LifeScan) blood glucose meter* (Fig. 12-1).

EQUIPMENT

1. SureStep meter
2. Penlet II or blood sampler device and lancets
3. Surestep meter test strips
4. Surestep meter control solution
5. Soap and water, washcloth, and towels
6. Disposable nonsterile gloves, sharps container, and an impermeable plastic trash bag (see *Infection Control*)

PROCEDURE

1. Explain the procedure to the patient/caregiver.
2. Assemble the equipment at a convenient work area.
3. Instruct the patient to wash his or her hands with soap and warm water before the finger stick. Rinse and dry.
4. Press the on/off button on the meter.
5. A code and number will appear on the display. Press the C button until the code number on the meter matches the code number on your current test strip package.
6. Remove the test strip from the vial or foil package. (Be

---

*Reference to specific products does not imply an endorsement by the author or Mosby, Inc.

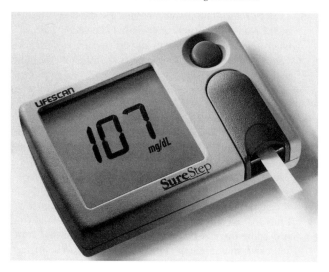

Fig. 12-1 The SureStep blood glucose meter. (Courtesy LifeScan, Milpitas, Calif.)

careful not to tear the strip. If you are using a vial, replace the cap immediately.)

7. **Control Solution Test:**
   a. After shaking the control solution vial, apply one drop of control solution to the pink test square on the test strip.
   b. Check to see that the confirmation dot on the back of the test strip has turned completely blue to ensure enough control solution has been applied
   c. Within 2 minutes after applying the control solution, insert the test strip into the meter, pink side up, and read the results (takes about 30 seconds to appear).
   d. Compare the control solution test result with the control range printed on the SureStep test strip package. When the control solution test result is within the control range, test the blood sample (repeat the procedure and/or contact the manufacturer if test results do not fall within or continue to be out of the control range).
   e. The meter automatically turns off within 2 minutes after control solution testing or 3 minutes after the meter

displays a blood glucose reading. To conserve energy, turn off the meter after solution and blood sample testing.

8. **Blood Sample Test:**
   a. Instruct the patient to always wash his or her hands with soap and water before performing this test. If using an alcohol wipe when cleansing the skin, let the area dry before obtaining the blood sample.
   b. Turn on the SureStep glucose meter. Symbols indicating to (1) apply blood to the test strip and (2) to insert the test strip into the meter will alternate on the display. You have 2 minutes to insert the test strip before the meter automatically turns off.
   c. Obtain a blood sample by pressing the lancet loaded Penlet II or a blood sampling device against the side of the finger (the harder you press, the deeper the puncture). Press the release button.
   d. Squeeze the finger to get a large, hanging drop of blood.
   e. Hold the test strip under the finger, and touch the drop of blood to the pink test square.
   f. After a few seconds, look at the confirmation dot on the back of the test strip. If it is completely blue, go on with the test.
   g. Slide the test strip into the test strip holder, pink side up. Insert the test strip within *2 minutes* to obtain an accurate result. Turn off the meter after obtaining the reading.
9. Provide patient comfort measures.
10. Notify the physician if blood glucose results are abnormal.
11. Clean the meter according to OSHA guidelines and manufacturer's recommendations. Discard disposable items according to *Standard Precautions*.

NURSING CONSIDERATIONS

Test results less than 60 mg/dl mean low blood glucose (hypoglycemia). Test results greater than 240 mg/dl mean high blood glucose (hyperglycemia). Recheck the reading to confirm the value. Contact the physician if the patient is symptomatic or has abnormal blood glucose readings 2 days in a row (consider obtaining physician's orders to make a next day home visit if glucose readings are abnormal upon admission and *always* when the patient is symptomatic).

Monitor the accuracy of the meter whenever a blood sample is drawn for laboratory testing. Evaluate the blood glucose level at the same time the sample is drawn, and compare the meter results with the laboratory readings. There should be no more than 10% to 15% variance with the laboratory readings.

Be aware that extremes in the hematocrit level can affect test results. Very high hematocrit levels (more than 60%) and very low hematocrit levels (less than 25%) can cause false results. Likewise, severe dehydration and excessive water loss may cause false low results. Consult with the physician as appropriate.

Instruct the patient/caregiver in home diabetic management, including self-blood glucose monitoring (SBGM). Ensure that the patient/caregiver operates his or her meter correctly, even if he or she has been using it for some time. If the patient cannot use a meter, instruct him or her how to visually read a reagent strip (be aware that a visual reading only provides a gross estimate of the patient's blood glucose level). Also, see the procedure for *Glucose and Ketone Urine Testing: Reagent Strip.*

Home health nursing staff should perform a quality care test at the beginning of each day to verify that their meters are working correctly. Home health nursing staff and patient/caregivers should perform a quality care test whenever they open a new vial of strips, if they should accidentally drop your meter or if they suspect an inaccurate reading.

Be aware that user errors are the most common reason for inaccuracies. The most common mistake is failing to get an appropriate amount of blood on the test strip.

Home health nursing staff should not leave their glucose meters in their cars overnight because extremes in temperature may damage the meters.

DOCUMENTATION GUIDELINES

Document the following on the visit report:
- The procedure and patient toleration
- Calibration or testing of the meter, as applicable
- Blood glucose results
- Any patient/caregiver instructions regarding home dia-

betic management, including the ability to perform a blood glucose test
- Physician notification of blood glucose results and any subsequent orders
- *Standard Precautions*
- Other pertinent findings

Document insulin administration on the medication record, as applicable.

Update the plan of care.

Blood Sampling

❖ Arterial Blood Gas Sampling

PURPOSE

- To obtain arterial blood specimen laboratory analysis

RELATED PROCEDURES

- Central Venous Catheter Care (see Chapter 7)
- Inserting a Winged-Tip Needle (see Chapter 7)
- Specimen Labeling and Transport

GENERAL INFORMATION

Arterial sampling is done to determine arterial blood gas status (pH, $PACO_2$, PAO_2, CO_2). The home health nurse should be certified to draw an arterial blood gas sample. Draw blood samples only from the radial artery. Notify the physician after three unsuccessful attempts to draw a blood sample.

EQUIPMENT

1. 3 cc syringe with a 1-inch, 23- or 25-gauge needle
2. 1000 U/ml heparin solution
3. Syringe cap
4. Bandage
5. 2- × 2-inch gauze pad
6. Laboratory requisition
7. Antiseptic wipes
8. Disposable nonsterile gloves, impermeable specimen

transport baggys marked with a biohazard sign, leak-proof and puncture-proof specimen transport container marked with a biohazard sign, sharps container, and an impermeable plastic trash bag (see *Infection Control*)

PROCEDURE

1. Explain the procedure to the patient/caregiver.
2. Assist the patient to a sitting or a supine position to access the radial artery.
3. Palpate the radial artery; feel the bounding pulse. Perform Allen's test to verify collateral circulation of the ulnar artery. (The ulnar artery is capable of supplying the blood flow to the hand if the radial artery is damaged or if it becomes damaged or occluded during the procedure.) If Allen's test is negative and if there is no collateral circulation of the ulnar artery, notify the physician, and do not perform the procedure in that arm. Allen's test is performed in the following manner:
    a. Instruct the patient to make a tight fist
    b. Apply direct pressure to both radial and ulnar arteries
    c. Instruct the patient to open his or her hand
    d. Release pressure over the ulnar artery, and observe the color of the fingers, thumbs, and hand
4. Clean the needle site with an antiseptic wipe in a circular motion, moving outward 3 or 4 cm from the needle site.

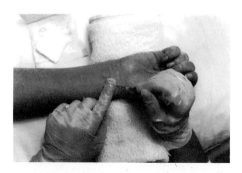

Fig. 12-2 Insertion of the needle for arterial puncture. (From Perry AG, Potter PA: *Clinical nursing skills and techniques,* ed 4, St Louis, 1998, Mosby.)

5. Prepare the syringe and the needle in the following manner:
    a. Flush with 0.5 ml of heparin solution to coat the inside of the syringe.
    b. Expel excess heparin
6. Insert the needle into the radial artery at a 45-degree angle with the bevel up (Fig. 12-2).
7. Obtain 2 to 3 ml of blood.
8. Apply a 2- × 2-inch gauze pad to the needle insertion site and withdraw the needle.
9. Apply pressure to the site for 5 to 10 minutes or until it no longer bleeds (Fig. 12-3). Cover with a bandage as needed.
10. Expel air bubbles from the syringe, and remove the needle.
11. Put a cap on the end of the syringe. Clean the syringe with antiseptic wipes as needed.
12. Roll the syringe to distribute the heparin
13. Label the specimen, and place it in a bag of ice. Double bag the specimen in a specimen baggy to prevent leakage during transport. Place the baggy in a leak-proof, puncture-proof container for transport.
14. Assess the needle site to ensure that there is no bleeding.
15. Provide patient comfort measures.
16. Clean and replace the equipment. Place the used needles and syringes in a sharps container. Discard disposable items according to *Standard Precautions.*
17. Fill out the laboratory requisition. Transport (use *Stan-*

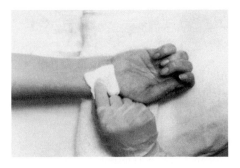

Fig. 12-3   Applying pressure to the puncture site. (From Perry AG, Potter PA: *Clinical nursing skills and techniques,* ed 4, St Louis, 1998, Mosby.)

dard Precautions) to the laboratory within 30 minutes of sampling.

NURSING CONSIDERATIONS

Clean air bubbles from the syringe after obtaining the sample because not taking this measure could result in falsely elevated PAO_2 and lower CO_2 levels.

Clean the syringe of excess heparin before the procedure because this could falsely decrease the PAO_2 and pH levels.

Copious secretions or suctioning within 10 minutes of the procedure could give a false reading.

The minimum recommended blood sample volume is 1 ml.

DOCUMENTATION GUIDELINES

Document the following on the visit report:
- The procedure and patient toleration
- Cardiopulmonary status
- Allen's test results
- Any home mechanical ventilator settings or oxygen liter flow
- Patient's temperature
- Length of time the pressure dressing is held to the needle site
- The type of laboratory test ordered by the physician; date and time the specimen was collected
- Designated laboratory for delivery
- Physician notification of laboratory test results and any subsequent orders
- *Standard Precautions*
- Other pertinent findings

Update the plan of care.

❖ Venous Blood Sampling

PURPOSE

- To obtain venous blood for laboratory testing

RELATED PROCEDURE

- Specimen Labeling and Transport

GENERAL INFORMATION

Do not draw blood from the patient's arm that has a shunt or intravenous therapy line. Gray-, blue-, and purple-topped test tubes should be gently inverted a couple of times after they are filled with the blood sample to prevent clotting. Notify the physician after three unsuccessful attempts to enter the vein.

EQUIPMENT

1. Vacutainer specimen tubes
2. Vacutainer holder and vacutainer needles or syringe large enough to hold the quantity of blood desired with a 19- to 21-gauge needle
3. Tourniquet
4. Bandage
5. 2- × 2-inch gauze pad
6. Laboratory requisition
7. Antiseptic wipes
 8. Disposable nonsterile gloves, impermeable specimen transport baggys marked with a biohazard sign, leak-proof and puncture-proof specimen transport container marked with a biohazard sign, sharps container, and an impermeable plastic trash bag (see *Infection Control*)

PROCEDURE

1. Explain the procedure to the patient/caregiver.
2. Assemble the equipment at a convenient work area. Determine the type of laboratory test requested by the physician, and obtain correct blood tubes for sampling.
3. Assist the patient to either a sitting or supine position for venipuncture.
4. Select the site for venipuncture.
5. Place the arm in a dependent position. Apply a tourniquet 6 to 8 inches above the site of venipuncture.
6. Cleanse the area with antiseptic wipes, moving the wipes in a circular motion 3 to 4 cm outward from the needle insertion site.
7. Fix the chosen vein with the thumb, and draw the skin taut immediately below the site before inserting the needle.
8. At approximately ½-inch below the venipuncture site, insert the needle with the bevel up at a 30-degree angle so that it enters the skin and then the vein (Fig. 12-4).
9. Observe for blood flow.
10. Lower the syringe so that it is almost parallel to the skin.
11. The following is the technique for using a syringe:
    a. Withdraw the desired amount of blood into the syringe.
    b. Release the tourniquet *before* removing the needle from

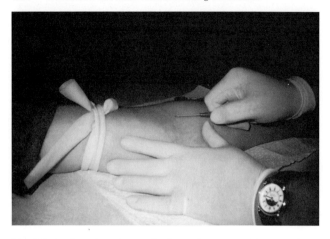

Fig. 12-4 Inserting the needle for venipuncture. (Photo courtesy Robyn Rice.)

      the vein to reduce the incidence of hematoma formation.

  c. Elevate the arm. Apply pressure to the area with a 2- × 2-inch gauze pad for approximately 2 to 4 minutes or longer if the patient is receiving anticoagulant therapy.

  d. Inject blood from the syringe into the proper vacutainer specimen tubes (Fig. 12-5).

  e. As needed, apply a bandage to the area.

12. The following is the technique for using a vacutainer:

  a. Insert the vacutainer specimen tube into the holder but not onto the 2-way vacutainer needle.

  b. Perform venipuncture as described.

  c. Gently push the vacutainer specimen tube against the end of the holder onto the 2-way needle; make sure that the 2-way needle completely pierces the rubber stopper of the specimen tube; the vacuum in the specimen tube will automatically draw up the blood sample (Fig. 12-6).

  d. If more than one sample is needed, gently withdraw the filled specimen tube from the holder; insert the next tube into the holder so that the needle completely pierces the rubber stopper.

  e. Release the tourniquet *before* the last tube is completely

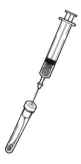

Fig. 12-5 Placing blood into the specimen tube. (From Perry AG, Potter PA: *Clinical nursing skills and techniques,* ed 3, St Louis, 1994, Mosby.)

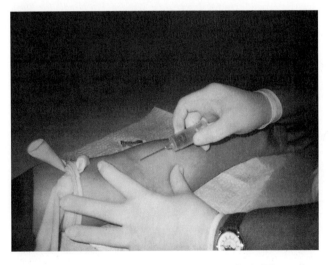

Fig. 12-6 Venipuncture using the vacutainer method. (Photo courtesy Robyn Rice.)

filled; this reduces the incidence of hematoma formation; allow the last tube to fill.

f. Elevate the arm; apply pressure to the area for approximately 2 to 5 minutes or *longer* if the patient is receiving anticoagulant therapy.

g. Apply a bandage to the area as needed.

13. Clean specimen tubes with antiseptic wipes as needed, and label them.

14. Place the specimen tube(s) in a plastic bag, and seal it. If refrigeration is required, place the specimen tube(s) on ice, and double bag the tube(s) to prevent leakage. Place in a specimen transport container for travel.

15. Provide patient comfort measures.

16. Clean and replace the equipment. Place the needles and syringes in a sharps container. Discard disposable items according to *Standard Precautions*.

17. Fill out the laboratory requisition, and transport the specimen tubes according to *Standard Precautions*.

 NURSING CONSIDERATIONS

See the procedures for *Inserting a Winged-Tip Needle for Blood Sampling* in Chapter 7 for fragile veins, and see procedures for specific *Central Venous Catheter Blood Sampling* in Chapter 7.

 DOCUMENTATION GUIDELINES

Document the following on the visit report:
- The procedure and patient toleration, including the condition of the venipuncture site
- The type of laboratory test ordered by the physician; date and time the specimen was collected
- Designated laboratory for delivery
- Physician notification of laboratory test results and any subsequent orders
- *Standard Precautions*
- Other pertinent findings

Update the plan of care.

Culture Collection

PURPOSE

• To obtain specimens for culture and laboratory analysis

RELATED PROCEDURES

• Specimen Labeling and Transport
• Suctioning (see Chapter 3)

GENERAL INFORMATION

Collect all cultures using aseptic principles. Sterile containers are required for all culture specimens except stool. If the patient is taking an antibiotic, note the drug and dosage on the laboratory requisition. A laboratory requisition must accompany all cultures.

❖ Throat

EQUIPMENT

1. Tongue blade
2. Culturette
3. Penlight or flashlight
4. Laboratory requisition
5. Disposable nonsterile gloves, impermeable specimen transport baggys marked with a biohazard sign, leakproof and puncture-proof specimen transport containers marked with a biohazard sign, and an impermeable plastic trash bag (see *Infection Control*)

PROCEDURE

1. Explain the procedure to the patient/caregiver.
2. Assemble the equipment at a convenient work area.
3. Assist the patient to a sitting or a lying-down position.
4. Remove the cap from the culture tube. Do not touch the cap stem or the inside of the culture tube. Remove the swab from the culture tube.
5. Instruct the patient to open his or her mouth as wide as possible and to say "Aahh." Depress the tongue with a

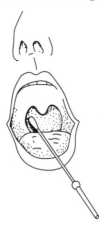

Fig. 12-7   Obtaining a throat culture.

tongue blade, and obtain a culture by moving the swab over the inflamed or purulent area (Fig. 12-7).
6. Return the swab to the culture tube. Replace the cap. Holding the cap down, crush the ampule at the bottom of the culture tube to release the culture medium fluid.
7. Label the culture tube, and seal it in a plastic baggy. Place the baggy in the specimen transport container for travel.
8. Offer oral care.
9. Provide patient comfort measures.
10. Clean and replace the equipment. Discard disposable items according to *Standard Precautions*.
11. Fill our the laboratory requisition, and transport the specimen according to *Standard Precautions*.

❖ Ova and Parasite

EQUIPMENT
1. Bedpan
2. Tongue blade
3. Parasite (PVA) and formalin kits or specimen cup
4. Laboratory requisition
🛑 5. Disposable nonsterile gloves, impermeable specimen transport baggys marked with a biohazard sign, leak-

proof and puncture-proof specimen transport container marked with a biohazard sign, and an impermeable plastic trash bag (see *Infection Control*)

PROCEDURE

1. Explain the procedure to the patient/caregiver.
2. Assist the patient onto the bedpan or into the bathroom.
3. Collect a specimen by using a tongue blade to obtain a small amount of stool and placing it in the specimen cup or in the PVA and formalin kit.
4. Perform perineal care as needed.
5. Label the specimen, and seal it in a plastic bag. Do **not** refrigerate for ova and parasite. Place the bag in a specimen transport container for travel.
6. Provide patient comfort measures.
7. Clean and replace the equipment. Discard disposable items according to *Standard Precautions*.
8. Fill out the laboratory requisition, and transport the specimen according to *Standard Precautions*.

❖ Sputum

GENERAL INFORMATION

Obtain a sputum specimen in the morning when the patient has more strength to expectorate. Sputum can be collected for culture by expectoration, as well as by naso-oropharyngeal, endotracheal, or tracheal suctioning.

EQUIPMENT

1. Sterile specimen cup (if for culture and sensitivity)
2. Laboratory requisition
3. Antiseptic wipes

4. Disposable nonsterile gloves, impermeable specimen transport baggys marked with a biohazard sign, leakproof and puncture-proof specimen transport container marked with a biohazard sign, and an impermeable plastic trash bag (see *Infection Control*)

PROCEDURE

1. Explain the procedure to the patient/caregiver.
2. Assemble the equipment at a convenient work area.
3. Instruct the patient to expectorate. Clarify the difference

between sputum and saliva, as well as the time of day to collect the specimen.

4. Instruct the patient to rinse the mouth with water. The patient should breathe deeply and then forcefully cough to expectorate lower respiratory secretions directly into the container.

5. For tracheostomy, the following is performed:
   a. Attach a sputum trap between the suction catheter and the suction tubing
   b. Suction the patient's stoma
   c. Remove the sputum trap, and close it according to the manufacturer's instructions

6. Offer oral hygiene as needed.

7. Label the specimen, and seal it in a plastic baggy. Place the baggy in a specimen transport container for travel.

8. Provide patient comfort measures.

9. Clean and replace the equipment. Discard disposable items according to *Standard Precautions.*

10. Fill out the laboratory requisition, and transport the specimen according to *Standard Precautions.*

❖ Stool

GENERAL INFORMATION

Obtain a culture with the first morning stool.

EQUIPMENT

1. Culturette or stool specimen cup
2. Tongue blade
3. Bedpan or container
4. Laboratory requisition

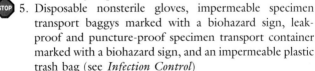

5. Disposable nonsterile gloves, impermeable specimen transport baggys marked with a biohazard sign, leak-proof and puncture-proof specimen transport container marked with a biohazard sign, and an impermeable plastic trash bag (see *Infection Control*)

PROCEDURE

1. Explain the procedure to the patient/caregiver.
2. Assemble the equipment at a convenient work area.
3. Assist the patient onto the bedpan or into the bathroom.
4. Collect a stool specimen using a tongue blade to obtain a

small amount of stool, to be placed in a specimen cup, or by swabbing stool with a swab culturette.

5. If you are using a specimen cup, replace the container cap.
6. If you are using a culturette, place the swab in the container. Hold the cap down, and crush the ampule at the bottom to disperse culture medium fluid.
7. Perform perineal care as needed.
8. Label the specimen and seal it in a plastic bag. Do **not** refrigerate stool specimen. Place in a specimen baggy. Place the baggy in the specimen transport container for travel.
9. Provide patient comfort measures.
10. Clean and replace the equipment. Discard disposable items according to *Standard Precautions*
11. Fill out the laboratory requisition, and transport the specimen according to *Standard Precautions.*

❖ Wound

GENERAL INFORMATION

Anaerobic cultures are not done with culturette specimens. Deep wounds should be aspirated by the physician using a syringe and sent to the laboratory in an anaerobic culture tube; otherwise, cleanse the wound with sterile normal saline to remove the debris before obtaining a specimen for culture.

EQUIPMENT

1. Culturette
2. Wound dressing and irrigation/cleansing solution as prescribed by the physician
3. Laboratory requisition
4. Disposable nonsterile gloves, impermeable specimen transport baggys marked with a biohazard sign, leakproof and puncture-proof specimen transport container marked with a biohazard sign, and an impermeable plastic trash bag (see *Infection Control*)

PROCEDURE

1. Explain the procedure to the patient/caregiver.
2. Position the patient to expose the wound. Drape the patient appropriately.
3. Apply nonsterile gloves, and remove the dressing.
4. Remove the cap and swab from the culturette; do not

Start

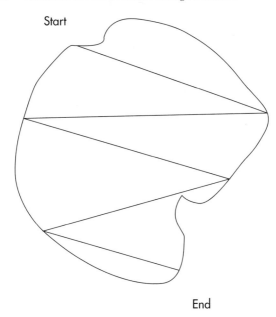

End

Fig. 12-8 Using a zigzag method to obtain a culture from a wound. (From Rice R: *Home health nursing practice: concepts and application*, ed 2, St Louis, 1996, Mosby.)

    touch the cap end, the swab, or inside the culturette container.
5. Swab across the wound using a zigzag method (Fig. 12-8).
6. Return the swab to the culturette (Fig. 12-9, *A*). Hold the cap end down, and crush ampule at the bottom to disperse the culture medium fluid (Fig. 12-9, *B*).
7. Discard the nonsterile gloves, and apply sterile gloves.
8. Clean and re-dress the patient's wound, using sterile technique.
9. Label the specimen, and seal it in a plastic bag.
10. Provide patient comfort measures.
11. Clean and replace the equipment. Discard disposable items according to *Standard Precautions*.
12. Fill out the laboratory requisition, and transport the specimen according to *Standard Precautions*.

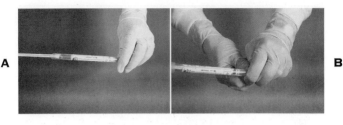

Fig. 12-9 **A,** Returning the swab to the culturette after obtaining a wound specimen. **B,** Crushing the ampule to disperse the culture medium fluid. (From Perry AG, Potter PA: *Clinical nursing skills and techniques,* ed 4, St Louis, 1998, Mosby.)

DOCUMENTATION GUIDELINES

Document the following on the visit report:
- The procedure and patient toleration
- Condition of the specimen site
- Appearance of the culture specimen (color, amount, etc.)
- The type of laboratory test ordered by the physician; date and time the specimen was collected
- Designated laboratory for delivery
- Physician notification of test results and any subsequent orders
- *Standard Precautions*
- Other pertinent findings

Update the plan of care.

Fecal Occult Blood

PURPOSE
• To detect the presence of blood in the stool

GENERAL INFORMATION
Ingestion of high doses of vitamin C (ascorbic acid) in excess of 250 mg each day has been associated with false negative readings. Be aware that certain oral medications may cause gastrointestinal irritation and bleeding. Ingestion of iron preparations, turnips, fish, rare meat, and poultry are associated with false positive readings.

EQUIPMENT
1. Reagent product and slide card
2. Tongue blade
3. Bedpan or container
4. Soap and warm water, basin, tissues, washcloth, and towels
 5. Disposable nonsterile gloves and an impermeable plastic trash bag (see *Infection Control*)

PROCEDURE
1. Explain the procedure to the patient/caregiver.
2. Assemble the equipment at a convenient work area.
3. Assist the patient to the bedpan or to the bathroom.
4. Wash the perineal area with soap and water as needed. Rinse and pat dry.
5. Obtain stool specimen in the bedpan or container.
6. Collect a small sample of the stool on the end of the tongue blade.
7. Follow the manufacturer's instructions for reagent testing.
8. Compare the results with the manufacturer's color chart and guidelines (blue is usually positive for occult blood).
9. Notify the physician of abnormal results.
10. Provide patient comfort measures
11. Clean and replace the equipment. Discard disposable items according to *Standard Precautions.*

DOCUMENTATION GUIDELINES

Document the following on the visit report:
- The procedure and patient toleration
- Color of stool
- Results obtained
- Physician notification of test results and any subsequent orders
- *Standard Precautions*
- Other pertinent findings

Update the plan of care.

Glucose and Ketone Urine Testing: Reagent Strip

PURPOSE

- To detect the presence of glucose or ketone in the urine

GENERAL INFORMATION

The renal threshold for glucose is 180 mg/ml. Ketones appear when fatty acids are used as energy. Abnormal glucose and ketone level results may occur in patients with diabetes or who are malnourished, fasting, or on low-carbohydrate diets.

EQUIPMENT

1. Glucose and ketone test strips
2. Test strip color chart
3. Specimen container
4. Watch with second hand or digital reading
5. Soap and warm water, basin, washcloth, and towels
6. Disposable nonsterile gloves and an impermeable plastic trash bag (see *Infection Control*)

PROCEDURE

1. Explain the procedure to the patient/caregiver.
2. Assemble the equipment at a convenient work area.

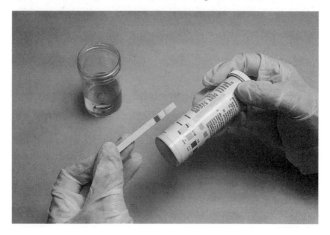

Fig. 12-10 Testing urine, using a reagent strip. (From Perry AG, Potter PA: *Clinical nursing skills and techniques*, ed 4, St Louis, 1998, Mosby.)

3. Assist the patient onto the bedpan or to the bathroom.
4. Wash the perineal area with soap and water to obtain a fresh urine specimen (collect a double-voided specimen if possible). Rinse and dry.
5. Immerse the end of the strip that is impregnated with chemical reagent into a fresh urine specimen.
6. Remove the strip from the container, and gently tap it against the side of the container.
7. Follow the manufacturer's instructions to time the strip for a specified number of seconds, and compare the color strip with the manufacturer's color chart (Fig. 12-10).
8. Notify the physician of abnormal results. (Ketones are reported as negative or as positive. Urine glucose is normally negligible and is reported as none, trace 1+, 2+, 3+, or 4+.) (See Table 12-1.)
9. Provide patient comfort measures.
10. Clean and replace the equipment. Discard disposable items according to *Standard Precautions.*

NURSING CONSIDERATIONS

Instruct the patient/caregiver to perform glucose and ketone urine testing when the patient has a fever, suspects that he or

Table 12-1   Miltistix

Test	When to read	Range of results
pH	Anytime	5 to 9
Protein	Anytime	(−) to +4 (72,000 mg/dl)
Glucose	10 seconds (qualitative)	(−) to +4
	30 seconds (quantitative)	(−) to +4 (270)
Ketones	15 seconds	(−) to +3 (large)
Blood	25 seconds	(−) to +3 (large)

From Perry AG, Potter PA: *Clinical nursing skills and techniques,* ed 4, St Louis. 1998. Mosby.

she may have an infection, or if self-blood glucose monitoring is not an option.

Notify the physician about abnormal results.

DOCUMENTATION GUIDELINES

Document the following on the visit report:
- The procedure and patient toleration
- Glucose and ketone test results
- Any patient/caregiver instructions and response to teaching, including the ability to test urine with reagent strips
- Physician notification of abnormal test results and any subsequent orders
- *Standard Precautions*
- Other pertinent findings

Update the plan of care.

Specimen Labeling and Transport

PURPOSE

- To identify laboratory specimen(s) with appropriate data
- To provide guidelines for delivering specimens to the laboratory for analysis according to *Standard Precautions*

EQUIPMENT

1. Tape or specimen label and biohazard labels
2. Plastic bags
3. Laboratory requisition
4. Antiseptic wipes
5. Disposable nonsterile gloves, impermeable specimen transport baggys marked with a biohazard sign, leak-proof and puncture proof cooler or container marked with a biohazard sign, and an impermeable plastic trash bag (see *Infection Control*)

PROCEDURE

1. Clarify with the physician the designated laboratory for the delivery of specimens.
2. Clarify with the designated laboratory, the color of the test tubes, a specimen collection container, and the patient data that is required to process the specimen.
3. Clean blood and body substances from outside of test tube(s) or specimen container(s) with antiseptic wipes as needed.
4. Label the specimen container in the following manner:
   a. Patient's name
   b. Test to be performed by the laboratory
   c. Time and date specimen was collected
   d. Initials of the person who collected the specimen
5. Place test tubes or the specimen container in a plastic baggy, and seal it to prevent possible leakage during transport. Place a biohazard label on the outside of the plastic baggy. Consider double bagging the specimen to prevent possible leakage when using ice to refrigerate the specimens or PRN as needed.

6. Place the specimen into a leak-proof, puncture-proof cooler or container.
7. Place the cooler or container on the floorboard of the car during transport.
8. Fill out the laboratory requisition, and transport the specimen.
9. Call the physician with the laboratory results as soon as they are available.
10. Discard disposable items according to *Standard Precautions.*

NURSING CONSIDERATIONS

Many specimens must be delivered to the laboratory within 30 minutes to 1 hour after sampling.

Consult with the laboratory concerning the type of container or test tube that should be used to collect the specimen and whether the specimen should be refrigerated by placing it on ice; also inquire about a time frame for deliveries.

Many laboratories provide courier services to pick up specimens at the patient's home.

DOCUMENTATION GUIDELINES

Document the following on the visit report:
- The type of laboratory test ordered by the physician; date and time the specimen was collected
- Designated laboratory for delivery
- *Standard Precautions*
- Other pertinent findings

Document physician notification of laboratory test results on the visit report or appropriate home health agency communiqué and any subsequent orders.

Update the plan of care.

Urine Collection

PURPOSE
- To obtain a urine specimen for laboratory analysis

RELATED PROCEDURES
- Ostomy Care (see Chapter 5)
- Specimen Labeling and Transport

❖ Midstream Urine Collection

EQUIPMENT
1. Urine collection kit
2. Bedpan or urinal
3. Laboratory requisition
4. Soap and warm water, basin, washcloth or disposable towelettes, and towels

 5. Disposable nonsterile gloves, impermeable plastic transport baggys marked with a biohazard sign, leak-proof and puncture-proof container marked with a biohazard sign, and an impermeable plastic trash bag (see *Infection Control*)

PROCEDURE
1. Explain the procedure to the patient/caregiver.
2. Assemble the equipment at a convenient work area.
3. Assist the patient onto the bedpan or to the bathroom
4. Wash the perineal area with soap and water. Rinse and dry.
5. Remove the contents from the midstream collection set.
6. Cleanse the urinary meatus with presaturated towelettes, using each towelette only once. (Retract the foreskin if applicable.)
7. Remove the lid from the specimen container by using only the tab. Do **not** touch the rim or underside of the lid.
8. Instruct the patient to release a small amount of urine into

the bedpan or urinal and then to finish emptying bladder into the specimen container.

9. Replace the lid, handling only the tab. Secure the lid tightly.
10. Perform perineal care as needed.
11. Label the specimen container, and seal it in a specimen baggy. Place the baggy in the specimen container for transport.
12. Provide patient comfort measures.
13. Clean and replace the equipment. Discard disposable items according to *Standard Precautions.*
14. Fill out the laboratory requisition, and transport the specimen.

❖ Routine Urine Collection

EQUIPMENT

1. Bedpan or urinal
2. Urine specimen container with lid
3. Laboratory requisition
4. Soap and warm water, basin, washcloth or disposable towelettes, and towels

 5. Disposable nonsterile gloves, impermeable specimen transport baggy marked with a biohazard sign, leak-proof and puncture-proof container marked with a biohazard sign, and an impermeable plastic trash bag (see *Infection Control*)

PROCEDURE

1. Explain the procedure to the patient/caregiver.
2. Assemble the equipment at a convenient work area.
3. Assist the patient onto the bedpan or to the bathroom.
4. Wash the perineal area with soap and water as needed. Rinse and dry.
5. Instruct the patient to urinate into the specimen container, bedpan, or urinal.
6. After the bedpan or urinal has been used, pour approximately 50 ml of urine into the urine specimen container, and seal it with a lid.
7. Follow steps *10* through *14* of the procedure for *Midstream Urine Collection.*

❖ Sterile Urine Specimen Collection from a Foley Catheter

EQUIPMENT

1. 12 cc syringe
2. 23-gauge needle
3. Clamp or rubber band
4. Sterile specimen container
5. Laboratory requisition
6. Antiseptic wipes
7. Soap and warm water, basin, washcloth or disposable towelettes, and towels
8. **STOP** Disposable nonsterile gloves, impermeable specimen transport baggy marked with a biohazard sign, leak-proof and puncture-proof specimen transport container marked with a biohazard sign, and an impermeable plastic trash bag (see *Infection Control*)

PROCEDURE

1. Explain the procedure to the patient/caregiver.
2. Assemble the equipment at a convenient work area.
3. Assist the patient to a supine position with the knees flexed and legs separated. Uncover the Foley catheter.
4. Wash the perineal area with soap and water as needed. Rinse and dry. Drape the patient for privacy.
5. Clamp or kink off the Foley catheter with a rubber band below the aspiration port. Wait 20 to 30 minutes so that the urine can accumulate in the catheter.
6. Clean the port with an antiseptic wipe.
7. Insert a 23-gauge needle at a 90-degree angle into the port (Fig. 12-11).
8. Aspirate urine into the syringe.

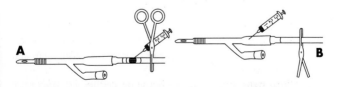

Fig. 12-11   Urine from a sterile catheter. **A,** Indwelling catheter with a specimen port. **B,** Indwelling catheter.

9. Inject the urine into a sterile specimen container.
10. Seal the sterile specimen container.
11. Unclamp or unkink the catheter to allow the urine to flow into the collection bag.
12. Perform perineal care as needed.
13. Label the specimen container, and seal it in a specimen baggy. Place the baggy in a specimen container for transport.
14. Provide patient comfort measures.
15. Clean and replace the equipment. Discard disposable items according to *Standard Precautions.*
16. Fill out the laboratory requisition, and transport the specimen.

❖ Sterile Urine Specimen from a Urostomy

EQUIPMENT

1. Sterile straight catheter (size specified by physician)
2. Sterile catheter tray
3. Sterile urine specimen container
4. Laboratory requisition
5. Soap and warm water, basin, washcloth, and towels
6. Disposable nonsterile and sterile gloves, impermeable specimen transport baggy marked with a biohazard sign, leak-proof and puncture-proof specimen transport container marked with a biohazard sign, and an impermeable plastic trash bag (see *Infection Control*)

PROCEDURE

1. Explain the procedure to the patient/caregiver.
2. Assemble the equipment at a convenient work area.
3. Position the patient in a supine position to expose the urostomy. Drape the patient for privacy.
4. Open the catheter tray, and set up a sterile field. Pour the antiseptic solution over cotton balls.
5. Don nonsterile gloves to remove the urostomy pouch and wash around the stoma with soap and water (leave the water on); use a spiral pattern working outward from the stoma. Pat dry.
6. Discard the nonsterile gloves and don sterile gloves to clean the stoma with cotton balls. Use one ball for each wipe.

7. Apply lubricant to the tip of the Foley catheter. Place the other end of the Foley catheter into the sterile urine specimen container for urine collection.

8. Insert the tip of the Foley catheter approximately 2 to 3 inches into the stoma, and collect urine into the sterile urine specimen container. Do **not** force the Foley catheter into the stoma.

9. Seal the sterile urine specimen container.

10. Reapply the urostomy pouch.

11. Label the specimen container, and seal it in a specimen baggy. Place the baggy in a specimen container for transport.

12. Provide patient comfort measures.

13. Clean and replace the equipment. Discard disposable items according to *Standard Precautions.*

14. Fill out the laboratory requisition, and transport the specimen.

DOCUMENTATION GUIDELINES

Document the following on the visit report:
- The procedure and patient toleration
- Date, time, and amount of urine collected
- Color and character of urine
- Designated laboratory for delivery
- Physician notification, if applicable
- *Standard Precautions*
- Other pertinent findings

Update the plan of care.

Urologic and Renal Care

Arteriovenous Fistula and Shunt Care

PURPOSE

- To prevent infection
- To maintain patency of the arteriovenous fistula or shunt
- To instruct the patient/caregiver in shunt care and precautions
- To promote self-care in the home

EQUIPMENT

1. 4- × 4-inch gauze dressing
2. Antiseptic wipes
3. Antimicrobial ointment
4. Elastic bandage
5. Cannula clamps
6. Hypoallergenic tape
7. Stethoscope

 8. Disposable nonsterile gloves and an impermeable plastic trash bag (see *Infection Control*)

❖ Shunt Dressing Change

PROCEDURE

1. Explain the procedure to the patient/caregiver.
2. Assemble the equipment at a convenient work area.
3. Assist the patient to a comfortable position to perform shunt care.
4. Remove the elastic bandage and dressing. Discard the dressing.
5. Remove the crust and any drainage from around the catheter exit sites with povidone iodine (Betadine) swabs.

6. Cleanse each end of the shunt with separate povidone swabs.
7. Apply a small amount of antimicrobial ointment around the cannula insertion sites—both arterial and venous.
8. Secure the shunt by taping connections with tabs at the ends of the tape to prevent tension on the shunt site when untaping.
9. Cover the shunt with a 4- × 4-inch gauze dressing.
10. Wrap the arm with an elastic bandage. Be sure not to constrict or kink the shunt. Leave the U-shaped portion of the shunt exposed to assess patency of the shunt (Fig. 13-1).
11. Secure the elastic bandage with fasteners.
12. Keep the cannula clamps (to control bleeding from accidental separation of the shunt) fastened on the outside of the elastic bandage at all times. (If the shunt should become accidentally separated, immediately clamp each shunt.)
13. Notify the physician of any signs of infection at the shunt site or of problems with the shunt.
14. Provide patient comfort measures.
15. Clean and replace the equipment. Discard disposable items according to *Standard Precautions.*

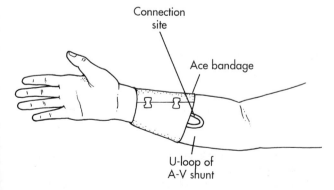

Connection site

Ace bandage

U-loop of
A-V shunt

Fig. 13-1   The AV shunt.

❖ Preserving Patency of the Arteriovenous Fistula

PROCEDURE

1. Follow steps *1* through *8* of the procedure for *Shunt Dressing Change*.

2. Assess patency of the arteriovenous (AV) fistula or shunt in the following way:
   a. Place the stethoscope over the suture line, and auscultate for a bruit (if patent, the fistula will sound like a full, bounding pulse)
   b. Gently palpate the shunt or fistula (palpation should elicit a bruit)
   c. Inspect the U-loop of the AV shunt for color and warmth (if patent, the cannula will be warm, and blood flow will be bright red; separation of blood or dark purple [black] blood indicates clotting)

3. Apply the dressing and elastic bandage as described in the procedure for *Shunt Dressing Change*.

4. Keep the cannula clamps (to control bleeding from accidental separation of the shunt) fastened on the outside of the elastic bandage at all times. (If the shunt should become separated, immediately clamp each shunt.)

5. Notify the physician if no bruit is heard, if the shunt accidentally separates or clots off, or if bleeding occurs.

6. Instruct the patient/caregiver in the following precautions:
   a. Look at the U-loop in the morning and evening to check for patency
   b. Never place restricting clothes or restraints around the fistula extremity
   c. Protect the arm with the shunt when turning or moving
   d. Clean catheter exit sites; reapply dressings and elastic bandages should they become loose or soiled
   e. Clamp off the catheter ends, and apply a pressure dressing to the site if bleeding occurs

7. Instruct the patient/caregiver to notify the physician and home health agency clinical supervisor if the following occur:
   a. U-loop becomes dark and cool

  b. Pain and bleeding or discoloration of the extremity occur(s)
  c. The shunt becomes accidentally separated
8. Follow steps *14* and *15* of the procedure for *Shunt Dressing Change*.

NURSING CONSIDERATIONS

Do not take blood pressures, perform venipunctures, or give injections on an arm with an AV fistula or shunt.

Consult with your fiscal intermediary regarding guidelines for reimbursement of home health services for patients with end stage renal dialysis (ESRD).

DOCUMENTATION GUIDELINES

Document the following on the visit report:
- The procedure and patient toleration
- Condition of catheter exit sites
- Patency of the AV fistula and shunt, including auscultatory findings from assessment of the fistula or shunt
- Any patient/caregiver instructions and response to teaching, including the ability to maintain the integrity of the shunt
- Physician notification, if applicable
- *Standard Precautions*
- Other pertinent findings

Update the plan of care.

Bladder Training

PURPOSE

- To assist the patient to regain control of micturition without a catheter
- To avoid urinary tract infections
- To manage urinary incontinence
- To prevent skin breakdown
- To improve body image and self-esteem
- To promote self-care in the home

RELATED PROCEDURES

- Bowel Training (see Chapter 5)
- Condom Catheter Care
- Indwelling Foley Catheter Insertion and Care
- Intake and Output (see Chapter 2)
- Skin Care (see Chapter 4)
- Intermittent Straight Catheterization

GENERAL INFORMATION

Urinary incontinence is defined as involuntary loss of urine that is sufficient to be considered a problem. The U.S. Department of Health and Human Services Urinary Incontinence Guideline Panel (1992) recommends the following step-wise process of patient management:

1. Question the patient about continence: where, when, and at what time do problems with incontinence occur.
2. Investigate the condition of patients who complain of incontinence.
3. Evaluate the patient by taking a history and by ordering a physical examination and a urinalysis. Patients who complain of urinary incontinence should be evaluated regarding the medication they are currently taking; the duration and characteristics of the incontinence; frequency, timing, and amount of continent and incontinent voids; symptoms of urinary tract infection; altered bowel or sexual function; and the use of pads, briefs, or other protective devices.
4. Identify the type of urinary incontinence: incontinence,

urge incontinence, overflow incontinence, or mixed incontinence.

5. Identify the need for further evaluation by a specialist.
6. Identify treatment options. The three major categories of treatment are behavioral, pharmacologic, and surgical. For most patients, behavioral techniques coupled with pharmacologic intervention are effective (Table 13-1).

Methods to encourage micturition include reflex stimulation: the patient strokes certain *trigger points,* such as the navel, hips, outer or inner aspect of the thighs, abdomen or buttocks, or the area around the sacrum or coccyx. In addition, the patient may be taught to lean forward while applying light pressure with clasped hands over the bladder area to increase bladder emptying.

EQUIPMENT

1. Bedpan, bedside commode, urinal, and toilet
2. Catheter clamp (if necessary, a spring-type clothespin or rubber bands may be used for the purpose of home improvisation)
3. Soap and warm water, basin, tissues, washcloth, and towels
4. Disposable nonsterile gloves and an impermeable plastic trash bag (see *Infection Control*)

❖ Bladder Training for Patients with an Indwelling Catheter

PROCEDURE

1. Explain the procedure to the patient/caregiver.
2. Assemble the equipment at a convenient work area.
3. Perform perineal care as needed.
4. Establish the following schedule for toileting:
   a. Clamp off the urinary catheter for 2 hours at a time to increase bladder tone (the catheter may also be clamped by kinking and securing with rubber bands)
   b. Unclamp the catheter at regular intervals; encourage the patient to push down with the abdominal muscles to completely empty the bladder
   c. Instruct the caregiver to continue to clamp and unclamp the catheter every 2 hours, until the patient is

Table 13-1 Drugs used to treat urinary incontinence

Drugs	Dosages	Mechanisms of action	Types of incontinence	Potential adverse effects
ANTICHOLINERGIC AND ANTISPASMODIC AGENTS				
Oxybutynin (Ditropan) Propantheline (Pro-Banthine)	2.5 to 5.0 mg tid 15 to 30 tid	Increase bladder capacity	Urge or stress with detrusor instability or hyperreflexia	Dry mouth, blurry vision, elevated intraocular pressure, delirium, constipation
Dicyclomine (Bentyl) Flavoxate (Urispas) Imipramine (Tofranil)	10 to 20 mg tid 100 to 200 mg tid 25 to 50 mg tid	Diminish involuntary bladder contractions		Above effects plus postural hypotension, cardiac conduction disturbances

Continued

From Kane RL, Ouslander JG, Abrass IB: *Essentials of clinical geriatrics,* ed 2, New York, 1989, McGraw-Hill.

Table 13-1 Drugs used to treat urinary incontinence—cont'd

Drugs	Dosages	Mechanisms of action	Types of incontinence	Potential adverse effects
ALPHA-ADRENERGIC AGONISTS				
Pseudoephedrine (Sudafed)	15 to 30 mg tid	Increase urethral smooth muscle contraction	Stress incontinence with sphincter weakness	Headache, tachycardia, elevation of blood pressure
Phenylpropanolamine (Ornade)	75 mg tid			All effects listed above
Imipramine (Tofranil)	25 to 50 mg tid			
CONJUGATED ESTROGENS*				
Oral (Premarin)	0.625 mg/day	Increase periurethral blood flow Strengthen periurethral tissues	Stress incontinence Urge incontinence associated with atrophic vaginitis	Endometrial cancer, elevated blood pressure, gallstones
Topical	0.5 to 1.0 g per application			

CHOLINERGIC AGONISTS†

Drug	Dosage	Action	Indication	Side Effects
Bethanechol (Urecholine)	10 to 30 mg tid	Stimulate bladder contraction	Overflow incontinence with atonic bladder	Bradycardia, hypotension, bronchoconstriction, gastric acid secretion

ALPHA-ADRENERGIC ANTAGONIST

Drug	Dosage	Action	Indication	Side Effects
Prazosin (Minipress)‡	1 to 2 mg tid	Relax smooth muscle of urethra and prostatic capsule	Overflow or urge incontinence associated with prostatic enlargement	Postural hypotension

From Kane RL, Ouslander JG, Abrass IB: *Essentials of clinical geriatrics*, ed 2, New York, 1989, McGraw-Hill.
*With prolonged use, cyclical administration with a progestational agent should be considered. Transdermal preparations are also available but have not been studied for treating incontinence.
†The efficacy of chronic bethanechol therapy is controversial.
‡May provide some symptomatic relief in patients who are unwilling or unable to undergo prostatectomy.

able to hold about 250 ml of urine and *feels* the urge to void

5. Remove the indwelling catheter once the patient has control of the bladder.
6. Instruct the patient in Kegel exercises to increase bladder tone.
7. Instruct the patient in methods of reflex stimulation as needed.
8. Instruct the patient/caregiver to keep an accurate record of fluid intake and output.
9. Provide patient comfort measures.
10. Clean and replace the equipment. Discard disposable items according to *Standard Precautions.*

NURSING CONSIDERATIONS

Encourage the patient to drink 8 to 10 glasses of water during the day, unless he or she is on a fluid restriction diet. (Hold fluids after 7 PM for problems with night incontinence. Avoid alcoholic beverages or beverages with caffeine.

Administer diuretics in the morning to prevent the patient from needing to void frequently at night.

Instruct the patient/caregiver to notify the home health agency's clinical supervisor or physician about complaints of abdominal discomfort or if the patient does not void at least 250 ml of urine within 8 hours after removal of the indwelling Foley catheter.

Consult with the physician and consider pharmacologic intervention to prevent urinary incontinence.

Long-term use of indwelling catheters can lead to secondary problems, such as infection. Intermittent catheterization may be appropriate for the management of acute or chronic urinary retention.

Institute a skin-care regimen for problems with incontinence.

❖ Bladder Training for Patients without an Indwelling Catheter

PROCEDURE

1. Explain the procedure to the patient/caregiver.
2. Perform perineal care as needed.
3. Instruct the patient to lean forward and push down with the abdominal muscles to help empty the bladder completely at each voiding.

4. Instruct patient in Kegel exercises to increase bladder tone.

5. Instruct the patient/caregiver to record voiding patterns to establish a bladder routine.

6. Plan a voiding schedule at regular intervals every 1½ or 2 hours as needed.

7. As appropriate, instruct the caregiver to assist the patient to the toilet or commode after meals, and naps, and before bed and or activity. Consider having the patient use a walker or cane.

8. If the patient demonstrates restlessness, assess the need to void. More frequent trips to the bathroom may be necessary if the patient's bladder capacity is small.

9. If night incontinence is a problem, the patient can be awakened once or twice by an alarm. (If the patient continues to lack control at night, consider having the patient use an external urinary collection device, and pad the bed.)

10. Encourage the patient to use the toilet in the bathroom as a part of independent activities of daily living (ADLs) whenever possible. (Use a bedpan or urinal only when absolutely necessary. Consider use of a bedside commode.)

11. Evaluate the bathroom for patient accessibility and safety:
    a. Consider installing a safety bar
    b. Ensure that the bathroom lighting is adequate at all times, especially at night
    c. Ensure that the distance to the toilet is no more than 40 feet from the living area
    d. Keep walkways to the bathroom clutter-free; remove throw rugs on the bathroom floor

12. Instruct the patient to wear nonrestrictive clothing that is easy to get in and out of quickly. Velcro fasteners may be substituted for difficult buttons or zippers. In some cases stockings or underwear may need to be eliminated for independent toileting. Instruct the patient to wear nonskid shoes when going to the bathroom.

13. Follow steps *7* through *10* of the procedure for *Bladder Training for Patients with an Indwelling Catheter.*

NURSING CONSIDERATIONS

Consult with the physician and consider pharmacologic intervention to manage urinary incontinence.

Institute a skin-care regimen for problems with incontinence.

DOCUMENTATION GUIDELINES

Document the following on the visit report:
- The procedure and patient toleration
- The condition of the patient's skin
- The patient's ability to remain continent of urine and void at scheduled intervals
- Any patient/caregiver instructions and response to teaching, including adherence to the bladder training program
- Physician notification, if applicable
- *Standard Precautions*
- Other pertinent findings

Update the plan of care.

Closed Urinary Drainage Management

PURPOSE
- To provide continuous drainage of the bladder
- To prevent infection
- To promote self-care in the home

RELATED PROCEDURES
- Bladder Instillation and Irrigation (see Chapter 9)
- Coudé Catheter Insertion
- Indwelling Foley Catheter Insertion and Care
- Intake and Output (see Chapter 2)
- Suprapubic Catheter Care

EQUIPMENT
1. Disposable closed urinary collection bag with drainage tubing
2. Hypoallergenic tape
3. Disposable nonsterile and sterile gloves and an impermeable plastic trash bag (see *Infection Control*)

PROCEDURE
1. Explain the procedure to the patient/caregiver.
2. Assemble the equipment at a convenient work area.
3. Assist the patient to a comfortable position.

4. After catheterization or bladder irrigation has been performed, insert the drainage tubing into the urinary catheter. (Take care not to contaminate the ends of the drainage tubing or the urinary catheter before insertion.)

5. Tighten the connections to prevent leakage or contamination of the system.

6. Attach the urinary collection bag to the bed frame to allow urine to drain with gravity and prevent backflow (Fig. 13-2). (Keep the drainage below the level of the patient's bladder.)

7. Apply tape to the drainage tubing, making tabs on the end of the tape. Tape the catheter to the thigh or lower abdomen, or coil and fasten the drainage tubing to the patient's gown with a safety pin through the tape tabs.

8. Place the urinary collection bag below the level of the hip when the patient sits in a chair or ambulates to prevent backflow. (Caution the patient not to step on the tubing when ambulating.)

9. Use sterile technique to change the urinary collection bag and drainage tubing at least every 30 days or when it is contaminated or heavily soiled.

10. Empty the collection bag when it is two-thirds full through the bottom outlet into an appropriate container that is used to collect, measure, or discard urine.

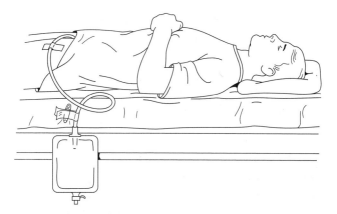

Fig. 13-2 Closed urinary drainage system.

11. If the drainage is dark or thick or contains mucus, report to the physician for possible bladder irrigation.
12. Provide patient comfort measures
13. Clean and replace equipment. Discard disposable items according to *Standard Precautions.*

NURSING CONSIDERATIONS

Instruct the patient/caregiver in home catheter management and precautions.
See the Patient Education Guidelines box, *Caring for the Urinary Catheter at Home,* on pp. 546-547.

DOCUMENTATION GUIDELINES

Document the following on the visit report:
- The procedure and patient toleration
- Intake and output, if ordered
- Patient's fluid and hydration status
- Color, odor, amount, and characteristics of the patient's urine
- Any patient/caregiver instructions and response to teaching
- Physician notification, if applicable
- *Standard Precautions*
- Other pertinent findings
Update the plan of care.

❖ Condom Catheter Care

PURPOSE

- To provide an external urinary drainage system as an adjunct to continence management
- To prevent skin irritation
- To instruct the patient/caregiver in condom catheter management
- To promote self-care in the home

RELATED PROCEDURE

- Closed Urinary Drainage Management

GENERAL INFORMATION

Condom catheters are also referred to as *external* or *Texas catheters.*

EQUIPMENT

1. Rubber condom sheath; condom, size as appropriate (small, medium, large, extra large)
2. Velcro or elastic sheath holder; hypoallergenic tape
3. Urinary collection bag and drainage tubing
4. Soap and warm water, basin, washcloth, and towels

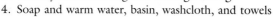

5. Disposable nonsterile gloves and an impermeable plastic trash bag (see *Infection Control*)

PROCEDURE

1. Explain the procedure to the patient/caregiver.
2. Assist the patient to a supine position. Place a towel or waterproof pad underneath the buttocks.
3. Wash the penis with soap and water, and dry it. If the patient is not circumcised, retract the foreskin and cleanse the meatus. Rinse and dry. Drape the patient for privacy.
4. Hold the penis at a 90-degree angle from the patient's body. Gently roll the condom over the penis.
5. Firmly (but not too tightly) secure the condom catheter with a sheath holder to completely encircle the penis at about 1 to 2 inches from the base.
6. Connect the condom catheter to the urinary catheter drainage system, and tape it to prevent tugging (Fig. 13-3).
7. Instruct the patient/caregiver in the following condom catheter management:
   a. Apply a new condom catheter every day
   b. Wash the penis, including under the foreskin if the patient is not circumcised, with soap and water at least daily
   c. If the patient is not circumcised, the foreskin must be pulled down over the head of the penis after cleaning to prevent swelling
   d. Do not put on the condom catheter if the penis becomes discolored or swollen; notify the home health agency clinical supervisor
8. Assist the patient to dress.
9. Provide patient comfort measures.
10. Clean and replace the equipment. Discard disposable items according to *Standard Precautions.*

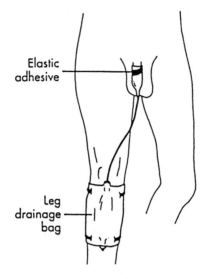

Fig. 13-3 The condom catheter.

NURSING CONSIDERATIONS

Never use adhesive tape to secure a condom catheter because circulation to the penis can be cut off, even if the urine flow is not impaired.

DOCUMENTATION GUIDELINES

Document the following on the visit report:
- The procedure and patient toleration
- Size of the condom catheter applied
- Condition of the skin on the penis
- Color, odor, amount, and characteristics of the patient's urine
- Any patient/caregiver instructions and response to teaching, including hygiene practices
- Physician notification, if applicable
- *Standard Precautions*
- Other pertinent findings

Update the plan of care.

Coudé Catheter Insertion

PURPOSE
- To relieve bladder distention or to empty bladder contents by bypassing an obstruction

RELATED PROCEDURE
- Closed Urinary Drainage Management

GENERAL INFORMATION
The Coudé catheter is a curved-tip urethral catheter that is generally used to catheterize males who have a urethral obstruction. The catheter's curved tip conforms more closely to the natural curve of the male urethra, allowing easier passage into the bladder. Coudé catheters are inserted much like any other urethral catheter, with one exception: the curved tip must be **facing** the direction of the urethral curve. Before inserting a Coudé catheter, but sure you know the anatomy of the male urethra (Fig. 13-4).

Most Coudé catheters are manufactured with a dark line that extends along the top surface of the catheter. This is the same surface that the curved tip faces. The line shows which direction the curved tip is pointing once it has passed into the urethra.

EQUIPMENT
1. Coudé catheter (size ordered by the physician)
2. Sterile catheter tray
3. Soap and warm water, basin, washcloth, and towels
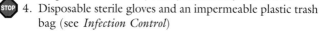 4. Disposable sterile gloves and an impermeable plastic trash bag (see *Infection Control*)

PROCEDURE
1. Explain the procedure to the patient/caregiver.
2. Assemble the equipment at a convenient work area.
3. Assist the patient to a supine position, with the knees flexed and separated. Place a towel or waterproof pad underneath the buttocks.
4. Wash the penis with soap and water. If the patient is not

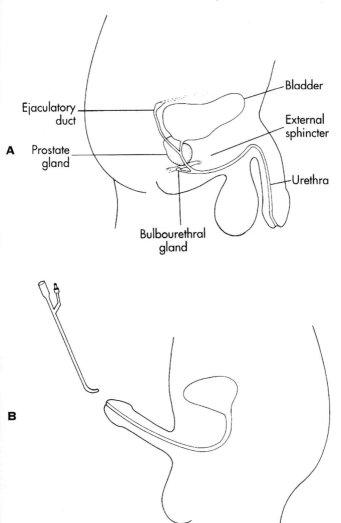

Fig. 13-4   A. Anatomy of male urethra. **B,** The Coudé catheter.

circumcised, retract the foreskin and cleanse the meatus. Rinse and dry. Drape the patient for privacy.

5. Open the catheter tray using sterile technique.
6. Don sterile gloves.
7. Place underpads from the tray beneath the patient's penis, about the scrotum, and across the thighs (plastic side down).
8. Drape the patient with a fenestrated towel.
9. Attach a sterile syringe to the sideport lumen of the catheter, and inject 5 to 10 ml of normal saline solution to test the integrity of the catheter balloon. Maintain sterility of the catheter. Deflate the balloon before insertion.
10. Open the antiseptic solution, and pour it over cotton balls.
11. Lubricate the tip of the catheter, or place the tip of the syringe that is filled with lubricant directly into the meatus and inject the lubricant into the urethra.
12. With the nondominant hand, hold the patient's penis upright at approximately a 90-degree angle to the patient's body.
13. If the patient is not circumcised, retract the foreskin, exposing the meatus.
14. With the dominant hand, use forceps to pick up a cotton ball and cleanse the glans from the meatus outward using antiseptic solution. Use a clean cotton ball for each stroke.
15. Insert the catheter tip into the meatus with the curve facing **upward.** As the catheter is advanced, the dark line on the catheter should continue to face upward. Make sure the patient's penis is held upright as the catheter is inserted and advanced.
16. Some resistance may be felt as the catheter tip meets the external sphincter. Slightly twisting the catheter from side to side while advancing it may help the catheter pass beyond this point. It may be necessary to withdraw the catheter a short distance, and attempt to readvance it slowly.
17. Once the urine begins to flow, advance the catheter another 4 to 5 inches to prevent inflating the balloon in the urethra.
18. Place the end of the catheter into the urine tray receptacle.
19. Inflate the balloon with 5 to 10 ml of normal saline solution. Gently pull back on the catheter to make sure that the balloon is inflated and will hold the catheter in place.

20. If the patient is not circumcised, pull the foreskin back over the meatus to prevent swelling.
21. Connect the catheter to the urinary catheter drainage system.
22. Assist the patient to dress.
23. Provide patient comfort measures.
24. Clean and replace the equipment. Discard disposable items according to *Standard Precautions.*

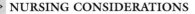 **NURSING CONSIDERATIONS**

Instruct the patient/caregiver in home catheter management and precautions. See the Patient Educations Guidelines box, *Caring for the Urinary Catheter at Home,* on pp. 546-547.

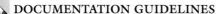 **DOCUMENTATION GUIDELINES**

Document the following on the visit report:
- The procedure and patient toleration
- Size of the catheter inserted and ml capacity of catheter balloon
- Amount of saline solution that was injected into the catheter balloon
- Color, odor, amount, and characteristics of the patient's urine
- Physician notification, if applicable
- *Standard Precautions*
- Other pertinent findings

Update the plan of care.

Indwelling Foley Catheter Insertion and Care

PURPOSE
- To empty the bladder
- To prevent infection
- To obtain urine specimens for laboratory evaluation
- To promote self-care in the home

RELATED PROCEDURES
- Bladder Instillation and Irrigation (see Chapter 9)
- Closed Urinary Drainage Management
- Intermittent Straight Catheterization: Sterile Technique

EQUIPMENT
1. Sterile Foley catheter (size ordered by the physician)
2. Sterile Foley catheter tray
3. Urinary collection bag and drainage tubing
4. Hypoallergenic tape
5. Soap and warm water, basin, washcloth, and towels
6. Disposable sterile gloves and an impermeable plastic trash bag (see *Infection Control*)

PROCEDURE
1. Explain the procedure to the patient/caregiver.
2. Assemble the equipment at a convenient work area.
3. Consider positioning the patient sideways on the bed with the legs separated and dangling over the side of the bed to better access the perineal area and the urethral meatus.
4. Prepare the patient, and open the contents of the sterile Foley catheter tray as described in the procedure for *Intermittent Straight Catheterization: Female* or *Male, Sterile Technique.*
5. Attach a sterile syringe to the sideport lumen of the catheter, and inject 5 to 10 ml of normal saline solution to test the integrity of the balloon. Maintain the sterility of the catheter. Deflate the balloon before insertion.
6. To insert the catheter, follow the procedures for *Intermittent Straight Catheterization: Female* or *Male, Sterile Technique.*

7. Attach a syringe to the sideport lumen of the catheter, and inject 5 to 10 ml of normal saline solution to inflate the balloon.
8. Gently pull the catheter to be sure the balloon is inflated and will hold the catheter in the bladder.
9. Connect the end of the catheter to the drainage tubing and the urinary collection bag. Be careful not to contaminate the end of the catheter or the drainage tubing.
10. Secure the catheter and drainage tubing to prevent tugging (Fig. 13-5).
11. Change the indwelling Foley catheter every 30 days to prevent infection and adhesions.
12. Always remember to deflate the balloon before discontinuing the catheter.
13. Provide patient comfort measures.
14. Clean and replace the equipment. Discard disposable items according to *Standard Precautions.*

NURSING CONSIDERATIONS

Instruct the patient/caregiver on home indwelling Foley catheter management, including signs and symptoms of urinary tract infection to report to the physician.

See the Patient Education Guidelines box, *Caring for the Urinary Catheter at Home,* on pp. 546-547.

DOCUMENTATION GUIDELINES

Document the following on the visit report:
- The procedure and patient toleration
- Size of the catheter that was inserted and ml capacity of balloon
- Amount of saline solution that was injected into the catheter balloon
- Color, odor, amount, and characteristics of the patient's urine
- Any patient/caregiver instructions and response to teaching
- Physician notification, if applicable
- *Standard Precautions*
- Other pertinent findings

Update the plan of care.

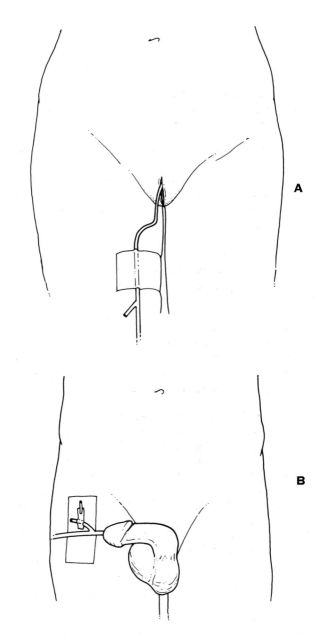

Fig. 13-5 Anchoring of Foley catheter. **A,** In female patient. **B,** In male patient. (From Phipps WJ, Long BC, Woods NF, Cassmeyer VL: *Medical-surgical nursing: concepts and clinical practice,* ed 4, St Louis, 1991, Mosby.)

Intermittent Straight Catheterization: Female

PURPOSE
- To empty the contents of the bladder
- To relieve bladder distention
- To obtain a specimen for laboratory sampling
- To instruct the patient/caregiver in clean technique to empty the bladder contents or to relieve distention at home
- To promote self-care in the home

RELATED PROCEDURES
- Bladder Instillation or Irrigation (see Chapter 9)
- Specimen Labeling and Transport (see Chapter 12)
- Urine Collection (see Chapter 12)

EQUIPMENT
1. Sterile catheter (size ordered by the physician)
2. Sterile catheter tray
3. Basin or appropriate container for urine collection
4. Soap and warm water, basin, washcloth, and towels
5. Disposable sterile gloves and an impermeable plastic trash bag (see *Infection Control*)

❖ Sterile Technique

PROCEDURE
1. Explain the procedure to the patient/caregiver.
2. Assemble the equipment at a convenient work area.
3. Assist the patient to a supine position, with knees flexed and separated. Place a towel or waterproof pad underneath the patient's buttocks.
4. Wash the perineal area with soap and water. Use downward strokes from front to back. Rinse and dry. Drape the patient for privacy.
5. Open the catheter tray, using sterile technique.
6. Open the sterile wrap to provide a sterile field.
7. Don sterile gloves.

8. Drape the patient with fenestrated towels (plastic side down).

9. Open the antiseptic solution, and pour it over the cotton balls.

10. Lubricate the tip of the catheter. Place the other end into the basin or into an appropriate container for urine collection.

11. With your nondominant hand, separate the labia to expose the urethral meatus. Maintain this position throughout the procedure.

12. With your dominant hand, pick up a cotton ball with the forceps, and cleanse the perineal area, starting from the clitoris and progressing downward past the vagina.

13. Use a clean cotton ball for each stroke. Cleanse directly over the urethral meatus with the last cotton ball.

14. With your dominant hand, gently insert the catheter tip into the urethral meatus (approximately 2 to 3 inches) until urine flows. Instruct the patient to breathe deeply to relax the perineal muscles and to overcome resistance to the entry.

15. Release the labia, and collect urine.

16. Pinch the catheter when the flow of urine ceases, and gently and slowly withdraw the catheter. (Do not remove more than 800 ml of urine at one time because this could precipitate shock.)

17. Place the urine specimen in a container for transport if laboratory evaluation is ordered. Otherwise, discard the urine.

18. Assist the patient to dress.

19. Provide patient comfort measures.

20. Clean and replace the equipment. Discard disposable items according to *Standard Precautions.*

❖ Clean Technique (For Self-Catheterization)

EQUIPMENT

1. Catheter (size ordered by the physician)
2. Basin or appropriate container for urine collection
3. Mirror and good lighting
4. Water-soluble lubricant
5. Soap and warm water, basin, washcloth, and towels
6. Impermeable plastic trash bag (see *Infection Control*)

PROCEDURE

1. Instruct the patient/caregiver in the following clean technique:
   a. Wash the hands thoroughly
   b. Assemble the equipment within easy reach
   c. Separate the labia to wash the genitalia with soap and water; use downward strokes from front to back; rinse and dry
   d. Lie or sit down with the knees flexed, or stand with one foot on the edge of the commode; place a towel or a waterproof pad underneath the buttocks if lying or sitting down
   e. Use a mirror to identify the labia, clitoris, urethral meatus, and vagina
   f. Lubricate the tip of the catheter
   g. With your nondominant hand, hold the labia apart with your index and ring fingers
   h. With your dominant hand, insert the tip of the catheter into the urethral meatus (approximately 2 to 3 inches) until urine flows
   i. Release the labia
   j. With your nondominant hand, place the drainage end of the catheter into the toilet or an appropriate container
   k. With your nondominant hand, pinch the catheter when the flow of urine ceases
   l. With your dominant hand, gently and slowly withdraw the catheter, keeping the tip held up to prevent the dribbling of urine
   m. Dispose of the urine
   n. Clean the catheters with soap and water, then boil them for 20 minutes; air dry the catheters on a clean paper towel; store the dry catheters in a plastic bag for future use
   o. Replace torn, hardened, or cracked catheters
   p. Clean and replace your equipment. Discard disposable items according to *Standard Precautions*

NURSING CONSIDERATIONS

Intermittent self-catheterization should be done at least 4 times a day and at bedtime.

Instruct the patient/caregiver that to prevent infections the bladder should not hold more than 1½ cups of urine at a time.

DOCUMENTATION GUIDELINES

Document the following on the visit report:
- The procedure and patient toleration
- Color, odor, amount, and characteristics of the patient's urine
- Catheter size
- Urine collected for laboratory analysis and designated laboratory for delivery, as appropriate
- Any patient/caregiver instructions and response to teaching, including the ability to perform straight catheterization using clean techniques
- Physician notification, if applicable
- *Standard Precautions*
- Other pertinent findings

Update the plan of care.

Intermittent Straight Catheterization: Male

PURPOSE
- To empty the contents of the bladder
- To relieve bladder distention
- To obtain a specimen for laboratory sampling
- To instruct the patient/caregiver in clean technique to empty the bladder contents or to relieve distention at home
- To promote self-care in the home

RELATED PROCEDURES
- Bladder Instillation and Irrigation (see Chapter 9)
- Specimen Labeling and Transport (see Chapter 12)
- Urine Collection (see Chapter 12)

❖ Sterile Technique

EQUIPMENT
1. Sterile catheter (size ordered by the physician)
2. Sterile catheter tray
3. Basin or appropriate container for urine collection

    4. Soap and warm water, basin, washcloth, and towels

 5. Disposable sterile gloves and an impermeable plastic trash bag (see *Infection Control*)

PROCEDURE

1. Explain the procedure to the patient/caregiver.
2. Assemble the equipment at a convenient work area.
3. Assist the patient to a supine position, with knees flexed and separated. Place a towel or waterproof pad underneath the patient's buttocks.
4. Wash the penis with soap and water. If the patient is not circumcised, retract the foreskin and cleanse the meatus. Rinse and dry. Drape the patient for privacy.
5. Open the catheter tray using sterile technique.
6. Open the sterile wrap to provide a sterile field.
7. Don sterile gloves.
8. Place towels from the tray beneath the penis, about the scrotum, and across the thighs (plastic side down).
9. Open the antiseptic solution, and pour it over the cotton balls.
10. Lubricate the tip of the catheter. Place the other end into the basin or into an appropriate container for urine collection.
11. With your nondominant hand, hold the penis upright approximately at a 90-degree angle to the patient's body. Retract the foreskin if the patient is not circumcised, and expose the meatus. Maintain this position throughout the procedure.
12. With your dominant hand, pick up a cotton ball with the forceps, and cleanse the glans with antiseptic solution from the meatus outward. Use a clean cotton ball for each stroke.
13. With your dominant hand, gently insert the catheter about 6 or 7 inches into the urethral meatus, advancing approximately 2 or 3 inches until urine flows.
14. Some resistance may be felt as the catheter tip meets the external sphincter. Instruct the patient to breathe deeply to relax the perineal muscles and overcome resistance to the entry. (Slightly twisting the catheter from side to side while advancing it may help the catheter pass beyond this point; or it may be necessary to withdraw the catheter a short distance and attempt to readvance it slowly.)

15. Collect the urine.
16. If the patient is not circumcised, place the foreskin back to its previous position to prevent swelling.
17. When the flow of urine ceases, pinch the catheter and gently and slowly withdraw it. (Do not remove more than 800 ml of urine at one time because this could precipitate shock.)
18. Place the urine specimen in a container for transport if laboratory evaluation is ordered. Otherwise, discard the urine.
19. Assist the patient to dress.
20. Provide patient comfort measures.
21. Clean and replace the equipment. Discard disposable items according to *Standard Precautions.*

❖ Clean Technique (For Self-Catheterization)

EQUIPMENT

1. Catheter (size ordered by the physician)
2. Basin or appropriate container for urine collection
3. Good lighting
4. Water-soluble lubricant
5. Soap and warm water, basin, washcloth, and towels
6. Impermeable plastic trash bag (see *Infection Control*)

PROCEDURE

1. Instruct the patient/caregiver in the following clean technique:
   a. Wash the hands thoroughly
   b. Assemble the equipment within easy reach
   c. Wash the penis with soap and water; if you are not circumcised, retract the foreskin, and wash the head of the penis with soap and water; rinse and dry
   d. Lie or sit down with the knees flexed, or stand in front of the toilet; place a towel or a waterproof pad underneath the penis if lying or sitting down
   e. Lubricate the tip of the catheter
   f. With your nondominant hand, hold your penis at a 90-degree angle to your body, and retract the foreskin if you are not circumcised
   g. With your dominant hand, slowly insert the lubricated catheter
   h. Once the urine begins to flow, advance the catheter an-

      other 2 to 3 inches to make sure that the catheter is in your bladder

  i. Place the drainage end of the catheter into the toilet or an appropriate container

  j. With your nondominant hand, pinch the catheter when the flow of urine ceases

  k. With your dominant hand, gently and slowly withdraw the catheter, keeping the tip held up to prevent the dribbling of urine

  l. If you are not circumcised, return your foreskin back into its previous position

  m. Dispose of the urine

  n. Clean the catheters with soap and water, then boil them for 15 minutes; air dry the catheters on a clean paper towel; store the dry catheters in a plastic bag for future use

  o. Replace torn, hardened, or cracked catheters

  p. Clean and replace your equipment. Discard disposable items according to *Standard Precautions*

NURSING CONSIDERATIONS

Intermittent self-catheterization should be done at least 4 times a day and at bedtime.

Instruct the patient/caregiver that to prevent infections, the bladder should not hold more than 1½ cups of urine at a time.

DOCUMENTATION GUIDELINES

Document the following on the visit report:
- The procedure and patient toleration
- Color, odor, amount, and characteristics of the patient's urine
- Catheter size
- Urine collected for laboratory analysis and designated laboratory for delivery, as appropriate
- Any patient/caregiver instructions and response to teaching, including the ability to perform straight catheterization using clean techniques
- Physician notification, if applicable
- *Standard Precautions*
- Other pertinent findings

Update the plan of care.

Nephrostomy Catheter Care

PURPOSE
- To promote drainage of the urine from the kidney when it is not possible or desirable that the urine flow through a ureter
- To prevent infection

RELATED PROCEDURES
- Closed Urinary Drainage Management
- Dressing Changes: Hydrocolloid Dressings and Transparent Adhesive Films (see Chapter 4)

EQUIPMENT
1. Sterile normal saline as prescribed by the physician
2. Sterile bladder irrigation set (solution container, asepto syringe, 4- × 4-inch gauze pads, drainage basin)
3. Antiseptic wipes
4. Sterile 4- × 4-inch gauze dressings
5. Transparent adhesive dressing (optional)
6. Hypoallergenic tape
7. Disposable nonsterile gloves and an impermeable plastic trash bag (see *Infection Control*)

PROCEDURE
1. Explain the procedure to the patient/caregiver.
2. Assemble the equipment at a convenient work area.
3. Position the patient to access the nephrostomy site. Drape the patient for privacy.
4. Cleanse around the nephrostomy catheter with antiseptic wipes (avoid using hydrogen peroxide and Betadine because these can promote skin irritation).
5. Examine the catheter exit site; report signs of redness or infection to the physician as needed.
6. Place the gauze dressing around the catheter; secure with tape (instead of a gauze dressing, a transparent adhesive film may be applied).
7. To clear a plugged catheter, do the following:
   a. Gently irrigate the catheter with 5 ml of sterile normal

saline (obtain physician guidelines); never force the irrigant into the catheter

b. Gently aspirate the installed irrigant, or allow the irrigant to flow back via gravity into the drainage basin

c. Discard the irrigation solution in the drainage basin into the toilet

8. Apply a catheter strap and leg bag for daytime drainage.
9. Apply tubing and a urinary collection bag for nighttime drainage.
10. Assist the patient to dress.
11. Provide patient comfort measures.
12. Clean and replace equipment. Discard disposable items according to *Standard Precautions*.

 NURSING CONSIDERATIONS

Sterile technique **is required** to prevent kidney infection.

Tape the catheter to the patient's skin to prevent it from becoming dislodged (to ensure continuous drainage, do not bend or kink the catheter).

Do not clamp the catheter unless ordered by the physician.

DOCUMENTATION GUIDELINES

Document the following on the visit report:

• The procedure and patient toleration
• The condition of the nephrostomy catheter exit site
• Patient's fluid and hydration status
• Color, odor, amount, and characteristics of the patient's urine
• Any patient/caregiver instructions and response to teaching
• Physician notification, if applicable
• *Standard Precautions*
• Other pertinent findings

Update the plan of care.

Pessary: Removal and Insertion

PURPOSE
- To support the uterus
- To reduce symptoms of pelvic relaxation, including urinary incontinence

EQUIPMENT
1. Pessary
2. Water-soluble jelly
3. Paper towels

 4. Disposable nonsterile gloves and an impermeable plastic trash bag (see *Infection Control*)

PROCEDURE
1. Explain the procedure to the patient/caregiver.
2. Assemble the equipment at a convenient work area.
3. Assist the patient to a supine position, with knees flexed and separated. Drape the patient for privacy.
4. To remove the pessary, do the following:
   a. Gently insert the fingers into the vagina
   b. Hook fingertips under the pessary rim and pull the pessary straight out
   c. Wash the pessary with soap and water, and dry with paper towels (switch to a new pessary every month or prn as needed)
5. To reinsert the pessary, do the following:
   a. Lubricate the rim of the pessary with water-soluble jelly
   b. Gently squeeze the pessary rim together, and reinsert the pessary toward the back of the vagina (the outside rim of the pessary should fit under the symphysis pubis)
   c. Check the placement of the pessary with the fingertips (the rim of the pessary should be smooth and circular, not wrinkled)
6. Provide patient comfort measures.
7. Clean and replace equipment. Discard disposable items according to *Standard Precautions*.

> **NURSING CONSIDERATIONS**

If the patient complains of pain or discomfort, re-position the
pessary as necessary.

> **DOCUMENTATION GUIDELINES**

Document the following on the visit report:
- The procedure and patient toleration
- Any vaginal discharge or foul order
- Any patient/caregiver instructions and response to teach-
  ing
- Physician notification, if applicable
- *Standard Precautions*
- Other pertinent findings

Update the plan of care.

Suprapubic Catheter Care

PURPOSE
- To empty the contents of the bladder
- To prevent infection and skin breakdown
- To collect a urine sample for laboratory analysis
- To instruct the patient/caregiver to clean and apply a dress-
  ing to the suprapubic catheter using clean technique
- To promote self-care in the home

RELATED PROCEDURES
- Bladder Instillation and Irrigation (see Chapter 9)
- Closed Urinary Drainage Management
- Specimen Collection and Transport (see Chapter 12)
- Urine Collection (see Chapter 12)

GENERAL INFORMATION
The suprapubic catheter is inserted into the bladder through
a permanent opening in the abdominal wall that has been surgically created to provide an alternate path for urine flow from
the bladder.

❖ Catheter Change

EQUIPMENT

1. Sterile catheter (size ordered by the physician)
2. Sterile catheter tray
3. Urinary collection bag and drainage tubing
4. Sterile 12 cc syringe
5. Sterile syringe with 10 ml normal saline solution
6. Soap and warm water, basin, washcloth, and towels

STOP 7. Disposable nonsterile and sterile gloves and an impermeable plastic trash bag (see *Infection Control*)

PROCEDURE

1. Explain the procedure to the patient/caregiver.
2. Assemble the equipment at a convenient work area.
3. Position the patient in a reclining position. Place a towel under the buttocks.
4. Perform perineal care as needed. Drape the patient for privacy.
5. Don nonsterile gloves.
6. Remove the old dressing to expose the suprapubic catheter.
7. Attach a 12 cc sterile syringe onto the sideport lumen of the catheter. Remove 5 to 10 ml of sterile normal saline solution or water to deflate the balloon.
8. Gently and slowly remove the catheter.
9. Gently wash the peristomal area with soap and water. Use a spiral pattern, beginning at the stoma site and working outward. Rinse and pat dry.
10. Inspect the stoma site for redness or drainage; report to the physician as appropriate.
11. Discard the catheter, syringe, and nonsterile gloves.
12. Open the catheter tray using sterile technique.
13. Open the sterile wrap to provide a sterile field.
14. Don sterile gloves.
15. Open the contents in the catheter tray.
16. Insert a sterile syringe on the sideport of the lumen at the end of the catheter. Inflate 5 to 10 ml of sterile normal saline solution to test the integrity of the balloon. Deflate the balloon before the insertion of the catheter.
17. Pour antiseptic solution over cotton balls.

18. Use the forceps to pick up the cotton balls, and cleanse the stoma and the surrounding area. Use one ball per wipe.
19. With the dominate hand, dip the catheter tip into the lubricant, and gently insert the catheter into the stoma until resistance is felt.
20. Inflate the bulb of the catheter with 5 to 10 ml of sterile normal saline solution or water.
21. Collect a urine specimen if ordered.
22. Connect the catheter to the urinary drainage system.
23. Dress the stoma as described in the procedure for *Suprapubic Catheter Care, Dressing Change: Clean Technique (Patient-Administered)*.
24. Assist the patient to dress.
25. Provide patient comfort measures.
26. Clean and replace the equipment. Discard disposable items according to *Standard Precautions*.

❖ Dressing Change: Clean Technique (Patient-Administered)

EQUIPMENT

1. Antiseptic ointment as prescribed the physician
2. 4- × 4-inch gauze dressing or drain sponge
3. Scissors
4. Hypoallergenic tape
5. Soap and warm water, basin, washcloth, and towels

PROCEDURE

1. Instruct the patient/caregiver in dressing change, using the following clean technique:
   a. Gather the equipment; wash the hands
   b. Sit or recline to expose the suprapubic catheter
   c. Remove and discard soiled dressing
   d. Gently clean the peristomal area with mild soap and water; use a spiral pattern, beginning at the stoma site and working outward; rinse and pat dry
   e. Inspect the stoma for redness or irritation, green or yellow drainage, foul odor, bleeding, urinary leakage or accidental catheter dislodgement; notify the physician and the home health agency clinical supervisor if you have any questions or concerns

   f. If the catheter accidentally comes out, cover the stoma with a clean 4- × 4-inch gauze dressing and secure it with tape until a new one can be inserted

   g. Apply a small amount of antiseptic ointment around the stoma

   h. Reapply a clean 4- × 4-inch gauze dressing or drain sponge, cut to the center on one side to fit around the catheter like a collar

   i. Tape the edges of the dressing to prevent it from coming loose

   j. Change the dressing daily; long-term suprapubic catheter dressing changes may be decreased to 3 to 4 times a week when your physician instructs you to do so

   k. Clean and replace your equipment. Discard disposable items according to *Standard Precautions.*

DOCUMENTATION GUIDELINES

Document the following on the visit report:
- The procedure and patient toleration
- Color, odor, amount, and characteristics of the patient's urine
- Catheter size
- Condition of the stoma site
- Urine collected for laboratory analysis and designated laboratory for delivery, as appropriate
- Any patient/caregiver instructions and response to teaching, including the ability to care for the suprapubic catheter using clean techniques
- Physician notification, if applicable
- *Standard Precautions*
- Other pertinent findings

Update the plan of care.

Urinary Pouch for Females

PURPOSE

- To provide drainage of the bladder using an external urine collection system
- To prevent skin irritation and breakdown

GENERAL INFORMATION

The female urinary pouch is designed to be worn externally. The pouch is primarily used for incontinent patients for whom an indwelling catheter is contraindicated. The pouch may also be used to collect a clean urine specimen.

The pouch has foam-backed synthetic skin. The pre-cut opening in the barrier may be enlarged as needed. The pouch also has an outlet that is used to drain urine. The outlet can be connected to tubing and a urine collection bag for nighttime management.

EQUIPMENT

1. Female urinary pouch (e.g., Hollister)
2. Disposable closed urinary collection bag with drainage tubing (optional)
3. Tube paste (e.g., Hollister Premium Paste)
4. Microporous adhesive tape
5. Skin prep wipes
6. Plastic sheet or towel
7. Nonsterile disposable gloves and an impermeable plastic trash bag (see *Infection Control*)

PROCEDURE

1. Explain the procedure to the patient/caregiver.
2. Assemble the equipment at a convenient work area.
3. Assist the patient to a supine position, with knees flexed and separated. Place a plastic sheet or towel underneath the buttocks to protect the linens. Drape the patient for privacy.
4. Cleanse the external genitalia with soap and water. Dry. Apply skin prep wipes to the external labia.
5. Separate the labia to examine the urethral meatus and periurethral floor.

6. Assess the size of the vulva opening, then release the labia.
7. As necessary, use scissors to enlarge the pouch opening so that it corresponds to the size of the vulva opening (review manufacturer's guidelines; do **not** cut beyond the lines indicated on the backing of the paper).
8. Make sure that the convenience drain cap on the pouch is closed.
9. Remove the protective paper from the skin barrier.
10. Apply a thin coat of paste around the pouch opening.
11. With the labia in a normal position, apply the pouch barrier to the perineum. Gently press the barrier against the perineum until it contacts the skin at all points.
12. To promote a good seal, apply pressure to the barrier for 1 minute.
13. Apply the microporous adhesive tape on the edge of the pouch for extra security.
14. Promote patient comfort measures.
15. Clean and replace equipment. Discard disposable items according to *Standard Precautions*.

NURSING CONSIDERATIONS

Remove the cap on the convenience drain to drain urine. Remove the cap on the convenience drain and attach tubing for continuous drainage into a urine collection bag.

Change the pouch about every 5 day or prn (empty the pouch before removing it; ease the skin barrier away from the skin in the direction of pubic hair growth).

Discontinue the use of the pouch with patient symptoms of fever or abnormal vaginal discharge.

DOCUMENTATION GUIDELINES

Document the following on the visit report:
- The procedure and patient toleration
- Patient's fluid and hydration status
- Color, odor, amount, and characteristics of the patient's urine
- Any patient/caregiver instructions and response to teaching
- Physician notification, if applicable
- *Standard Precautions*
- Other pertinent findings

Update the plan of care.

Patient Education Guidelines

Caring for the Urinary Catheter at Home

When caring for a urinary catheter at home, remember the following:

1. Unless your physician tells you otherwise, drink 8 to 10 glasses of water a day to keep your urine clear and yellow.
2. Tell your nurse if your urine changes color. Remember that certain medicines and vitamins can change the color of urine.
3. If your catheter accidentally comes out or leaks, place a towel or waterproof pad underneath you to protect the bed or chair. Do not attempt to reinsert the catheter.
4. If urine does not flow into your drainage bag for 6 to 8 hours, check to make sure the drainage tubing isn't twisted or bent; this will block the flow of urine. If the tubing is not twisted or bent, notify your nurse or home health agency's clinical supervisor.
5. Keep the drainage bag below the level of your bladder to prevent a backflow of urine and possible infection. **Never** raise the drainage bag above the stomach.
6. Avoid tugging or pulling on the drainage tubing; this could cause bleeding and trauma. Likewise, be careful not to step on the tubing when ambulating. Walk with the drainage tubing coiled in your hand and the drainage bag held below your bladder.
7. Tape the catheter to your thigh or pin it to the sheet to prevent tugging. A catheter leg strap should be used for permanent catheters. Leave enough slack in the tubing so that it is comfortable.

Patient Education Guidelines—cont'd
Caring for the Urinary Catheter at Home

8. Clean the skin around your catheter with soap and water at least once a day to remove clots, secretions, and drainage. Pat dry. Cleanliness and good personal care are **important** in preventing infection and skin breakdown. Always wash your hands before and after performing catheter care.

9. Clean your urinary collection bag or leg bag with soap and water at least every week if you plan to reuse it. Soak the bag in a solution of 1 part white vinegar to 3 parts tap water for 30 minutes. Then empty the bag, and air dry. Store the bag in a clean plastic bag until you are ready to use it.

10. Call and notify your nurse or the on-call home health agency clinical supervisor if the following should occur:
    • Your catheter comes out or leaks
    • Your urine is bloody, discolored, or cloudy
    • No urine has drained from the catheter after 6 to 8 hours
    • Abdominal pain, elevated temperature, or a burning sensation when you urinate
    • Catheter supplies are needed

11. Go to the emergency room if you experience acute abdominal pain or discomfort caused by the catheter.

Dermal Wound Care Products

Product	Manufacturer	Comments
PHYSIOLOGIC SOLUTIONS		Isotonic solutions used in wound irrigation and mechanical debridement; no chemical or antiseptic action
Normal saline	Generic	
Ringer's lactate	Generic	
ANTISEPTIC SOLUTIONS		
Acetic acid	Generic	Known to inhibit growth of *Pseudomonas aeruginosa*, *Trichomonas vaginalis*, and *Candida albicans*; strong concentrations may destroy fibroblasts; dilute to 0.25%
Alcohol/ethanol	Generic	Use only on iodine-sensitive patients
Povidone iodine	Generic	Can be absorbed through any body surface except adult intact skin; dries skin; may destroy fibroblasts unless properly diluted to < 1%
Dakin's (diluted sodium hypochlorite)	Generic	Controls odor; may interfere with coagulation; solution unstable; replace every day

Continued

Product	Manufacturer	Comments
ASEPTIC SOLUTIONS		
Hydrogen peroxide	Generic	Use only on wounds with necrotic debris; can separate new epithelium from underlying tissue; do not use in abdominal cavity because gas may invade capillaries and lymphatics; slightly warms wound, enhancing vasodilation and decreasing inflammation; in strong concentrations, shown to destroy fibroblasts; dilute to < 3%
Zephiran chloride (benzalkonium)	Generic	Inactivated by soaps; rinse wound thoroughly with normal saline solution before use; reported to enhance growth of some *Pseudomonas* species; do not cover with occlusive dressings
DETERGENT SOLUTIONS		
Cara Klenz	Carrington Labs	Isotonic solutions used in wound irrigation and mechanical debridement; no antiseptic action
Saflens	Calgon-Vestal-Merck	
Constant-Clens	Sherwood Medical	
COTTON DRESSINGS (GAUZE)		
Fine-mesh gauze	Generic	Approximately 41-47 thread count in a 4- × 4-inch pad; capillary beds rarely grow into the interstices of fine mesh and are not damaged when dressing is removed

Wide-mesh gauze	Generic	Approximately 30-39 thread count in a 4- × 4-inch pad; used in mechanical debridement because coarse weave allows necrotic debris to adhere to dressing for removal

COTTON DRESSINGS (IMPREGNATED)

Adaptic	Johnson & Johnson	Drying out adversely affects wound healing
Melolite	Smith-Nephew	
Mesalt	Scott Health Care	
Scarlet-Red	Cheesbrough-Ponds	
Zeroform	Sherwood Medical	
Vaseline gauze	Cheesbrough-Ponds	

COMBINATION DRESSINGS

Viasorb	Cheesbrough-Ponds	Provide nonadherent, absorbent layer within a transparent membrane
Polymen	Ferris	
Nu-Derm	Johnson & Johnson	

COTTON DRESSINGS (PASTE BANDAGE)

Unna boot	Miles Pharmaceuticals	Cotton mesh, impregnated with zinc oxide, calamine (Unna boot), and gelatin; dries to provide extremity with compression and support; no gaps should be left in bandage, otherwise edema will accumulate
Viscopaste	Smith-Nephew	

Continued

Product	Manufacturer	Comments
EXUDATE ABSORPTIVE DRESSINGS		
Bard Absorption	Bard Home Health	Absorb and wick up bacteria and exudates
Debrisan	Johnson & Johnson	
DuoDerm Granules	ConvaTec	
DuoDerm Paste	ConvaTec	
Hydra-Gran	Baxter	
Hydron	Bioderm Sciences	
Algosteril	Johnson & Johnson	
Kaltostat	Calgon-Vestal-Merck	May be used in conjunction with prescribed solution for copious-draining wounds; is not the treatment of choice for wound management because gauze may leave particles and fibers in the wound
Sorbsan	Dow Hickman	
Wound Exudate	Hallister	
Absorber Gauze	Generic	
FOAM DRESSINGS		
Allevyn	Smith-Nephew	Avoid using in wounds with dry eschar
Epi-Lock	Calgon-Vestal-Merck	
Lyofoam	Ultra Labs	
Primaderm	Absorbent Cotton Corporation	
Synthaderm		

HYDROCOLLOID DRESSINGS

Product	Company	
Comfeel Pressure Relief Dressing	Kendall	Dressing change required about every 4 to 7 days or PRN for leakage; relatively impermeable to gas and vapor exchange; use with caution in deep, full-thickness wounds because it may foster anaerobic infection
Comfeel Ulcer Care Dressing	Kendall	
Cutinova Hydro	Beiersdorf Medical	
Duoderm and Duoderm CGF	ConvaTec	
Hydropad	Baxter	
Intact	Bard Home Health	
Johnson & Johnson Ulcer Dressing	Johnson & Johnson	
Restore	Hollister	
Tegasorb	3M	
Ultec	Sherwood Medical	

HYDROGEL DRESSINGS

Product	Company	
Intrasite gel	Smith-Nephew	Available in gel or sheet gel form; normalize wound humidity; sterile as packaged
Vigilon	Bard Home Health	
Geliperm	E. Furgera & Co.	
Nugel	Johnson & Johnson	
Elastogel	Southwest Technologies	

Continued

Product	Manufacturer	Comments
HYDROPHILIC POWDER DRESSINGS		
Chronicure	ABS LifeScience	Hydrophilic powder dressing that becomes a gel when contact is made with the wound surface
Multidex	Lange Medical Products	
TOPICAL DEBRIDING AGENTS		
Debrisan	Johnson & Johnson	Absorb wound drainage and bacteria
DuoDerm Paste	ConvaTec	Physiologic debrider
Elase	Parke-Davis	Indicated for slough and eschar
Santyl	Knoll	Indicated for slough and eschar
Silvadine Cream	Marion Labs	Physiologic debrider with antimicrobial properties; bacterial and fungicidal action maintained for about 12 hours; change twice each day
Travase	Flint Labs	Indicated for eschar; moisten only with sterile water or saline; not appropriate for pregnant women
TOPICAL MOISTURIZERS		
Carrington Gel	Carrington Labs	Available in gel, granulate, or sheet form
Dermagran	Dermasciences	
DuoDerm Paste	ConvaTec	
Geliperm Wet	E. Furgera & Co.	
Second Skin	Spence	

TRANSPARENT FILL (ADHESIVE)

Acuderm	Acme United	Semipermeable; dressing change required about every 4 to 7 days or PRN; may be used to protect skin against friction
Bio-Occlusive	Johnson & Johnson	
Ensure	Deseret	
Opraflex	Professional Medical Products	
Op-Site	Smith-Nephew	
Polyskin	Kendall	
Tegaderm	3-M	
Uniflex	Acme United	

TRANSPARENT FILL (NONADHESIVE)

Jobskin	Jobst	Clings to superficial open wounds without the need of adhesive; topicals may be applied to the dressing; removal—when the dressing falls off or by flushing with normal saline solution
Omiderm	Dermatological Research Laboratories (D.R. Labs)	

MISCELLANEOUS (TRADITIONAL)

Karaya	Generic	Absorbent, adhesive, and hydrophilic properties; promotes wound bed
Insulin	Generic	Enhances protein synthesis by skin; observe for hypoglycemia; apply at meal times

Continued

Product	Manufacturer	Comments
MISCELLANEOUS (TRADITIONAL)—cont'd		
Stomahesive	ConvaTec	Useful in debriding thick, hard necrotic tissue
Sugar	Generic	Hypertonic sugar solutions absorb moisture and debris, which may enhance wound healing; use with caution because sugar may provide a medium for bacterial growth
MISCELLANEOUS (CONTEMPORARY)		
Biobrane	Woodruff Labs	Silicone membrane coated with collagen and hydrophilic peptide; drying and sticking to wound bed may damage healthy tissue; often used for burns
Procurren	Curatec	Platelet-derived formula containing growth factors to increase healing of severe and chronic wounds

Laboratory Values

Test	Reference range	
	Conventional values	SI units*
BLOOD, PLASMA, OR SERUM VALUES		
Acetoacetate plus acetone	0.30-2.0 mg/dl	3-20 mg/l
Acetone	Negative	Negative
Acid phosphate	Adults: 0.10-0.63 U/ml (Bessey-Lowry)	28-175 nmol/s/L
	0.5-2.0 U/ml (Bodansky)	
	1.0-4.0 U/ml (King-Armstrong)	
	Children: 6.4-15.2 U/L	
Activated partial thromboplastin time (APTT)	30-40 sec	30-40 sec
Adrenocorticotropic hormone (ACTH)	6 AM 15-100 pg/ml	10-80 ng/L
	6 PM <50 pg/ml	<50 ng/L
Alanine aminotransferase (ALT)	5-35 IU/L	5-35 U/L
Albumin	3.2-4.5 g/dl	35-55 g/L
Alcohol	Negative	Negative
Aldolase	Adults: 3.0-8.2 Sibley-Lehninger U/dl	22-59 mU/L at 37° C
	Children: approximately 2 × adult values	
	Newborns: approximately 4 × adult values	

Aldosterone	Peripheral blood:	
	Supine: 7.4 ± 4.2 ng/dl	0.08-0.3 nmol/L
	Upright: 1-21 ng/dl	0.14-0.8 nmol/L
	Adrenal vein: 200-800 ng/dl	
Alkaline phosphatase	Adults: 30-85 ImU/ml	
	Children and adolescents:	
	<2 years: 85-235 ImU/ml	
	2-8 years: 65-210 ImU/ml	
	9-15 years: 60-300 ImU/ml (active bone growth)	
	16-21 years: 30-200 ImU/ml	
Alpha-aminonitrogen	3-6 mg/dl	2.1-3.9 mmol/L
Alpha-1-antitrypsin	>250 mg/dl	
Alpha fetoprotein (AFP)	<25 ng/ml	
Ammonia	Adults: 15-110 μg/dl	47-65 μmol/L
	Children: 40-80 μg/dl	
	Newborns: 90-150 μg/dl	

Continued

Modified from Pagana KD, Pagana TJ: *Diagnostic testing and nursing implications*, ed 3, St Louis, 1994, Mosby.

*The use of the System of International Units (SI) was recommended at the 30th World Health Assembly in 1977 to implement an international language of measurement. Because this system is being adopted by numerous laboratories, many of the common values are expressed in both conventional and SI units. SI units are calculated by multiplying the conventional unit by a number factor. The SI measurement system uses *moles* as the basic unit for the amount of a substance, *kilograms* for its mass, and *meter* for its length.

| | Reference range | |
Test	Conventional values	SI units*
BLOOD, PLASMA, OR SERUM VALUES—cont'd		
Amylase	56-190 IU/L	25-125 U/L
	80-150 Somogyi units/ml	
Angiotensin-converting enzyme (ACE)	23-57 U/ml	
Antinuclear antibodies (ANA)	Negative	
Antistreptolysin O (ASO)	Adults: ≤160 Todd units/ml	
	Children:	
	Newborns: similar to mother's value	
	6 months-2 years: ≤50 Todd units/ml	
	2-4 years: ≤160 Todd units/ml	
	5-12 years: ≤200 Todd units/ml	
Antithyroid microsomal antibody	Titer <1:100	
Antithyroglobulin antibody	Titer <1:100	
Ascorbic acid (vitamin C)	0.6-1.6 mg/dl	23-57 μmol/L
Aspartate aminotransferase (AST, SGOT)	12-36 U/ml	0.10-0.30 μmol/s/L
	5-40 IU/L	5-40 U/L
Australian antigen (hepatitis-associated antigen, HAA)	Negative	Negative
Barbiturates	Negative	Negative

Base excess	Men: −3.3 to +1.2	0 ± 2 mmol/L
	Women: −2.4 to +2.3	0 ± 2 mmol/L
Bicarbonate (HCO$_3^-$)	22-26 mEq/L	22-26 mmol/L
Bilirubin		
Direct (conjugated)	0.1-0.3 mg/dl	1.7-5.1 μmol/L
Indirect (unconjugated)	0.2-0.8 mg/dl	3.4-12.0 μmol/L
Total	Adults and children: 0.1-1.0 mg/dl	5.1-17.0 μmol/L
	Newborns: 1-12 mg/dl	
Bleeding time (Ivy method)	1-9 min	
Blood count (see Complete blood count)		
Blood gases (arterial)		
pH	7.35-7.45	
Pco$_2$	35-45 mm Hg	4.7-6.0 kPa
HCO$_3^-$	22-26 mEq/L	21-28 nmol/L
Po$_2$	80-100 mm Hg	11-13 kPa
O$_2$ saturation	95%-100%	
Blood urea nitrogen (BUN)	5-20 mg/dl	3.6-7.1 mmol/L
Bromide	Up to 5 mg/dl	0-63 mmol/L
Bromosulfophthalein (BSP)	<5% retention after 45 min	
CA 15-3	<22 U/ml	
CA-125	0-35 U/ml	
CA 19-9	<37 U/ml	

Continued

Test	Reference range	
	Conventional values	SI units*
BLOOD, PLASMA, OR SERUM VALUES—cont'd		
C-reactive protein (CRP)	<6 μg/ml	
Calcitonin	<50 pg/ml	<50 pmol/L
Calcium (Ca)	9.0-10.5 mg/dl (total)	2.25-2.75 mmol/L
	3.9-4.6 mg/dl (ionized)	1.05-1.30 mmol/L
Carbon dioxide (CO_2) content	23-30 mEq/L	21-30 mmol/L
Carboxyhemoglobin (COHb)	3% of total hemoglobin	
Carcinoembryonic antigen (CEA)	<2 ng/ml	0.2-5 μg/L
Carotene	50-200 μg/dl	0.74-3.72 μmol/L
Chloride (Cl)	90-110 mEq/L	98-106 mmol/L
Cholesterol	150-250 mg/dl	3.90-6.50 mmol/L
Clot retraction	50%-100% clot retraction in 1-2 hours, complete retraction within 24 hours	
Complement	C_3: 70-176 mg/dl	0.55-1.20 g/L
	C_4: 16-45 mg/dl	0.20-0.50 g/L
Complete blood count (CBC)		
Red blood cell (RBC) count	Men: 4.7-6.1 million/mm^3	
	Women: 4.2-5.4 million/mm^3	
	Infants and children: 3.8-5.5 million/mm^3	
	Newborns: 4.8-7.1 million/mm^3	

Hemoglobin (Hgb)	Men: 14-18 g/dl	8.7-11.2 mmol/L
	Women: 12-16 g/dl (pregnancy: >11 g/dl)	7.4-9.9 mmol/L
	Children: 11-16 g/dl	1.74-2.56 mmol/L
	Infants: 10-15 g/dl	
	Newborns: 14-24 g/dl	2.56-3.02 mmol/L
Hematocrit (Hct)	Men: 42%-52%	
	Women: 37%-47% (pregnancy: >33%)	
	Children: 31%-43%	
	Infants: 30%-40%	
	Newborns: 44%-64%	
Mean corpuscular volume (MCV)	Adults and children: 85-95 μ^3	80-95 fl
	Newborns: 96-108 μ^3	
Mean corpuscular hemoglobin (MCH)	Adults and children: 27-31 pg	0.42-0.48 fmol
	Newborns: 32-34 pg	
Mean corpuscular hemoglobin concentration (MCHC)	Adults and children: 32-36 g/dl	0.32-0.36
	Newborns: 32-33 g/dl	

Continued

Test	Reference range		
	Conventional values	SI units*	
BLOOD, PLASMA, OR SERUM VALUES—cont'd			
White blood cell (WBC) count	Adults and children >2 years: 5000-10,000/mm^3		
	Children ≤2 years: 6200-17,000/mm^3		
	Newborns: 9000-30,000/mm^3		
Differential count			
Neutrophils	55%-70%		
Lymphocytes	20%-40%		
Monocytes	2%-8%		
Eosinophils	1%-4%		
Basophils	0.5%-1%		
Platelet count	150,000-400,000/mm^3		
Coomb's test			
Direct	Negative	Negative	
Indirect	Negative	Negative	
Copper (Cu)	70-140 µg/dl	11.0-24.3 µmol/L	
Cortisol	6-28 µg/dl (AM)	170-635 nmol/L	
	2-12 µg/dl (PM)	82-413 nmol/L	

CPK isoenzyme (MB)	<5% total	
Creatinine	0.7-1.5 mg/dl	<133 µmol/L
Creatinine clearance	Men: 95-104 ml/min	<133 µmol/L
	Women: 95-125 ml/min	
Creatinine phosphokinase (CPK)	5-75 mU/ml	12-80 units/L
Cryoglobulin	Negative	Negative
Differential (WBC) count (see CBC)		
Digoxin	Therapeutic level: 0.5-2.0 ng/ml	40-79 µmol/L
	Toxic level: >2.4 ng/ml	>119 µmol/L
Erythrocyte count (see Complete blood count)		
Erythrocyte sedimentation rate (ESR)	Men: up to 15 mm/hour	
	Women: up to 20 mm/hour	
	Children: up to 10 mm/hour	
Ethanol	80-200 mg/dl (mild to moderate intoxication)	17-43 mmol/L
	250-400 mg/dl (marked intoxication)	54-87 mmol/L
	>400 mg/dl (severe intoxication)	>87 mmol/L
Euglobulin lysis test	90 min-6 hours	
Fats	Up to 200 mg/dl	

Continued

| | Reference range | |
Test	Conventional values	SI units*
BLOOD, PLASMA, OR SERUM VALUES—cont'd		
Ferritin	15-200 ng/ml	15-200 µg/L
Fibrin degradation products (FDP)	<10 µg/ml	
Fibrinogen (factor I)	200-400 mg/dl	5.9-11.7 µmol/L
Fibrinolysis/euglobulin lysis test	90 min-6 hours	
Fluorescent treponemal antibody (FTA)	Negative	Negative
Fluoride	<0.05 mg/dl	<0.027 mmol/L
Folic acid (Folate)	5-20 µg/ml	14-34 mmol/L
Follicle-stimulating hormone (FSH)	Men: 0.1-15.0 ImU/ml	
	Women: 6-30 ImU/ml	
	Children: 0.1-12.0 ImU/ml	
	Castrate and postmenopausal: 30-200 ImU/ml	
Free thyroxine index (FTI)	0.9-2.3 ng/dl	
Galactose-1-phosphate uridyl transferase	18.5-28.5 U/g hemoglobin	
Gammaglobulin	0.5-1.6 g/dl	
Gamma-glutamyl transpeptidase (GGTP)	Men: 8-38 U/L	5-40 U/L at 37° C
	Women: <45 years: 5-27 U/L	
Gastrin	40-150 pg/ml	40-150 ng/L

Glucagon	50-200 pg/ml	14-56 pmol/L
Glucose, fasting (FBS)	Adults: 70-115 mg/dl	3.89-6.38 mmol/L
	Children: 60-100 mg/dl	
	Newborns: 30-80 mg/dl	
Glucose, 2-hour postprandial (2-hour PPG)	<140 mg/dl	
Glucose-6-phosphate dehydrogenase (G-6-PD)	8.6-18.6 IU/g of hemoglobin	
Glucose tolerance test (GTT)	Fasting: 70-115 mg/dl	
	30 min: <200 mg/dl	
	1 hour: <200 mg/dl	
	2 hours: <140 mg/dl	
	3 hours: 70-115 mg/dl	
	4 hours: 70-115 mg/dl	
Glycosylated hemoglobin	Adults: 2.2%-4.8%	
	Children: 1.8%-4.0%	
	Good diabetic control: 2.5%-6%	
	Fair diabetic control: 6.1%-8%	
	Poor diabetic control: >8	
Growth hormone	<10 ng/ml	<10 µg/L
Haptoglobin	100-150 mg/dl	16-31 µmol/L

Continued

Test	Reference range		SI units*
	Conventional values		
BLOOD, PLASMA, OR SERUM VALUES—cont'd			
Hematocrit (Hct)	Men: 42%-52%		
	Women: 37%-47% (pregnancy: >33%)		
	Children: 31%-43%		
	Infants: 30%-40%		
	Newborns: 44%-64%		
Hemoglobin (Hgb)	Men: 14-18 g/dl		8.7-11.2 mmol/L
	Women: 12-16 g/dl (pregnancy: >11 g/dl)		7.4-9.9 mmol/L
	Children: 11-16 g/dl		
	Infants: 10-15 g/dl		
	Newborns: 14-24 g/dl		
Hemoglobin electrophoresis	Hgb A_1: 95%-98%		
	Hgb A_2: 2%-3%		
	Hgb F: 0.8%-2%		
	Hgb S: 0		
	Hgb C: 0		
Hepatitis B surface antigen (HB_sAG)	Nonreactive		Nonreactive

Heterophil antibody	Negative	Negative
HLA-B27	None	None
Human chorionic gonadotropin (HCG)	Negative	Negative
Human placental lactogen (HPL)	Rise during pregnancy	
5-Hydroxyindoleacetic acid (5-HIAA)	2.8-8.0 mg/24 hours	
Immunoglobulin quantification	IgG: 550-1900 mg/dl	5.5-19.0 g/L
	IgA: 60-333 mg/dl	0.6-3.3 g/L
	IgM: 45-145 mg/dl	0.45-1.5 g/L
Insulin	4-20 µU/ml	36-179 pmol/L
Iron (Fe)	60-190 µg/dl	13-31 µmol/L
Iron-binding capacity, total (TIBC)	250-420 µg/dl	45-73 µmol/L
Iron (transferrin) saturation	30%-40%	
Ketone bodies	Negative	Negative
Lactic acid	0.6-1.8 mEq/L	0.4-1.7 µmol/s/L
Lactic dehydrogenase (LDH) isoenzymes	90-200 ImU/ml	
	LDH-1: 17%-27%	
	LDH-2: 28%-38%	
	LDH-3: 19%-27%	
	LDH-4: 5%-16%	
	LDH-5: 6%-16%	
Lead	120 µg/dl or less	<1.0 µmol/L

Continued

BLOOD, PLASMA, OR SERUM VALUES—cont'd

Test	Reference range		
	Conventional values	SI units*	
Leucine aminopeptidase (LAP)	Men: 80-200 U/ml		
	Women: 75-185 U/ml		
Leukocyte count (see Complete blood count)			
Lipase	Up to 1.5 units/ml	0-417 U/L	
Lipids			
Total	400-1000 mg/dl	4-8 g/L	
Cholesterol	150-250 mg/dl	3.9-6.5 mmol/L	
Triglycerides	40-150 mg/dl	0.4-1.5 g/L	
Phospholipids	150-380 mg/dl	1.9-3.9 mmol/L	
Lithium	Therapeutic level: 0.8-1.2 mEq/L		
Long-acting thyroid-stimulating hormone (LATS)	Negative	Negative	
Magnesium (Mg)	1.6-3.0 mEq/L	0.8-1.3 mm/L	
Methanol	Negative	Negative	
Mononucleosis spot test	Negative	Negative	
Nitrogen, nonprotein	15-35 mg/dl	10.7-25.0 mmol/L	
Nuclear antibody (ANA)	Negative	Negative	
5'-Nucleotidase	Up to 1.6 U	27-233 nmol/s/L	

Osmolality	275-300 mOsm/kg	
Oxygen saturation (arterial)	95%-100%	0.95-1.00 of capacity
Parathormone (PTH)	<2000 pg/ml	
Partial thromboplastin time, activated (APTT)	30-40 sec	
P_{CO_2}	35-45 mm Hg	7.35-7.45
pH	7.35-7.45	
Phenylalanine	Up to 2 mg/dl	<0.18 mmol/L
Phenylketonuria (PKU)	Negative	Negative
Phenytoin (Dilantin)	Therapeutic level: 10-20 µg/ml	
Phosphatase (acid)	0.10-0.63 U/ml (Bessey-Lowry)	0.11-0.60 U/L
	0.5-2.0 U/ml (Bodansky)	
	1.0-4.0 U/ml (King-Armstrong)	
Phosphatase (alkaline)	Adults: 30-85 ImU/ml	20-90 U/L
	Children and adolescents:	
	<2 years: 85-235 ImU/ml	
	2-8 years: 65-210 ImU/ml	
	9-15 years: 60-300 ImU/ml (active bone growth)	
	16-21 years: 30-200 ImU/ml	
Phospholipids (see Lipids)		

Continued

Test	Reference range	
	Conventional values	SI units*

BLOOD, PLASMA, OR SERUM VALUES—cont'd

Test	Conventional values	SI units*
Phosphorus (P, PO$_4$)	Adults: 2.5-4.5 mg/dl	0.78-1.52 mmol/L
	Children: 3.5-5.8 mg/dl	1.29-2.26 mmol/L
Platelet count	150,000-400,000/mm^3	
Po$_2$	80-100 mm Hg	
Potassium (K)	3.5-5.0 mEq/L	3.5-5.0 mmol/L
Progesterone	Men, prepubertal girls, and postmenopausal women: <2 ng/ml	6 nmol/L
	Women, luteal: peak >5 ng/ml	>16 nmol/L
Prolactin	2-15 ng/ml	2-15 µg/L
Prostate-specific antigen (PSA)	<4 ng/ml	
Protein (total)	6-8 g/dl	55-80 g/L
Albumin	3.2-4.5 g/dl	35-55 g/L
Globulin	2.3-3.4 g/dl	20-35 g/L
Prothrombin time (PT)	11.0-12.5 sec	11.0-12.5 sec
Pyruvate	0.3-0.9 mg/dl	34-103 µmol/L
Red blood cell count (see Complete blood count)		

Red blood cell indexes (see Complete blood count)		
Reticulocyte count	Adults and children: 0.5%-2% of total erythrocytes	
	Infants: 0.5%-3.1% of total erythrocytes	
	Newborns: 2.5%-6.5% of total erythrocytes	
Rheumatoid factor	Negative	Negative
Rubella antibody test	HAI titer: > 1:10-1:20	
Salicylates	Negative	
	Therapeutic: 20-25 mg/dl (to age 10 years; 25-30 mg/dl)	1.4-1.8 mmol/L
	Toxic: >30 mg/dl (after age 60 years: >20 mg/dl)	>2.2 mmol/L
Schilling test (vitamin B_{12} absorption)	8%-40% excretion/24 hours	
Serologic test for syphilis (STS)	Negative (nonreactive)	
Serum glutamic oxaloacetic transaminase (SGOT, AST)	12-36 U/ml	0.10-0.30 μmol/s/L
Serum glutamic-pyruvic transaminase (SGPT, ALT)	5-40 IU/L	0.05-0.43 μmol/s/L
	5-35 IU/L	

Continued

Test	Reference range	
	Conventional values	SI units*
BLOOD, PLASMA, OR SERUM VALUES—cont'd		
Sickle cell	Negative	
Sodium (Na⁺)	136-145 mEq/L	136-145 mmol/L
Sugar (see Glucose)		
Syphilis (see Serologic test for syphilis, Fluorescent treponemal antibody, Venereal Disease Research Laboratory)		
Testosterone	Men: 300-1200 ng/dl	10-42 nmol/L
	Women: 30-95 ng/dl	1.1-3.3 nmol/L
	Prepubertal boys and girls: 5-20 ng/dl	0.165-0.170 nmol/L
Thymol flocculation	Up to 5 U	
Thyroglobulin antibody (see Antithyroglobulin antibody)		
Thyroid-stimulating hormone (TSH)	1-4 µU/ml	5 m U/L
	Neonates: <25 µIU/ml by 3 days	

Thyroxine (T_4)	Murphy-Pattee:	50-154 nmol/L
	neonates: 10.1-20.1 µg/dl	
	1-6 years: 5.6-12.6 µg/dl	
	7-10 years: 4.9-11.7 µg/dl	
	>10 years: 4-11 µg/dl	
	Radioimmunoassay: 5-10 µg/dl	
Thyroxine-binding globulin (TBG)	12-28 µg/ml	129-335 nmol/L
Toxoplasmosis antibody titer	1:16-1:256 generally prevelant	
Transaminase (see Serum glutamic-oxaloacetic transaminase, Serum glutamic pyruvic transaminase)		
Triglycerides	40-150 mg/dl	0.4-1.5 g/L
Triiodothyronine (T_3)	110-230 ng/dl	1.2-1.5 nmol/L
Triiodothyronine (T_3) resin uptake	25%-35%	
Tubular phosphate reabsorption (TPR)	80%-90%	
Urea nitrogen (see Blood urea nitrogen		
Uric acid	Men: 2.1-8.5 mg/dl	0.15-0.48 mmol/L
	Women: 2.0-6.6 mg/dl	0.09-0.36 mmol/L
	Children: 2.5-5.5 mg/dl	

Continued

| | Reference range | |
Test	Conventional values	SI units*
BLOOD, PLASMA, OR SERUM VALUES—cont'd		
Venereal Disease Research Laboratory (VDRL)	Negative	Negative
Vitamin A	20-100 g/dl	0.7-3.5 μmol/L
Vitamin B₁₂	200-600 pg/ml	148-443 pmol/L
Vitamin C	0.6-1.6 mg/dl	23-57 μmol/L
Whole blood clot retraction (see Clot retraction)		
Zinc	50-150 μg/dl	
URINE VALUES		
Acetone plus acetoacetate (ketone bodies)	Negative	Negative
Addis count (12-hour)	Adults: WBCs and epithelial cells: 1.8 million/12 hours RBCs: 500,000/12 hours Hyaline casts: Up to 5000/12 hours	

Albumin	Children: WBCs: <1 million/12 hours RBCs: <250,000/12 hours Casts: >5000/12 hours Protein: <20 mg/12 hours Random: ≦8 mg/dl	Negative
Aldosterone	24-hour: 10-100 mg/24 hours 2-16 µg/24 hours	10-100 mg/24 hr 5.5-72 nmol/24 hours
Alpha-aminonitrogen	0.4-1.0 g/24 hours	28-71 nmol/24 hours
Amino acid	50-200 mg/24 hours	
Ammonia (24-hour)	30-50 mEq/24 hours 500-1200 mg/24 hours	30-50 nmol/24 hours
Amylase	≦5000 Somogyi units/24 hours 3-35 IU/hour	6.5-48.1 U/hr
Arsenic (24-hour)	<50 µg/L	<0.65 mol/L
Ascorbic acid (vitamin C)	Random: 1-7 ng/dl 24-hour: >50 mg/24 hours	0.06-0.40 mmol/L >0.29 mmol/24 hours
Bacteria	None	None
Bence Jones protein	Negative	Negative
Bilirubin	Negative	Negative

Continued

Test	Reference range		SI units*
	Conventional values		
URINE VALUES—cont'd			
Blood or hemoglobin	Negative		Negative
Borate (24-hour)	<2 mg/L		<32 µmol/L
Calcium	Random: 1 + turbidity		1 + turbidity
	24-hour: 1-300 mg (diet dependent)		
Catecholamines (24-hour)	Epinephrine: 5-40 µg/24 hours		<55 nmol/24 hours
	Norepinephrine: 10-80 µg/24 hours		<590 nmol/24 hours
	Metanephrine: 24-96 µg/24 hours		0.5-8.1 µmol/24 hours
	Normetanephrine: 75-375 µg/24 hours		140-250 mmol/24 hours
Chloride (24-hour)	140-250 mEq/24 hours		Amber-yellow
Color	Amber-yellow		>1.025
Concentration test (Fishberg test)	Specific gravity: >1.025		>850 mOsm/L
	Osmolality: 850 mOsm/L		0-0.4 µmol/24 hours
Copper (CU) (24-hour)	Up to 25 µg/24 hours		150-460 nmol/24 hours
Coproporphyrin (24-hour)	100-300 µg/24 hours		

Creatine	Adults: <100 mg/24 hours or <6% creatinine
	Pregnant women: ≤12%
	Infants <1 year: equal to creatinine
	Older children: ≤30% of creatinine
Creatinine (24-hour)	15-25 mg/kg body wt/24 hours
	0.13-0.22 nmol/kg^{-1} body wt/24 hours
Creatinine clearance (24-hour)	Men: 90-140 ml/min
	Women: 85-125 ml/min
	90-140 ml/min
	85-125 ml/min
Crystals	Negative
	Negative
Cystine or cysteine	Negative
	Negative
Delta-aminolevulinic acid (ΔALA)	1-7 mg/24 hours
	10-53 µmol/24 hours
Epinephrine (24-hour)	5-40 µg/24 hours
Epithelial cells and casts	Occasional
	Occasional
Estriol (24-hour)	>12 mg/24 hours
Fat	Negative
	Negative
Fluoride (24-hour)	<1 mg/24 hours
	0.053 mmol/24 hours
Follicle-stimulating hormone (FSH) (24-hour)	Men: 2-12 IU/24 hours
	Women:
	During menses: 8-60 IU/24 hours
	During ovulation: 30-60 IU/24 hours
	During menopause: >50 IU/24 hours

Continued

Test	Reference range		
	Conventional values		SI units*
URINE VALUES—cont'd			
Glucose	Negative		Negative
Granular casts	Occasional		Occasional
Hemoglobin and myoglobin	Negative		Negative
Homogentisic acid	Negative		Negative
Human chorionic gonadotropin (HCG)	Negative		Negative
Human placental lactogen (HPL)	Levels rise progressively with pregnancy		
Hyaline casts	Occasional		Occasional
17-Hydroxycorticosteroids (17-OCHS) (24-hour)	Men: 5.5-15.0 mg/24 hours		8.3-25 μmol/24 hours
	Women: 5.0-13.5 mg/24 hours		5.5-22 μmol/24 hours
	Children: lower than adult values		
5-Hydroxyindoleacetic acid (5-HIAA, serotonin) (24-hour)	Men: 2-9 mg/24 hours		10-47 μmol/24 hours
	Women: lower than men		
Ketones (see Acetone plus acetoacetate)			
17-Ketosteroids (17-KS) (24-hour)	Men: 8-15 mg/24 hours		21-62 μmol/24 hours
	Women: 6-12 mg/24 hours		14-45 μmol/24 hours

	Children:	
	12-15 yr: 5-12 mg/24 hours	
	<12 yr: <5 mg/24 hours	
Lactose (24-hour)	14-40 mg/24 hours	41-116 µm
Lead	<0.08 g/ml or <120 g/24 hours	0.39 µmol/L
Leucine aminopeptidase (LAP)	2-18 U/24 hours	
Magnesium (24-hour)	6.8-8.5 mEq/24 hours	3.0-4.3 mmol/24 hours
Melanin	Negative	Negative
Odor	Aromatic	Aromatic
Osmolality	500-800 mOsm/L	38-1400 mmol/kg water
pH	4.6-8.0	4.6-8.0
Phenolsulfonphthalein (PSP)	15 min: at least 25%	At least 0.25
	30 min: at least 40%	At least 0.40
	120 min: at least 60%	At least 0.60
Phenylketonuria (PKU)	Negative	Negative
Phenylpyruvic acid	Negative	Negative
Phosphorus (24-hour)	0.9-1.3 g/24 hours	29-42 mmol/24 hours
Porphobilinogen	Random: negative	Negative
	24-hour: up to 2 mg/24 hours	

Continued

| | Reference range | |
Test	Conventional values	SI units*
URINE VALUES—cont'd		
Porphyrin (24-hour)	50-300 mg/24 hours	25-100 nmol/24 hours
Potassium (K^+) (24-hour)	25-100 mEq/24 hours	
Pregnancy test	Positive in normal pregnancy or with tumors producing HCG	Positive in normal pregnancy or with tumors producing HCG
Pregnanediol	After ovulation: >1 mg/24 hours	
Protein (albumin)	Random: ≤8 mg/dl	>0.05 g/24 hours
	10-100 mg/24 hours	
Sodium (Na^+) (24-hour)	100-260 mEq/24 hours	100-260 nmol/24 hours
Specific gravity	1.010-1.025	1.010-1.025

Steroids (see 17-Hydroxycorticosteroids, 17-Ketosteroids)		
Sugar (see Glucose)		
Titratable acidity (24-hour)	20-50 mEq/24 hours	20-50 mmol/24 hours
Turbidity	Clear	Clear
Urea nitrogen (24-hour)	6-17 g/24 hours	0.21-0.60 mmol/24 hours
Uric acid (24-hour)	250-750 mg/24 hours	1.48-4.43 mmol/24 hours
Urobilinogen	0.1-1.0 Ehrlich U/dl	0.1-1.0 Ehrlich U/dl
Uroporphyrin	Negative	Negative
Vanillylmandelic acid (VMA) (24-hour)	1-9 mg/24 hours	
Zinc (24-hour)	0.20-0.75 mg/24 hours	<40 μmol/day

Internet Resources for Home Health Nurses

Sandra Lindquist • Donna Musser

Aging organizations and agencies
Web site:
http://www.aoa.dhhs.gov/aoa/webres/home-org.htm

Aids Action Council
1875 Connecticut Ave. NW #700
Washington, DC 20009-5740
Phone: (202) 986-1300

Al-Anon Family Group Headquarters, Inc.
1600 Corporate Landing Parkway
Virginia Beach, VA 23454-5617
Phone: (888) 4AL-ANON
E-mail: WSO@al-anon.org
Web sites: http://www.al-anon.alateen.org/ (main home page)
http://www.al-anon.alateen.org/alalist_usa.html (links to
state organizations)
(For meeting information in the United States and Canada,
call (888) 4AL-ANON between 8 AM and 6 PM ET Monday-
Friday. You can also use this number to locate electronic
meetings.)

Alcoholics Anonymous
World Services, Inc.
P.O. Box 459
New York, NY 10163
Phone: (212) 870-3400
Web sites: http://www.alcoholics-anonymous.org/
http://www.alcoholics-anonymous.org/ectroff.html (main
offices by state)

Allergy and Asthma Network/Mothers of Asthmatics, Inc.
2751 Prosperity Ave., Suite 150
Fairfax, VA 22031
Toll free: (800) 878-4403
Phone: (703) 641-9595
Fax: (703) 573-7794
E-mail: aanma@aol.com
Web site: http://www.aanma.org

Alliance of Genetic Support Groups
4301 Connecticut Ave., NW
Suite 404
Washington, DC 20008
Phone: (202) 966-5557
Fax: (202) 966-8553
Toll free: (800) 336-GENE
E-mail: info@geneticalliance.org
Web site: http://www.geneticalliance.org

The Alzheimer's Association National Headquarters
919 N. Michigan Ave., Suite 1000
Chicago, IL 60611-1676
Phone: (312) 335-8700
Toll free: (800) 272-3900
Fax: (312) 335-1110
E-mail: info@alz.org
Web sites: http://www.alz.org/us/index.htm
http://www.alz.org/chapters/index.htm (local chapters in all
states)

American Academy of Allergy, Asthma and Immunology
Online Communications Department
611 E. Wells St.
Milwaukee, WI 53202
Toll free: (800) 822-2762
Web site: http://www.aaaai.org/

American Association for Continuity of Care
638 Prospect Ave.
Hartford, CT 06105
Phone: (860) 586-7525
Fax: (860) 586-7550
Web site: http://www.continuityofcare.com/

American Association of Diabetes Educators
100 W. Monroe St.
Fourth Floor
Chicago, IL 60603-1901
Phone: (312) 424-2426
E-mail: aade/aade@aadenet.org
Web site: http://www.aadenet.org/

American Association of Retired Persons (AARP)
National Headquarters
601 E. St. NW
Washington, DC 20049
Toll-free: (800) 424-3410
Web sites: http://www.aarp.org/ (main home page)
http://www.aarp.org/statepages/ (regional and state home pages)

American Cancer Society
271 W. 125th St.
New York, NY 10027-4424
Phone: (212) 663-8800
Toll free: (800) ACS-2345
Web sites: http://www.cancer.org/
http://www.cancer.org/bottomdivisions.html (to locate local chapters)

American Diabetes Association
National Office
1660 Duke St.
Alexandria, VA 22314
Toll free: (800) DIABETES or (800) 342-2383
Web sites: http://www.diabetes.org/
http://www.diabetes.org/ada/states.asp (to locate local information)

American Foundation for AIDS Research
120 Wall St.
Thirteenth Floor
New York, NY 10005
Phone: (212) 806-1600
Fax: (212) 806-1601
Web site: http://www.amfar.org/

American Heart Association
National Center
7272 Greenville Ave.
Dallas, TX 75231
Toll free: (800) AHA-USA1
Women's health information: (888) MY-HEART
Web sites: http://www.americanheart.org/
http://www.americanheart.org/affilil/ (to locate local chapter)

American Juvenile Arthritis Organization
1330 W. Peachtree St.
Atlanta, GA 30309
Phone: (404) 872-7100
Arthritis answers: (800) 283-7800
Web site: http://www.arthritis.org/ajao/

American Lung Association
Toll free: (800) LUNG-USA or (800) 586-4872
Web site: http://www.lungusa.org/index.html

American Nurses Association
600 Maryland Ave., SW
Suite 100 West
Washington, DC 20024
Phone: (202) 651-7000
Toll free: (800) 274-4ANA
Fax: (202) 651-7001
Web sites: http://www.nursingworld.org
http://www.nursingworld.org/affil/index.htm (links to numerous affiliated nursing organizations)

American Paralysis Association
500 Morris Ave.
Springfield, NJ 07081
Phone: (973) 379-2690
Toll free: (800) 225-0292
Fax: (973) 912-9433
E-mail: paralysis@aol.com
Web site: http://www.apacure.com/

The American Parkinson Disease Association, Inc.
1250 Hylan Blvd., Suite 4B
Staten Island, NY 10305-1946
Toll free: (800) 223-2732
Referral center: (888) 400-2732
E-mail: apda@admin.con2.com
Web sites: http://www.apdaparkinson.com/
http://www.apdaparkinson.com/I&ctr.htm (for referrals)
http://www.apdaparkinson.com/chaploc.htm (to locate referrals)

American Red Cross National Headquarters
Attn: Public Inquiry Office
11th Floor
1621 N. Kent St.
Arlington, VA 22209
Phone: (703) 248-4222
E-mail: info@usa.redcross.org
Web sites: http://www.redcross.org
http://www.redcross.org/where/where.html (to locate local services)

American Tinnitus Association
P.O. Box 5
Portland, OR 97207-0005
Phone: (503) 248-9985
Fax: (503) 248-0024
Web site: http://www.ata.org/

Anxiety Disorders Association of America
11900 Parklawn Drive, Suite 100
Rockville, MD 20852
Phone: (301) 231-9350
Web site: http://www.adaa.org/

Arthritis Foundation
National Office
1330 W. Peachtree St.
Atlanta, GA 30309
Phone: (404) 872-7100
Arthritis answers: (800) 283-7800
Web sites: http://www.arthritis.org
http://www.arthritis.org/offices/ (to locate local
chapters/offices)

Arthritis National Research Foundation
200 Oceangate, Suite 44
Long Beach, CA 90802
Phone: (800) 588-CURE (2873)
Web site: http://www.curearthritis.org/

Assisted Living Federation of America
10300 Eaton Place, Suite 400
Fairfax, VA 22030
Phone: (703) 691-8100
Fax: (703) 691-8106
E-mail: lc@alfa.org
Web site: http://www.alfa.org/

Asthma and Allergy Foundation of America
1125 Fifteenth St., NW, Suite 502
Washington, DC 20005
Phone: (202) 466-7643
Fax: (202) 466-8940
E-mail: info@aafa.org
Web sites: http://www.aafa.org/
http://www.aafa.org/chap sg.html (to locate local chapters)

Cancer Information Services
National Cancer Institute
Phone: (800) 4-CANCER or (800) 422-6237
Web site: http://cis.nci.nih.gov/

Centers for Disease Control and Prevention
1600 Clifton Road, NE
Atlanta, GA 30333
Phone: (404) 639-3311
E-mail: netinfo@cdc.gov
Web site: http://www.cdc.gov/

Center for Disease Control NPIN
P.O. Box 6003
Rockville, MD 20849-6003
Toll free: (800) 458-5231
TTY: (800) 243-7012
International: (301) 562-1098
International TTY: (301) 588-1589
Fax: (888) 282-7681
International fax: (301) 562-1050
E-mail: pubs@cdcnpin.org
Web site: http://www.cdcnpin.org/

Children's Hospice International
2202 Mt. Vernon Avenue, Suite 3C
Alexandria, VA 22301
Phone: (703) 684-0330
Fax: (703) 684-0226
Web site: http://www.chionline.org/

Children of Aging Parents
1609 Woodbourne Road, #302A
Levittown, PA 19057
Phone: (800) 227-7294
Web site:
http://www.careguide.net/careguide.cgi/caps/capshome.html/

Choices in Dying
National Office
1035 30th St., NW
Washington, DC 20007
Phone: (202) 338-9790
Fax: (202) 338-0242
Toll free: (800) 989-WILL (9455)
Web site: http://www.choices.org/

The Cooley's Anemia Foundation, Inc.
129-09 26th Ave., #203
Flushing, NY 11354
Toll free: (800) 522-7222
Phone: (718) 321-CURE (2873)
Fax: (718) 321-3340
E-mail: ncaf@aol.com
Web site: http://www.thalassemia.org/

Crohn's and Colitis Foundation of America, Inc.
386 Park Ave. South
17th Floor
New York, NY 10016-8804
Phone: (212) 685-3440
Toll free: (800) 932-2423
Fax: (212) 779-4098
E-mail: info@ccfa.org
Web site: http://www.ccfa.org/

Cystic Fibrosis Foundation
6931 Arlington Road
Bethesda, MD 20814
Phone: (301) 951-4422
Toll free: (800) FIGHT-CF
Fax: (301) 951-6378
E-mail: info@cff.org
Web site: http://www.cff.org/

Dystonia Medical Research Foundation
1 East Wacker Drive
Chicago, IL 60601-1905
Phone: (312) 755-0198
Toll free: (800) 377-DYST
Fax: (312) 803-0138
E-mail: dystonia@dystonia-foundation.org
Web site: http://www.dystonia-foundation.org/

Easter Seals Society
230 W. Monroe St.
Suite 1800
Chicago, IL 60606
Phone: (312) 726-6200
Toll free: (800) 221-6827
TDD: (312) 726-4258
Fax: (312) 726-1494
E-mail: info@easter-seals.org
Web sites: http://www.easter-seals.org/
http://www.easter-seals.org/cservices2/home.html (to find
local in-home services)
http://www.easter-seals.org/html/services.html (to locate
local services)

Environmental Protection Agency
401 M St., SW
Washington, DC 20460-0003
Phone: (202) 260-2090
Web site: http://www.epa.gov

Endometriosis Association International Headquarters
8585 N. 76th Place
Milwaukee, WI 53223
Phone: (414) 355-2200
Toll free: (800) 992-3636
Fax: (414) 355-6065
E-mail: endo@endometriosisassn.org
Web site: http://www.endometriosisassn.org/

Epilepsy Foundation
4351 Garden City Drive
Landover, MD 20785
Phone: (301) 459-3700
Toll free: (800) EFA-1000
Fax: (301) 577-4941
E-mail: info@efa.org
Web site: http://www.efa.org/

Family Caregiver Alliance
425 Bush St., Suite 500
San Francisco, CA 94108
Phone: (415) 434-3388
Fax: (415) 434-3508
E-mail: info@caregiver.org
Web site: http://www.caregiver.org

Foundation Fighting Blindness
Executive Plaza I, Suite 800
11350 McCormick Road
Hunt Valley, MD 21031-1014
Phone: (800) 683-5551
(410) 785-1414
(410) 785-9687
Toll free: (888) 394-3937
Web site: http://www.blindness.org/

Health Care Financing Administration (HCFA)
7500 Security Blvd.
Baltimore, MD 21244
Phone: (410) 786-3000
Web site: http://www.hcfa.org (information on Medicare,
Medicaid, and managed care)

Health Information (on just about anything with multiple
links)
Web site: http://www.heathfinder.org

Hemlock Society
P.O. Box 101810
Denver, CO 80250-1810
Phone: (303) 639-1202
Toll free: (800) 247-7421
Fax: (303) 639-1224
E-mail: hemlock@privateI.com
Web site: http://www2.privatei.com/hemlock/index.html

Hepatitis Information Network
Web site: http://www.hepnet.com

Home Medical Equipment information:
Consumer Fraud Pamphlet
Medicare and Home Medical Equipment
(Information provided by U.S. Department of Health and
  Human Services, Health Care Financing Administration,
  U.S. Government Printing Office: 1992-332-525,
  October, 1996)
Web site: http://www.medicare.gov/consumerfraud.html

Hospice Association of America
228 Seventh St., SE
Washington, DC 20003
Phone: (202) 546-4759
Fax: (202) 547-9559
Web site: http://www.nahc.org/HAA/home.html

Huntington's Disease Society of America
158 W. 29th St., Seventh Floor
New York, NY 10001-5300
Phone: (800) 345-HDSA or (212) 242-1968
E-mail: curehd@idt.net
Web site: http://www.hdsa.mgh.harvard.edu.hdsamain.nclk/

Joint Commission on Accreditation of Healthcare
Organizations
1 Renaissance Blvd.
Oakbrook Terrace, IL 60181
Phone: (630) 792-5000
Fax: (630) 792-5005
Web site: http://www.jcaho.org/

Juvenile Diabetes Foundation International
120 Wall St.
New York, NY 10005-4001
Phone: (212) 785-9500
Toll free: (800) JDF-CURE
Fax: (212) 785-9595
E-mail: info@jcfcure.org
Web sites: http://www.jdfcure.org/
http://www.jdfcure.org/chapters/index.html (to find a local
chapter)

Leukemia Society of America
600 Third Ave.
New York, NY 10016
Phone: (212) 573-8484
Information resource center: (800) 955-4LSA
Web sites: http://www.leukemia.org/
http://www.leukemia.org/docs/aboutlsa/chap docs/
   fs finder.html (to locate local chapters)

Lupus Foundation of America
1300 Piccard Drive, Suite 200
Rockville, MD 20850-4303
Phone: (301) 670-9292
Toll free: (800) 558-0121
E-mail: LupusInfo@aol.com
Web sites: http://www.internet-plaza.net/lupus (main home
page)
http://www.internet-plaza.net/lupus/info/help.html (to
locate local chapter)

March of Dimes
Birth Defects Foundation
National Office
1275 Mamaroneck Ave.
White Plains, NY 10605
Phone: (914) 428-7100
Web site: http://www.modimes.org

Mended Hearts, Inc.
7272 Greenville Ave.
Dallas, TX 75231-4596
Phone: (800) AHA-USA1 (ask for Mended Hearts)
Fax: (214) 706-5231
E-mail: dbonham@heart.org
Web sites: http://www.mendedhearts.org/
http://www.mendedhearts.org/localchapters.html (to locate
a local chapter)

Mental Health Net
570 Metro Place North
Dublin, OH 43017
Phone: (614) 764-0143
Fax: (614) 764-0362
E-mail: webmaster@cmhc.com
Web site: http://www.cmhc.com

Multiple Sclerosis Association of America National
Headquarters
706 Haddonfield Road
Cherry Hills, NJ 08002
Toll free: (800) LEARN-MS or (800) 532-7667
Fax: (609) 661-9797
E-mail: msaa@msaa.com
Web site: http://www.msaa.com/

Muscular Dystrophy Association
National Headquarters
3300 E. Sunrise Drive
Tucson, AZ 85718
Toll free: (800) 572-1717
E-mail: mda@mdausa.org
Web site: http://www.mdausa.org/

Myasthenia Gravis Foundation of America
222 S. Riverside Plaza
Suite 1540
Chicago, IL 60606
Phone: (312) 258-0522
Toll free: (800) 541-5454
Fax: (312) 258-0461
E-mail: myastheniagravis@msn.com
Web site: http://www.med.unc.edu/mgfa/welcome.htm

National Alliance for the Mentally Ill
200 N. Glebe Road, Suite 1015
Arlington, VA 22203-3754
Toll free helpline: (800) 950-NAMI (6264)
Front desk: (703) 524-7600
Fax: (703) 524-9094
TDD: (703) 516-7991
Web site: http://www.nami.org

National Arthritis and Musculoskeletal and Skin Diseases
Information Clearinghouse
National Institutes of Health
1 AMS Circle
Bethesda, MD 20892-3675
Phone: (301) 495-4484
TTY: (301) 565-2966
Fax: (301) 718-6366
E-mail: namsic@mail.nih.gov
Web site: http://www.nih.gov/niams/healthinfo/info.htm

National Association for Down Syndrome
P.O. Box 4542
Oak Brook, IL 60522
Web site: http://www.nads.org/

National Association for Home Care
228 Seventh St., SE
Washington, DC 20003
Phone: (202) 547-7424
Fax: (202) 547-3540
Web site: http://www.nahc.org/

National Association for Sickle Cell Disease
3345 Wilshire Blvd., Suite 1106
Los Angeles, CA 90010-1880
Phone: (213) 736-5455
Toll free: (800) 421-8453
Web site: http://www.cdc.gov/nccdphp/nccdhome.htm

National Center for Chronic Disease Prevention and Health
Promotion
Centers for Disease Control and Prevention
1600 Clifton Road, NE
Atlanta, GA 30333
E-mail: ccdinfo@cdc.gov
Web site: http://www.cdc.gov/nccdphp/nccdhome.htm

The National Clearinghouse for Alcohol and Drug
Information
P.O. Box 2345
Rockville, MD 20847-2345
Phone: (800) 729-6686
Fax: (301) 468-6433
E-mail: info@health.org
Web site: http://www.health.org/

National Clearinghouse on Child Abuse and Neglect
Information, National Center on Child Abuse and Neglect
300 C St., SW
Washington, DC 20447
Phone: (703) 385-7565
Toll free: (800) 394-3366
BBS: (800) 877-8800
Fax: (703) 385-3206
E-mail: nccanch@calib.com
Web site: http://www.calib.com/nccanch/

National Committee to Prevent Child Abuse
200 S. Michigan Ave., 17th Floor
Chicago, IL 60604-4357
Phone: (312) 663-3520
Toll free: (800) 55-NCPCA or (800) 835-2671
Fax: (312) 939-8962
Web site: http://www.childabuse.org/

The National Council on the Aging, Inc.
409 Third St., SE, Suite 200
Washington, DC 20024
Phone: (202) 479-6653
(202) 479-6654
(202) 479-6674
Fax: 202-479-0735
Web site: http://www.ncoa.org/

National Depressive and Manic-Depressive Association
730 N. Franklin St., Suite 501
Chicago, IL 60610-3526
Phone: (800) 826-3632
Fax: (312) 642-7243
E-mail: myrtis@aol.com
Web site: http://www.ndmda.org/
http://www.ndmda.org/chapdir.htm (to locate a chapter near you)

National Diabetes Information Clearinghouse (NDIC)
1 Information Way
Bethesda, MD 20892-3560
E-mail: ndic@info.niddk.nih.gov
Web site:
http://www.niddk.nih.gov/health/diabetes/ndic.htm

The National Down Syndrome Society
666 Broadway, Eighth Floor
New York, NY 10012-2317
Phone: (212) 460-9330
Toll free: (800) 221-4602
Web site: http://www.ndss/org/

National Headache Foundation
428 W. St. James Place, Second Floor
Chicago, IL 60614
Toll free: (800) 843-2256
Web site: http://www.headaches.org/

National Hemophilia Foundation
116 W. 32nd St., 11th Floor
New York, NY 10001
Phone: (212) 328-3700
Fax: (212) 328-3777
HANDI phone: (800) 42-HANDI
HANDI fax: (212) 328-3799
E-mail: info@hemophilia.org
HANDI e-mail: handi@hemophilia.org
Web site: http://www.hemophilia.org/

National Information Center on Deafness
Gallaudet University
800 Florida Ave., NE
Washington, DC 20002-3695
Phone: (202) 651-5051
Phone (TTY): (202) 651-5052
Fax: (202) 651-5054
E-mail: nicd@gallux.gallaudet.edu
Web site: http://www.gallaudet.edu/~nicd/

National Institute of Mental Health
5600 Fishers Lane, Room 7C-02, MSC 8030
Bethesda, MD 20892-8030
E-mail: nimhinfo@mail.nih.gov
Web site: http://www.nimh.nih.gov/home.htm

National Institute of Neurological Disorders and Stroke
P.O. Box 5801
Bethesda, MD 20824
Web site: http://www.ninds.nih.gov/

National Heart, Lung, and Blood Institute
NHLBI Information Center
P.O. Box 30105
Bethesda, MD 20824-0105
Phone: (301) 251-1223
E-mail: NHLBIIC@dgsys.com
Web site: http://www.nhlbi.nih.gov/nhlbi/infcntr/
    infocent.htm

National Hospice Association
1901 North Moore St., Suite 901
Arlington, VA 22209-1714
Phone: (703) 243-5900
Fax: (703) 525-5762
Web site: http://www.nho.org/
http://www.nho.org/database.htm (how to find a hospice)

National Kidney Foundation
30 E. 33rd St.
New York, NY 10016
Toll free: (800) 622-9010
Web site: http://www.kidney.org/

National Marfan Foundation
382 Main St.
Port Washington, NY 11050
Phone: (800) 8-MARFAN or (516) 883-8712
Fax: (516) 883-8040
E-mail: staff@marfan.org
Web site: http://www.marfan.org/

National Neurofibromatosis Foundation
95 Pine St., 16th Floor
New York, NY 10005
Phone: (212) 344-NNFF
Web site: http://www.nf.org/

National Organization for Rare Disorders
P.O. Box 8923
New Fairfield, CT 06812-8923
Phone: (203) 746-6518
Fax: (203) 746-6481
Web site: http://www.nord-rdb.com/~orphan/

National Osteoporosis Foundation
1150 17th St. NW, Suite 500
Washington, DC 20036-4603
Web site: http://www.nof.org/

National Parkinson Foundation, Inc.
Bob Hope Parkinson Research Center
1501 NW Ninth Ave.
Bob Hope Road
Miami, FL 33136-1494
Phone: (305) 547-6666
Toll free: (800) 327-4545
Fax: (305) 243-4403
E-mail: mailbox@npf.med.miami.edu
http://www.parkinson.org
http://www.parkinson.org/chapters.htm (to locate local
chapters)

National Reye's Syndrome Foundation
P.O. Box 829
Bryan, OH 43506-0829
Toll free: (800) 233-7393 (U.S. only)
Web site: http://www.bright.net/~reyessyn/index.html

National Spinal Cord Injury Association
8300 Colesville Road
Suite #551
Silver Spring, MD 20910
Toll free: (800) 962-9629
Fax: (301) 588-9414
Web site: http://www.spinalcord.org/

National Stroke Association
96 Inverness Drive East, Suite I
Englewood, CO 80112-5112
Phone: (303) 649-9299
Fax: (303) 649-1328
Web site: http://www.stroke.org/

National Tuberous Sclerosis Association
8181 Professional Place, Suite 110
Landover, MD 20785-2226
Phone: (800) 225-6872
Fax: (301) 459-0394
Web site: http://www.ntsa@ntsa.org/

National Voluntary Health Agencies
1925 K St. NW, Suite 510
Washington, DC 20006
Phone: (202) 467-5913
Toll free: (800) 654-0845
Fax: (202) 467-4280
E-mail: nvhainfo@
Web site: http://www.nvha.org/

Obsessive-Compulsive Foundation, Inc.
P.O. Box 70
Milford, CT 06460-0070
Phone: (203) 878-5669
Fax: (203) 874-2826
E-mail: info@ocfoundation.org
Web site: http://www.ocfoundation.org/

Occupational Safety and Health Administration (OSHA)
U.S. Department of Labor
200 Constitution Ave., N.W.
Washington, DC 20210
Web site: http://www.osha.gov/

Outcome and Assessment Information Set (OASIS) provides
information on the following:
- Core items of a comprehensive assessment for an adult
  home care patient
- Forms the basis for measuring patient outcomes for pur-
  poses of outcome-based quality improvement (OBQI)
- Web site: http://www.hcfa.gov/medicare/hsqub/oasis/
  hhoview.htm

Paralyzed Veterans of America
Communication Program
801 18th St., NW
Washington, DC 20006
Phone: (202) 872-1300
Toll free: (800) 424-8200
Web site: http://www.pva.org/

Parkinson's Disease Foundation
William Black Medical Building
Columbia-Presbyterian Medical Center
710 W. 168th St.
New York, NY 10032-9982
Phone: (212) 923-4700
Toll-free: (800) 457-6676
Fax: (212) 923-4778
E-mail: info@pdf.org
Web site: http:www.parkinsons-foundation.org/

Prevent Blindness America
500 E. Remington Road
Schaumberg, IL 60173
Phone: (847) 843-2020
Toll free: (800) 331-2020
E-mail: info@preventblindness.org
Web site: http://www.blindness.org/

Shriner's Hospitals for Crippled Children
2900 Rocky Point Drive
Tampa, FL 33607
Phone: (813) 281-0300
Fax: (813) 281-8113
Web site: http://shriners.com/hospitals/index.html

Sickle Cell Disease Association of America
4601 Market St.
Philadelphia, PA 19139
Phone: (215) 471-8686
Fax: (215) 471-7441
Web site: http://www.sickle.qpg.com/

Sudden Infant Death Syndrome Alliance
1314 Bedford Ave., Suite 210
Baltimore, MD 21208
Phone: (410) 653-8226
Fax: (410) 653-8709

The Society for Ambulatory Care Professionals (SACP)
1 North Franklin
Chicago, IL 60606
Phone: (312) 422-3900
Fax: (312) 422-4577
E-mail: sacpinfo@aha.org
Web site: http://www.sacp-net.org/

United Cerebral Palsy Associations
1660 L St., NW, Suite 700
Washington, DC 20036
Toll free: (800) 872-5827
Fax: (800) 776-0414
E-mail: ucpnatl@ucpa.org
Web site: http://www.ucpa.org/

United Ostomy Association
19772 MacArthur Blvd.
Suite 200
Irvine, CA 92612-2405
Phone: (714) 660-8624
Toll free: (800) 826-0826
Fax: (714) 660-9262
E-mail: uoa@deltanet.com
Web site: http://www.uoa.org/

The Wound Care Institute, Inc.
1541 NE 167th St.
North Miami Beach, FL 33162
Phone: (305) 919-9192
Fax: (305) 944-6260
E-mail: Tamara@Woundcare.org
Web site: http://woundcare.org/
(WCI is a tax exempt, nonprofit organization involved in the
advancement of wound healing and diabetic foot care)

BIBLIOGRAPHY AND SELECTED REFERENCES

CHAPTER 1

American Health Consultants,VRE, MRSA: Hospitals starting to send nasty new bugs to home care, *Homecare Education Management* 2(2):16-19, 1997.

Association for Professionals in Infection Control and Epidemiology, Inc: *APIC infection control and applied epidemiology: principles and practice,* 1996, St Louis, Mosby.

Backinger CL: Analysis of needlestick injuries to health care workers providing home care, *Am J Infect Control* 22(5):300-306, 1994.

Bissell W: *Conversation with Ms. Bissell, NIOSHA health compliance division, regarding current OSHA recommendations for managing health care worker exposure to bloodborne pathogens,* April, 1998, Washington, DC.

Callaghan I: Bacterial contamination of nurses' uniforms: a study, *Nurs Stand* 139(1):37-42, 1998.

Centers for Disease Control and Prevention: Update: Universal precautions for prevention of transmission of human immunodeficiency virus, hepatitis B virus, and other blood borne pathogens in health care settings, *MMWR* 37:377-382, 1988.

Centers for Disease Control and Prevention: Human immunodeficiency virus transmission in household settings—United States, *MMWR* 43(19):347-356, 1994.

Centers for Disease Control and Prevention: Guidelines for preventing the transmission of tuberculosis in health care facilities, *Federal Registrar* 59(208):54242-54303, 1994.

Centers for Disease Control and Prevention: Recommendations for preventing the spread of vancomycin resistance, *MMWR: Recommendations and Reports* 44(RR-12):7-10, 1995.

Centers for Disease Control and Prevention: *The abc's of safe and healthy child care: an online handbook for child care providers,* Washington, DC, 1996, US Department of Health and Human Services.

Centers for Disease Control and Prevention: The role of bcg vaccine in the prevention and control of tuberculosis in the United States: a joint statement by the Advisory Council for the Elimination of Tuberculosis and the Advisory Committee on Immunization Practices (ACIP), *MMWR: Recommendations and Reports* 45(RR-4):1-18, 1996.

Centers for Disease Control and Prevention: Immunization of health care workers: recommendations of the Advisory Committee on Immunization Practices (ACIP) and the Hospital Infection Control Practices Advisory Committee (HICPAC), *MMWR: Recommendations and Reports* 46(RR-18), 1997.

Herrick S, Loos KM: Designing an infection control program, *Home Care Provider* 1(3):153-156, 1996.

Hospital Infection Control Practices Advisory Committee: 1996 guidelines for isolation precautions in hospitals, *Infect Control Hosp Epidemiol* 17(1):53-80, 1996.

Free KW: Infection control and safety: client education in the home, *Home Healthc Nurse* 14(12):957-959, 1996.

Lynch P et al: Implementing and evaluating a system of generic infection precautions: body substance isolation, *Am J Infect Control* 18(1):243-246, 1990.

Magruder C, Hamilton G: Management of tuberculosis in home health care, *Home Health Care Manage Prac* 10(3):9-20, 1998.

Moscati R, Mayrose J, Fincher L, Jehle D: Comparison of normal saline with tap water for wound irrigation, *Am J Emerg Med* 16(4):379-381, 1998.

Occupational Safety and Health Administration: 29 CFR Part 1910.1030. *Occupational exposure to bloodborne pathogens: final rule,* Washington DC, 1991, US Department of Labor.

Occupational Safety and Health Administration: Guidelines for preventing the transmission of tuberculosis in health-care facilities, *Federal Registrar* 58(195):52810-52854, 1993.

Occupational Safety and Health Administration: *Occupational exposure to bloodborne pathogens, OSHA 3127 (revised),* Washington DC, 1996, US Department of Labor.

Occupational Safety and Health Administration: 29 CFR part 1910: occupational exposure to tuberculosis: proposed rule, *Federal Registrar* 17:54160-54308, 1997.

Ralph IG: Infectious medical waste management: a home care responsibility, *Home Healthc Nurse* 11(3):25-33, 1993.

Rice R: Infection control in the home. In R Rice, editor: *Home health nursing practice: concepts and application,* ed 2, St Louis, 1996, Mosby.

Roll D: Shielding eyes against bloodborne pathogens, *Occupational Health and Safety* 66(3):54-55, 1997.

Roop J: Implementation of a hepatitis B vaccine program: a how to guide for home care providers, *Home Healthc Nurse* 11(4):24-30, 1997.

Rosenheimer L: Establishing a surveillance system for infections acquired in home healthcare, *Home Healthc Nurse* 13(3):20-26, 1995.

Valenti WM: Infection control, human immunodeficiency virus, and home health care: risk to caregivers, *Am J Infect Control* 23(2):78-81, 1995.

CHAPTER 2

Abbot D et al: Guidelines for measurement of blood pressure, follow-up, and lifestyle counseling, *Can J Public Health* 85(Suppl 2):S29-35, 1994.

Benesh L, Szigeti E, Ferraro R, Gullucks J: Tools for assessing chronic pain in rural elderly women, *Home Healthc Nurse* 15(3):207-211, 1997.

Buckwalter K: How to unmask depression, *Geriatr Nurs* 11(4):179-181, 1990.

Bulau J, Dellasega C: Home health nurse's assessments of cognition, *Appl Nurs Res* 5(3):127-133, 1992.

Elnitsky C, Alexy B: Identifying health status and health risks of older rural residents, *J Com Health Nurs* 15(2):61-75, 1998.

Feldman CB: Caring for feet: patients and nurse practitioners working together, *Nurse Pract Forum* 9(2):87-93, 1998.

Inaba-Roland K, Maricle R: Assessing delirium in the acute care setting, *Heart Lung* 21(1):48-55, 1992

Jubeck M: Are you sensitive to the cognitive needs of the elderly? *Home Healthc Nurse* 10(5):20-25, 1992.

Lazarre M, Ax S: Assessment: patients, chronic heart failure, and home care, *Caring* 16(6):20-24, 1997.

Ludwig LM: Cardiovascular assessment for home health care nurses. Part I. Initial cardiovascular assessment, *Home Healthc Nurse* 16(7):450-456, 1998.

Nikitow DP: Ten strategies for repositioning patients, *Chiropractic Journal* 11(10):16-54, 1997.

Perry M, Anderson G: Assessment and treatment strategies for depressive disorders commonly encountered in primary care settings, *Nurse Pract* 12(1):25-36, 1992.

Rice R, Wiersema L: The patient with chronic wounds. In R Rice, editor: *Home health nursing practice: concepts and application*, ed 2, St. Louis, 1996, Mosby. Note: see also Chapter 4 bibliography for further wound care references.

Roper M: Back to basics: assessing orthostatic vital signs, *Am J Nurs* 96(8):43-46, 1996.

Rutledge DR, Donaldson NE: Pain assessment and documentation. Part I. Overview and application in adults, *Online J Clin Innovations* 1(5):1-37, 1998.

Rutledge DR, Donaldson NE: Pain assessment and documentation. Part II. Special populations of adults, *Online J Clin Innovations* 1(6):1-29, 1998.

Saba VK: Temperature-pulse-respiration. In VK Saba, editor: *Home health classification (HHCC) of nursing diagnoses and interventions*, Washington, DC, 1994, Author.

Swanson B, Cronin-Stubbs D, Colletti M: Dementia and depression in persons with AIDS: causes and care, *J Psychosoc Nurs* 28(10):33-39, 1990.

CHAPTER 3

Barr DM: The Unna boot as a treatment for venous ulcers, *The Nurse Practitioner* 21(7):55-64, 1996.

Carroll P: Using pulse oximetry in the home, *Home Healthc Nurse* 15(2):89-95, 1997.

Carroll P: Closing in on safer suctioning, *RN* 61(5):22-27, 1998.

Dean B: Evidence-based suction management in accident and emergency: a vital component of airway care, *Acc Emerg Nurs* 5(2):92-98, 1998.

Ferrick KJ et al: Inadvertent AICD inactivation while playing bingo, *Am Heart J* 121(1):206-207, 1991.

Findeis A, Larson J, Gallo A, Shekleton M: Caring for individuals using home ventilators: an appraisal by family caregivers, *Rehabilitat Nurs* 19(10):6-11, 1994.

Fitch MI, Ross E: Living at home on a ventilator, *CACCN* 9(1):87-99, 1998.

Fowler S, Knapp-Spooner C, Donohue D: The abcs of tracheostomy care, *J Pract Nurs* 459(1):44-48, 1995.

Gallauresi BA: Device errors. Pulse oximeters, *Nursing* 28(9):31, 1998.

Godden J, Hiley C: Managing the patient with a chest drain: a review, *Nurs Stand* 12(32):35-39, 1998.

Grap MJ: Protocols for practice: applying research at the bedside—pulse oximetry, *Critical Care Nurse* 189(1):94-99, 1998.

Higgins CA: The AICD: a teaching plan for patients and families, *Crit Care Nurse* 10(6):69-74, 1991.

McCloskey JC, Bulechek GM: Chest physiotherapy. In JC McCloskey, GM Bulechek, editors: *Nursing interventions classification (NIC),* ed 2, St Louis, 1996, Mosby.

McCloskey JC, Bulechek GM: Airway suctioning. In JC McCloskey, GM Bulechek, editors: *Nursing interventions classification (NIC),* ed 2, St. Louis, 1996, Mosby.

O'Donahue W et al: Long-term mechanical ventilation—guidelines for management in the home and at alternate community sites, *Chest* 90(1):15, 1986. *Classic reading.

O'Donahue WJ Jr: Guidelines for the use of nebulizers in the home and at domiciliary sites: report of a consensus conference, *Chest* 110(1):814-820, 1996.

Pettinicchi TA: Trouble shooting chest tubes, *Nursing* 28(3):58-59, 1998.

Rice R: The patient with CHF. In R Rice, editor: *Home health nursing practice: concepts and application,* ed 2, St Louis, 1996, Mosby.

Rice R: The patient with COPD. In R Rice, editor: *Home health nursing practice: concepts and application,* ed 2, St Louis, 1996, Mosby.

Rice R: The ventilator-dependent patient. In R Rice, editor: *Home health nursing practice: concepts and application,* ed 2, St Louis, 1996, Mosby.

Ridley PO, Myers C, Braimbridge MV: Open tube drainage of empyema thoracis, *Prof Nurse* 5(2):73-76, 1989.

Rokosky JM: Misuse of metered-dose inhalers: helping patients get it right, *Home Healthc Nurse* 15(1):13-21, 1997.

Ryan D: How to guides: BIPAP ventilation, *Care Crit Ill* 14(1):4, 1998.

Van der Palen J, Klein JJ, Kerkhoff HM, van Herwarrden CLA, Seydel E: Evaluation of the long-term effectiveness of three instruction modes for inhaling medicines, *Patient Educ Couns* 32 (Suppl):S87-S95, 1997.

CHAPTER 4

Anthony D, Barnes J, Unsworth J: An evaluation of current risk assessment scales for decubitus ulcer in general inpatients and wheelchair users, *Clin Rehabilit* 12(2):136-142, 1998.

Bale S, Jones V: *Wound care nursing—a patient-centered approach,* Philadelphia, 1997, Bailliere Tindall.

Bergstrom N et al: *Pressure ulcer treatment. Clinical practice guideline. Quick reference guide for clinicians, No. 15,* AHCPR Pub. No. 95-0653, Rockville, Md, 1994, US Department of Health and Human Services, Public Health Service, Agency for Health Care Policy and Research.

Barr JE, Cuzzell JZ: Wound care clinical pathway: a conceptual model, *Ostomy Wound Manage* 42(7):18-24, 1996.

Chesney PJ, Burgess IF: Lice: resistance and treatment, *Contemp Pediatr* 15(11), 181-192, 1998.

Cuzzell JZ: The RYB color code, *Home Health Focus* 1(1):6, 1994.

Forsman KE: Pediculosis and scabies, *Postgrad Med* 98(6):89-100, 1995.

Gilchrist B: Innovations in leg ulcer care, *J Wound Care* 7(3):151-152, 1998.

Green K: Leg ulcers: holistic care, *Practice Nurse* 13(6):324-325, 1997.

Healthcare Financing Administration: *Home health insurance manual,* Pub. No. 11, Washington, DC, June 1998 (with periodic updates/addendums), US Department of Health and Human Services, Author.

Hicks LEM, Lewis DJ: Management of chronic, resistive scabies: a case study, *Geriatr Nurs* 13(4):230-237, 1995.

Hollinworth H, Kingston JE: Using a non-sterile technique in wound care, *Prof Nurse* 13(4):226- 229, 1998.

Jones M, Davey J, Champion A: Dressing wounds, *Nurs Stand* 12(39):47-56, 1998.

Miller M: Wound care: the role of debridement in wound healing, *Community Nurse* 2(9):52-55, 1996.

O'Hare L: A strategy for wound management, *Practice Nurse* 16(3):157-158, 1998.

Panel on the Prediction and Prevention of Pressure Ulcers in Adults: *Pressure ulcers in adults: prediction and prevention. Quick reference guide for clinicians,* AHCPR Publication No. 92-0050, Rockville, Md, 1992, US Department of Health and Human Services, Public Health Service, Agency for Health Care Policy and Research.

Pigott KG: Protocols. Lice and scabies, *Lippincott's Primary Care Practice* 1(1):93-96, 1997.

Rice R, Wiesema L: The patient with chronic wounds. In R Rice, editor: *Home health nursing practice: concepts and application,* ed 2, St Louis, 1996, Mosby.

Rudolph DM: Pathophysiology and management of venous ulcers, *J WOCN* 25(5):248-255, 1998.

Thomas S: Assessment and management of wound exudate, *J Wound Care* 6(7):327-330, 1997.

Williams RL, Armstrong DG: Wound healing: new modalities for a new millennium, *Clin Podiatr Med Surg* 15(1):117-128, 1998.

CHAPTER 5

Amir I, Sharma R, Bauman WA, Korsten MA: Bowel care for individuals with spinal cord injury: comparison of four approaches, *J Spinal Cord Med* 21(1):21-24, 1998.

Arrowsmith H: Nursing management of patients receiving gastrostomy feeding, *Br J Nurs* 5(5):268-273, 1996.

Black P: Stoma care after hospital discharge, *Community Nurse* 1(6):24-26, 1995.

Borwell B: Colostomies and their management, *Nurs Stand* 8(45):49-56, 1994.

Corless R: Caring for a homosexual man: understanding a colostomy formation, *Br J Nurs* 1(10):501-506, 1992.

Eisenberg PG: Gastrostomy and jejunostomy tubes: a nurse's guide to tube feeding. Part 2. *RN* 57(11):54-60, 1994.

Frankel EH, Enow NB, Jackson KC II, Kloiber LL: Techniques and procedures. Methods of restoring patency to occluded feeding tubes, *Nutr Clin Pract* 13(3):129-131, 1998.

Grosso-Haacker M: Coping with an ostomy, *Ostomy Wound Manage* 33:43-46, 1991.

Krasner KD: What's wrong with this stoma? *Am J Nurs* 4:47-56, 1990.

Leidy NK: Structural model of stress, psychosocial resources and symptomatic experiences in chronic physical illness, *Nurs Res* 39(4):230-235, 1990.

MacDonald K: Colostomy irrigation: an option worth considering, *Prof Nurse* 7(1):15-19, 1991.

CHAPTER 6

Anonymous: Perspective. Guidelines for hearing aid fitting for adults, *Am J Audiol* 7(1):17-23, 1998.

Brown EW: "Eh? You say you don't need a hearing aid?" *Medical Update* 21(9):2, 1998.

Carden RG: The ins and outs of contact lenses, *RN* 48(2):48-50, 1995.

Cataract Management Guideline Panel: *Management of cataract in adults. Clinical practice guideline. Quick reference guide for clinicians, No. 4,* AHCPR Pub. No. 93-0543, Rockville, Md, 1994, US Department of Health and Human Services, Public Health Service, Agency for Health Care Policy and Research.

Cleary ME: Helping the person who is visually impaired: concerns, questions, remedies, and resources, *J Ophthalmic Nurs Technol* 14(5):205-211, 1995.

Herth K: Integrating hearing loss into one's life, *Qualitative Health Res* 8(2):207-223, 1998.

Larsen PD, Hazen SE, Martin JLH: Elder care. Assessment and management of sensory loss in elderly patients, *AORN Journal* 65(92):432-437, 1997.

McConnell EA: Clinical do's and don'ts. Caring for a patient who has a vision impairment, *Nursing* 26(5):28, 1996.

Smith H: Support for patients with recent visual impairment, *Nursing Times* 93(12):52-54, 1997.

Tolson D: Age-related hearing loss: a case for nursing intervention, *J Adv Nurs* 26(6):1150-1157, 1997.

CHAPTERS 7 AND 8

Alderman C: Chemotherapy by catheter, *Nurs Stand* 12(28):25-27, 1998.

Andris DA, Krzywda EA: Central venous access: clinical practice issues, *Nurs Clin North Am* 32(4):719-740, 1997.

Angeles T: Removing a nontunneled central catheter, *Nursing* 28(5):52-53, 1998.

Bard Access Systems: *Groshong central venous catheters,* Salt Lake City, 1994, Author.

Bard Access Systems: *Hickman, Leonard, and Broviac catheters,* Salt Lake City, 1994, Author.

Centers for Disease Control and Prevention: Transmission of hepatitis C virus infection associated with home infusion therapy for hemophilia, *MMWR* 46(26):597-600, 1997.

Galica LA: Parenteral nutrition, *Nurs Clin North Am* 32(4):705-717, 1997.

Hadaway L: *Vascular access devices,* New York, 1997, National Association of Vascular Access Devices.

Hayden S: *Midline catheters and peripherally inserted central catheters,* St. Louis, 1996, Mosby.

Intravenous Nursing Society: Revised intravenous nursing standards of practice, Belmont, Ma, 1998, Author.

Lee W, Vallino L: Intravenous insertion site protection, *J Intravenous Nurs* 19(4):194-197, 1996.

Marx M: The management of the difficult peripherally inserted central venous catheter removal, *J Intravenous Nurs* 18(5):246-249, 1995.

McConnell EA: Clinical do's and don'ts. Administering parenteral nutrition, *Nursing* 28(7):18, 1998.

PSA of America Healthcare: *Infusion policy and procedure manual,* Norcross, North Carolina, 1999, PSA Healthcare.

Todd J: Peripherally inserted central catheters, *Prof Nurse* 13(5):297, 299-302, 1998.

Trask K: The challenges of teaching universal precautions to multicultural, diverse patients and their family members, *J Intravenous Nurs* 18(6S):S32-S37, 1995.

Welker D: Troubleshooting vascular access devices, St. Paul, Minn., 1994, SIMS Deltec, Inc.

CHAPTER 9

Abd-E-Maebound K et al: Rectal suppository: common sense and mode of insertion, *Lancet* 338(8770):798-800, 1991.

Beyea SC, Nicoll LH: Back to basics: administering IM injections the right way, *Am J Nurs* 96(1):34-35, 1996.

Campbell J: Injections, *Professional Nurse* 19(3):455-458, 1995.

Carr N: Make love, not warfarin: oral anticoagulation management: nurse-led clinic, *Nursing Times* 94(25):39, 1998.

Centers for Disease Control and Prevention: Screening for tuberculosis and tuberculosis infection in high-risk populations and the use of preventative therapy for tuberculosis infection in the United Sates, *MMWR* 39(RR-8):1-2, 1994.

Covington TP, Trattler MR: Bull's-eye! Finding the right target for IM injections, *Nursing* 27(10):62-63, 1997.

Dalton E, Dragg L, MacLean S: IM injection volume limit. Administering IM injections the right way, *Am J Nurs* 96:13, 1996.

Gilbert V, Gobbi M: Making sense of bladder irrigation, *Nursing Times* 85(16):40-42, 1989.

Hadley SA, Chang M, Rogers K: Effect of syringe size on bruising following subcutaneous heparin injection, *Am J Crit Care* 5(4):271-276, 1996.

Hussar DA: Helping your patient follow his drug regimen, *Nursing* 25(10):62-64, 1995.

Lennard TA, Corsolini T: Soft tissue anatomy and injection techniques, *Phys Med Rehabilit* 10(3):461-472, 1996.

Long C, Holmes N, Ismeurt R: The tuberculin skin test, *Home Healthc Nurse* 11(3):13-18, 1993.

McConnell EA: Clinical do's and don'ts: how to instill nose drops, *Nursing* 23(7):18, 1993.

Peragallo-Dittko V: Research for practice. Rethinking subcutaneous injection technique, *Am J Nurs* 97:71-72, 1997.

Rothstein MS: Guidelines for the use of topical medications, *J Enterostomal Therapy* 10(6):203-206, 1983.

Schmelzer M, Wright KB: Enema administration: techniques used by experienced registered nurses, *Gastroenterol Nurs* 19(4):137-139, 1996.

Segbefia IL, Mallet L: Are your patients taking their medications correctly? If not, try this blue print for success, *Nursing* 27(4):58-60, 1997.

Self TH: Warfarin interactions: how various drugs and disorders alter anticoagulant effects, *J Crit Illness* 13(6):356-358, 1998.

CHAPTER 10

Agency for Health Care Policy and Research: *Treatment of pressure ulcers,* Rockville, Md, 1994, Author.

American Association of Diabetes Educators: Position statement. Medical nutrition therapy for people with diabetes mellitus, *Diabetes Educ* 21:17-18, 1995.

American Diabetes Association: Nutrition recommendations and principles for people with diabetes mellitus, *Diabetes Care* 21(suppl 1):S32-S35, 1998.

American Dietetic Association, Consultant Dietitians in Health Care Facilities: *Inservice manual,* ed 3, 1996, Author.

American Dietetic Association, Consultant Dietitians in Health Care Facilities: Nutrition care of the older adult, 1998, Author.

American Dietetic Association: *Handbook of clinical dietetics,* ed 2, 1992, Author.

American Dietetic Association: *Manual of clinical dietetics,* ed 5, 1996.

American Dietetic Association, Morrison Health Care, Inc: *Medical nutrition therapy across the continuum of care,* Supplement 1, 1997, Author.

American Dietetic Association, Morrison Health Care, Inc: *Medical nutrition therapy across the continuum of care,* 1996, Author.

American Dietetic Association: Position of the ADA: The role of registered dietitians in enteral and parenteral nutrition support, *J Am Diet Assoc* 97:302-304, 1997.

American Medical Directors Association: *Pressure ulcers. Clinical practice guidelines.* Columbia, Md, 1996, Author.

Brand JC, Snow BJ, Nabhan GP, Truswell AS: Plasma glucose and insulin responses to traditional Pima Indian meals, *Am J Clin Nutr* 51:416-421, 1990.

Chidester JC, Spangler AA: Fluid intake in the institutionalized elderly, *J Am Diet Assoc* 97:23-28, 1997.

Dantone JJ: *Bridging the gap diet manual,* ed 2, Grenada, Miss., 1997, Nutrition Education Resources. E-mail: jojo@dixie-net.com

Delahanty M: Clinical significance of medical nutrition therapy in achieving diabetes outcomes and the importance of the process, *J Am Diet Assoc* 98:28-30, 1998.

Donahoe M, Rogers RM: Nutritional assessment and support in chronic obstructive pulmonary disease, *Clin Chest Med* 11:487-504, 1990.

Egbert AM: The dwindles: failure to thrive in older patients, *Geriatrics* 48(7):63-69, 1993.

Expert Panel on Detection, Evaluation, and Treatment of High Blood Cholesterol in Adults: Summary of the second report of the National Cholesterol Education Program (NCEP) expert panel on detection, evaluation, and treatment of high blood cholesterol in adults, *JAMA* 269:3015-3023, 1993.

Frantz RA, Gardner S: Elderly skin care: principles of chronic wound care, *J Geron Nurs* 12(1): 35-47, 1994.

Gallagher PM, Meleady R, Shields DC et al: Homocysteine and risk of premature coronary heart disease. Evidence of a common gene mutation, *Circulation* 94:2154-2158, 1996.

Gilmore SA, Robinson G, Posthauer MA, Raymond J: Clinical indicators associated with unintentional weight loss and pressure ulcers in elderly residents of nursing facilities, *J Am Diet Assoc* 95:984-992, 1995.

Guthrie DW, Guthrie RA: *Nursing management of diabetes mellitus,* 1997.

Guthrie DW, Guthrie RA: *The diabetes sourcebook,* ed 3, 1997.

Harris JA, Benedict FG: *A biometric study of basal metabolism in man,* Washington, DC, 1919, Carnegie Institution of Washington.

Haskell WL, Alderman EL, Fair JM et al: Effects of intensive multiple risk factor reduction on coronary atherosclerosis and clinical cardiac events in men and women with coronary artery disease, The Stanford Coronary Risk Intervention Project (SCRIP), *Circulation* 89:975-990, 1994.

Howard L, Malone M: Clinical outcomes of geriatric patients in the United States receiving home parenteral and enteral nutrition, *Am J Clin Nutr* 66:1364-1370, 1997.

Jamison MS: Failure to thrive in older adults, *J Gerontol Nurse* 23(2):8-13, 1997.

Joint National Committee on Detection, Evaluation, and Treatment of High Blood Pressure: The fifth report of the Joint National Committee on Detection, Evaluation, and Treatment of High Blood Pressure (JNCV), *Arch Intern Med* 153:154-182, 1993.

Morrison HI, Schaubel D, Desmeules M, Wigle DT: Serum folate and risk of fatal coronary heart disease, *JAMA* 275:1893-1896, 1996.

Nelson J K et al: *Mayo Clinic diet manual,* ed 7, 1994.

Oster G, Thompson D: Estimating effects of reducing dietary saturated fat intake on the incidence and costs of coronary heart disease in the United States, *J Am Diet Assoc* 96:127-131, 1996.

Posthauer ME, Dorse B, Foiles RA et al: ADA's definitions for nutrition screening and nutrition assessment, *J Am Diet Assoc* 94(8):838-839, 1994.

Posthauer MA et al: Identifying patients at risk: ADA's definitions for nutrition screening and nutrition assessment, *J Am Diet Assoc* 94:838-839, 1994.

Shimon I, Almog S, Vered Z et al: Improved left ventricular function after thiamin supplementation in patients with congestive heart failure, *Am J Med* 98:485-490, 1995.

The Diabetes Control and Complications Trial Research Group: Nutrition interventions for intensive therapy in the diabetes control and complications trial, *J Am Diet Assoc* 93:768-772, 1993.

White JV, editor: *The role of nutrition in chronic disease care,* Washington, DC, 1997, Nutrition Screening Initiative.

Wolever TMS et al: Beneficial effects of low-glycemic index diets in overweight NIDDM subjects, *Diabetes Care* 15:562-564, 1992.

CHAPTER 11

Acute Pain Management Guideline Panel: *Acute pain management: operative or medical procedures and trauma. Clinical practice guideline,* AHCPR Pub. No. 92-0032. Rockville, Md, 1992, US Department of Health and Human Services, Public Health Service, Agency for Health Care Policy and Research.

Ascough A: Nursing practice in chronic and cancer pain, *Assignment* 4(3):3-9, 1998.

Bauer NA: The 4 rights of compression therapy for patients with chronic venous insufficiency and venous ulceration, *Home Healthc Nurse* 16(7):443-449, 1998.

Brand P: Coping with a chronic disease: the role of the mind and spirit, *Patient Educ Couns* 26(1-3):107-112, 1995.

Cullum N, Fletcher AW, Nelson EA, Sheldon TA: Compression bandages and stockings in the treatment of venous leg ulcers (Issue No. 3), Oxford, 1998, The Cochrane Library.

Cornely HZ: Functional outcome difference using a rollar walker versus a two-wheeled rolling walker, *Phys Ther Case Reports* 1(2):104-106, 1998.

Dale J: Venous leg ulcers: compression therapy, *Prof Nurse* 13(100):715-720, 1998.

Hanson LC, Danis M, Garrett J: What is wrong with end-of-life care? Opinions of bereaved family members, *J Geriatr Soc* 45(11):1339-1344, 1997.

Jacox A, Carr DB, Payne R et al: *Management of cancer pain. Clinical practice guideline No. 9,* AHCPR Publication No. 94-0592, Rockville, Md, 1994, US Department of Health and Human Services, Public Health Service, Agency for Health Care Policy and Research.

Ledbetter AK: Cast care. In MK Elkin et al, editors: *Nursing interventions and clinical skills,* St Louis, 1996, Mosby.

Management of Cancer Pain Panel: *Management of cancer pain,* AHCPR Pub No. 94-0592, Rockville, Md, 1992, US Department of Health and Human Services, Public Health Service, Agency for Health Care Policy and Research.

McConnell EA: Providing cast care, *Nursing* 23(1):19, 1993.

Rice R, Rappl L: The patient receiving rehabilitation services. In R Rice, editor: *Home health nursing practice: concepts and application,* ed 2, St Louis, 1996, Mosby.

Mourad L: *Orthopedic disorders,* St Louis, 1991, Mosby.

Schwenzer KJ: How to offer comfort and symptom relief to the dying patient: algorithms for effective pain management, *J Crit Illness* 13(6):381-386, 389-392, 1998.

Ufema J: Insights on death & dying. Pain management: worlds apart, *Nursing* 28(9):20-22, 1998.

Urinary Incontinence Guideline Panel: *Urinary incontinence in adults. Quick reference guide for clinicians,* AHCPR Pub. No. 92-0041k, Rockville, Md, 1992, US Department of Health and Human Services, Agency for Health Care Policy and Research, Public Health Service.

CHAPTER 12

Also see section on Chapter 1.

Harding KA: Comparison of four glucose monitors in a hospital medical surgical setting, *Clin Nurse Spec* 7(1):13-16, 1993.

Juchniewicz J: Selecting a QA glucose meter, *Am J Nurs* 4:81-82, 1993.

Kestel F: Using blood glucose meters: what you and your patient need to know. Part I. *Nurs 93* 3:34-40, 1993.

McKee L: Diagnosing infection in wound care, *Practice Nurse* 15(9):533-534, 536, 1998.

Mead M: Stool culture, *Practice Nurse* 16(3):170, 1998.

Michielsen WJS et al: A simple and efficient urine sampling method for bacteriological examination in elderly women, *Age & Aging* 26(6):493-495, 1997.

Tagg PI: Patient education. How to collect a urine specimen: females, *The Nurse Practioneer* 21(11):135, 1996.

Tagg PI: Patient education. How to collect a urine specimen: males, *The Nurse Practioneer* 21(11):136, 1996.

Zaloga GP: Reagent testing: bedside testing of gastrointestinal tract specimens. Part 2. *Consultant* 33(70):80-82, 1993.

Zelmanovitz T, Gross JL, Oliveria J, de Azevedo MJ: Proteinuria is still useful for the screening and diagnosis of overt diabetic nephropathy, *Diabetes Care* 21(7):1076-1079, 1998.

CHAPTER 13

Bear M, Dwyer JW, Benveneste D, Jett K, Dougherty M: Home-based management of urinary incontinence: a pilot study with both frail and independent elders, *J WOCN* 24(3):163-171, 1997.

Beckman NJ: An overview of urinary incontinence in adults: assessments and behavioral interventions, *Clin Nurse Specialist* 9(5):241-247, 274, 1995.

Binard JE, Persky L, Lockhart JL, Kelley B: Intermittent catheterization the right way! (Volume vs. time-directed), *J Spinal Cord Med* 19(3):194-196, 1997.

Colley W: Practical procedures for nurses. Catheter care—1: No. 13.6, *Nursing Times* 94(24):17-23, 1998.

Colley W: Practical procedures for nurses. Catheter care—2: No. 13.7, *Nursing Times* 94(25):24-30, 1998.

Edwards M: The care of older women with uterine prolapse, *Prof Nurse* 11(6):379-383, 1996.

Giannantoni A, Scivoletto G, Di Stasi SM, Silecchia A, Finazzi-Agro E, Micali I, Castellano V: Clean intermittent catheterization and prevention of renal disease in spinal cord injury patients, *Spinal Cord* 36(1):29-32, 1998.

Haas M: The long way to self-catheterizing with a zip, *Urolog Nurs* 17(1):35-36, 1997.

Houston K: The patient with bladder dysfunction. In R Rice, editor: *Home health nursing practice: concepts and application,* ed 2, St Louis, 1996, Mosby.

McConnell EA: How to apply a self-adhesive condom catheter, *Nursing* 24(11):26, 1994.

McConnell EA. Clinical do's and don'ts. Maintaining a closed urinary drainage system, *Nursing* 27(10):22, 1997.

McHahon-Parkes K: Management of suprapubic catheters, *Nursing Times* 94(25):49-51, 1998.

Moore S, Newton M, Yancy R: How to irrigate a nephrostomy tube, *Am J Nurs* 93(7):63-67, 1993.

Sampsell CM, Burns PA, Dougherty MC, Newman DK, Thomas KK, Wyman JF: Continence for women: evidence-based practice, *J Obstet Gynecol Neonatal Nurs* 26(4):375-385, 1997.

Stelling JD, Hale A: Protocol for changing condom catheters in males with spinal cord injury, *Nursing* 13(2):28-34, 1996.

Index

Notes

Notes

Notes

Notes

Notes

Notes